'We have waited a long time for this. We have had books on the history of Chinese medicine by sinologists who rarely understand the needs and focus of practitioners. And we have had decades of references to "traditional" Chinese medicine by practitioners who often know little about the history of our medicine, or who focus only on specific parts of it. Here at last is the best of both worlds – a work by an experienced practitioner with a passion for history. Brilliantly written, comprehensive, engrossing, practical and erudite, this book is a treasure.'

– *Peter Deadman, founder of* The Journal of Chinese Medicine

'*Acupuncture and Chinese Medicine* is a masterstroke, a scholarly treatise without the parched dryness that normally characterises this type of work. Buck succeeds in creating a captivating narrative that is accessible, whilst still giving justice to the rich history of ideas that have continuously developed into the medicine practised today. This book is a must-have for any practitioner of Chinese medicine wishing to understand the bedrock on which they are standing.'

– *Nigel Ching, author and principal teacher at the Acupuncture Academy, Copenhagen*

'Charlie has managed to compile in an easy-to-read form a comprehensive and extensive journey through the history of Chinese medicine, herbs and acumoxa. It is a combination of well-researched information from a range of texts in Chinese and English (a really useful bibliography is given) interspersed clearly with his own considerations developed over years of practice. Knowing how this wonderful medicine has come to its current position as the main medical modality to offer a different explanation of function and treatment from modern biomedicine is a must for all scholars of medicine, be it Chinese or Western.'

– *Felicity Moir, Chinese Medicine Course Leader, University of Westminster, UK of related interest*

**Developing Internal Energy for
Effective Acupuncture Practice**
**Zhan Zhuang, Yi Qi Gong and the Art
of Painless Needle Insertion**
Ioannis Solos
ISBN 978 1 84819 183 9
eISBN 978 0 85701 144 2

**An Illustrated Handbook of Chinese Qigong
Forms from the Ancient Texts**
Compiled by Li Jingwei and Zhu Jianping
ISBN 978 1 84819 197 6

The Compleat Acupuncturist
**A Guide to Constitutional and
Conditional Pulse Diagnosis**
Peter Eckman
Foreword by William Morris
ISBN 978 1 84819 198 3
eISBN 978 0 85701 152 7

Pricking the Vessels
Bloodletting Therapy in Chinese Medicine
Henry McCann
Foreword by Heiner Fruehauf
ISBN 978 1 84819 180 8
eISBN 978 0 85701 139 8

Daoist Meditation
**The Purification of the Heart Method of Meditation
and Discourse on Sitting and Forgetting (Zuò Wàng Lùn)
by Si Ma Cheng Zhen**
Translated and with a commentary by Wu Jyh Cherng
Foreword by Eva Wong
ISBN 978 1 84819 211 9
eISBN 978 0 85701 161 9

ACUPUNCTURE AND CHINESE MEDICINE

Roots of Modern Practice

Charles Buck

Foreword by Barbara Kirschbaum

SINGING
DRAGON

LONDON AND PHILADELPHIA

First published in 2015
by Singing Dragon
an imprint of Jessica Kingsley Publishers
73 Collier Street
London N1 9BE, UK
and
400 Market Street, Suite 400
Philadelphia, PA 19106, USA

www.singingdragon.com

Library of Congress Cataloging in Publication Data
Buck, Charles, 1955- author.
  Acupuncture and Chinese medicine : roots of modern practice / Charles Buck ; foreword by Barbara Kirschbaum.
      p. ; cm.
  Includes bibliographical references and index.
  ISBN 978-1-84819-159-4 (alk. paper)
  I. Title.
  [DNLM: 1. Acupuncture Therapy--history--China. 2. Medicine, Chinese Traditional--history--China. WZ 70 JC6]
  RM184
  615.8'920951--dc23
                        2014015065

British Library Cataloguing in Publication Data
A CIP catalogue record for this book is available from the British Library

ISBN 978 1 84819 159 4
eISBN 978 0 85701 133 6

Printed and bound in Great Britain

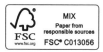

CONTENTS

FOREWORD

Reading this book as a practitioner of Chinese medicine has rekindled the enthusiasm I felt when I first began my study of Chinese medicine. Many of the well-known concepts are discussed in the context of the historical development of Chinese medicine, how these ideas came into being, and who the people were who developed them. Encountering this narrative can help us to feel part of the thread that has connected doctors of Chinese medicine over many centuries.

We work with this ancient medical tradition in the Western medical world and in modern times, in an intellectual context that is governed by the laws of the modern occidental version of 'rationality'. Today's practitioners work in an environment that demands a vault of justifications, explanations and endless citations of recent research on the treatment of symptoms and disease by Chinese medicine, and hopes to win the sympathy of the communities of thinkers who hold differing opinions on approaches to medicine.

In the modern world rationality presents itself in a narrow way, as an ability to collect and process exact facts about reality using a specific approach to logic. The impressive accomplishments of modern science, especially of natural and medical science, lead us to believe in a rationality that aims to explain everything and that discounts things that are not measurable. New theories in physics could show that 'realness or reality' has basically no substantial reality. Reality reveals itself as potentiality, as an 'as well as'. Complexity, relationships and the web of the functions of the natural world have turned out to be less amenable to linear logic. Although insights into these deficiencies have been accepted in the world of science, this paradigm shift has as yet to be incorporated into the theory and practice of modern medicine. This is one reason why it is interesting to study the approaches used by great thinkers of the past who aimed to understand human health and disease by using a holistic systems model.

Of course the model 'man as machine' is useful in medicine when an urgent repair is needed – let's say, someone is revived after cardiac arrest. A multitude of factors come together when somebody falls ill – these might include nutritional factors and emotional, environmental or climatic considerations. In dealing with chronic and complex diseases, the current biomedical model cannot always provide the answers and, too often, the sick person is reduced to a collection of signs and symptoms, which results in the prescription of a simple chemical agent that hopefully takes it all away. In simple situations this approach does save many lives, and so we should be grateful for the fact that science can provide these cures. At the same time, the complexity of all the factors contributing to ill health is often overlooked. Interventions are made to address each issue, often without taking note of their connection within the entire organism – a beta-blocker to counter high blood pressure, a statin to lower blood cholesterol, a drug to raise serotonin levels in mood disorders. Of course, a similar style of symptom treatment can also be seen in the community of the practitioners of Chinese medicine in the West – ginseng for more energy, lycium berries for better eyesight and so on. To quote the author:

> Given a better understanding of the roots of Chinese medicine we can gain a more reliable sense of what the tradition contains and what it has been about; this serves to counter some of the false assumptions that continue to exist. In particular, there is an urgent need to rise beyond notions of this medicine as a quaint, folksy and primitive play medicine that one might turn to in desperation. Indeed, the evidence is increasingly showing that it can help patients who cannot be treated safely or effectively with current biomedicine.

Although China's medical tradition is complex, multifaceted and always ready to adapt to current circumstances, it never loses sight of the relationship that exists between human beings and all the factors that influence their minds and bodies.

How might perceptions of health and illness and medicine's approach to treatment alter were Chinese medicine to be placed side-by-side with biomedical care? For one thing we could anticipate increased research on acupuncture and Chinese herbal medicine, but perhaps even more crucially, I believe the result would be a much greater appreciation of the seriousness of the historical legacy that underlies this medicine. Once this medicine's background is more widely understood, an increased acceptance of professional acupuncture, Chinese medicine and holistic medicine into general healthcare would ensue.

So often one is asked, 'Do I have to believe in acupuncture for it to work?' – it seems that there are believers and non-believers. The truth of the scientist is different from the faith of the believer, but ultimately they are looking for answers to the same question. In medicine the issue is, how can we cure and what is the cure? Such questions represent our twofold relationship towards reality. First there is the critical-rational position whereby man tries to understand the diversity of the world (in German we use the word *begreifen*, which means to get a grip, to touch it) with its own conceptualised thinking. An alternative path to understanding the world may come through meditation and by devoting attention to reflection on phenomena in a manner that tries to penetrate down to the essential essence of reality. Both positions are possible and both are tenable; indeed they can mutually complement each other. They represent two kinds of knowledge – the knowledge you can get a grip on and understand, and the knowledge that comes through reflection on the connections and relationships between things. There is the outer view: perception as an outside observer that requires the separation of the observer and the observed. In medicine this might mean accessing a certain level of reality by using histology techniques to examine a tissue biopsy under the microscope. Or there is the inner view, which is characteristically holistic and might be exemplified by Chinese medicine's pathways that link together top and bottom, and inside and outside, or that connect the adverse effect of sadness on the function of the lungs. Safety, effectiveness and experience in relation to the treatment of a human being entails having the capacity to include both, to focus on the outer view as well as on the inner view.

Working as a Chinese medicine specialist in an oncology ward I encounter on a daily basis the outer view, a world of cellular-biochemical-pharmacologic-based medicine that is applied to everyone with a particular histology report independent of the specific characteristics of the person who is ill due to a cancerous growth. Experience – for example, in the treatment of breast cancer – is on the one hand based on reproducible results published in research papers, and on the other hand also depends on the experience of the physician. Doctors feel on solid ground because they are adhering to the currently accepted guidelines laid down for the treatment of a specific cancer. In this manner they feel safe, secure within the realms of biomedicine.

How does that sense of safety and security of the practitioner of Chinese medicine arise? Is it sufficient to explain the health or illness by *yin* and *yang*, by evoking the concept of *qi* and the many other historical doctrines of the East Asian oriental medical tradition? I believe that the safe harbour for the acupuncturist and Chinese herbalist lies in the extended history and tradition of Chinese medicine, in its long experience. When writing a prescription or applying acupuncture, this is done in the knowledge that one is following in the footsteps of countless famed Chinese physicians who have transmitted their experience, theories and practical knowledge orally or in written works. Modern practitioners repeat something that doctors over centuries have done before. So the practitioner's sense of security rests in the knowledge and experience provided by historical scripts and writings alongside the fact that science is increasingly also helping to validate the tradition.

For this reason it is highly recommended for acupuncturists and Chinese medicine practitioners to acquaint themselves with the historical tradition, and to seek to understand the different strands of medical thought that have developed over the centuries. In this wonderful book Charles Buck has compiled the most important aspects of this in an easily accessible and readable manner. Reading this book, one becomes aware of the evolution of different schools of thought that orientated themselves on the needs of the time. China's doctors were not deluded or operating outside the real world; with characteristic pragmatism they were very much in it, and thus under the influence of political, social and economic realities that played a role in health and illness. The development and progress of Chinese medicine is not one that has evolved from a causal, analytical, rational way of thinking, but from the pressing demands of the specific time. Charles gives an example of this in Chapter 3 on the development of medicine in the Han dynasty:

In just a few years the Qin dynasty crumbled, as Shi Huang-di himself succumbed to his longevity medicines, making way for the foundation of the Han dynasty in −201 and the start of a prolonged era of peace and good government. Life became progressively more civilised and well organised as the Han dynasty progressed... Now that the threats to life from war, famine and strife had been reduced, medicine moved up the agenda for the *shi* classes. The results of this movement to create an improved professional medicine were summarised in the *Neijing*, most of which was compiled between −150 and +100 on the basis of earlier texts and what appears to have been deliberate and systematic medical investigation. Recent textual analysis indicates that the *Suwen*, the older part of the *Neijing*, was compiled by about 30 scholars from roughly 200 older writings.

Following Chinese medical history in this book, one learns how the great and famous doctors in each dynasty tried to find an answer for actual epidemic diseases as well as for lifestyle problems. This book guides us through the centuries, acquainting us with brilliant and creative doctors of Chinese medicine, giving an insight into their view of the inner and outer reality of society and the individual with common illnesses of their time. Interestingly enough one notices that most of those discussions on the causes of disease remain valid in modern times.

So why is the study of the historical tradition important for the student and the practitioner of this medicine? Quite simply, careful study of the different schools of thought that have been developed throughout history and that have shaped contemporary practice will sharpen our ability to really know Chinese medical thinking, and may eventually allow one to think outside of the box. The better we know the full scope of the tradition, the better placed we are to sense which aspects of it apply to our patients in clinic. If we only understand one style, our thinking is unavoidably limited. Further, as new medical problems arise, such as the increasing resistance to treatment by antibiotics, we can look backward to ways that past masters approached the difficulties.

For clarity, our teachers generally teach us the current standard model of practice that enables us to begin functioning as generalist practitioners. But it is only when we possess the wider knowledge of the many models of thought that we become really adept and accurate diagnosticians, able to write precise treatment plans and prescriptions for the person rather than for the disease. Suppose somebody has contracted a cold and is feverish but does not sweat. You might diagnose an externally contracted wind-cold disease, and then consult the *Shang Han Lun* for the right treatment. However, with wider understanding one might also consider a prescription from Ye Tian-shi when a warm-heat pathogen has caused a cold with a sore throat, and reached the nutritive and blood levels, resulting in macules and papules. Leaning on the diverse knowledge found in the historical tradition allows our thinking to be broad and divergent.

Chapter 5 on the Song dynasty describes the life of the famous paediatrician Qian Yi. He looked for a suitable treatment for children's diabetes and created a modification of the ancient *Shang Han Lun* prescription *jingui shenqi wan*. In doing so he devised the well-known *yin*-nourishing formula *liu wei dihuang wan*. The *yin*-nourishing and kidney-strengthening schools that developed in the subsequent Jin-Yuan and Ming dynasties regarded this formula as the basis for nourishment of the *yin*. Today this prescription, and its numerous standard variations, is used all over the world. Knowing the historic origin of this prescription as a long-term support treatment for children with diabetes, one understands much better its composition of mild and nourishing herbs.

As well as the common side effects of loose bowels and appetite loss, some cancer chemotherapy patients experience a feeling of severe inner coldness, a chill in the bones, but also feeling hot at the same time. Often this is combined with nausea or headaches. When I asked an oncologist about this, he was at a loss to explain these symptoms, and murmured something about the immune system and side effects. Unsure what to do to help these patients I knew I had to consult more experienced doctors. History provided the answer. Ming dynasty physician Wu You-xing (1582–1652), who encountered an epidemic in 1641–1642 in his neighbourhood, wrote a discussion on warm epidemics (*wen yi lun*), which focused on epidemic and warm diseases. His formula *da yuan yin* (Reach the Source Drink) was used to vent the pathogenic influences lurking in the half exterior, half interior level. Dr Wu applied this prescription when foul turbidity had entered the body and lodged in a place internally called the 'membrane source' (discussed in the book). Such foul turbidity creates dampness and compresses the *yang qi* in the interior. In some cases the chemotherapeutic medication caused foul turbidity in my patients, which in turn set off the nausea and the changing heat and cold sensations. Due to the weakened constitution of the patients, I modified the prescription and they fared well on this.

So, acquiring increased knowledge of classical and pre-modern theories of this medicine is often a key part of finding the right treatment for our patients. The many different schools that came forward with models of how they were perceiving reality at their time leads one away from the temptation to apply a reductionist approach. Not every case of diarrhoea is due to a spleen *qi* deficiency, and not every breast cancer is due to a stagnation of liver *qi*. Considering the environment, the seasonal influences, eating habits and the emotional state was incorporated in the process of diagnosis, and so the doctors in ancient and present times devised the correct steps of treatment, which was never detached from the current circumstances. Therefore the thinking of pathology and functions of points or herbs would alter, because doctors were influenced by the time period they lived in. One finds that in relation to economic circumstances and natural catastrophes or epidemics the doctors tried to find an answer to the threat of illness occurring due to this. This valuable book helps guide us to an understanding that medicine is always a reflection of the times we live in.

Reading this carefully researched book by Charles Buck leads one back to the source and makes one understand about the continuity of the development of

Chinese medicine. The book also rekindles the memory of one's first encounters with the study of Chinese medicine. It is, by turns, gripping and fascinating, and at times the read engages like a novel. Revealing the pragmatic, and at times non-pragmatic, character of Chinese medicine, each single chapter brings you back to its roots. Routine and a busy practice sometimes leads one towards a too pragmatic approach in diagnosis and treatment, and one easily loses the connection with the many threads that Chinese medicine encompasses.

This book supplies us with a diversity of information, describing the development of Chinese medicine throughout history in relation to the demands that a particular time dictated. We can better understand the quite pragmatic approach to healthcare that we encounter in this medicine that is applied in the treatment of particular symptoms or diseases. Yet within that we learn, too, that human beings were never perceived without their connection to the workings of the universe.

I highly recommend this book, because after reading it, one holds still for a moment and reflects a little longer before applying a treatment.

Barbara Kirschbaum
Hamburg, May 2014

ACKNOWLEDGEMENTS

Throughout my life I have been inspired my many teachers, beginning, aged seven, with my science mentor, Donald Clark. My love for Chinese medicine has been kept alight by the many great people I have had the privilege to have learned from, including Dr J.D. van Buren, Giovanni Maciocia, Dr Ted Kaptchuk and Barbara Kirschbaum. Inspiration has come too from the numerous people I have learned from in our worldwide community of Chinese medicine, in particular Dr Li Lin, Bob Flaws, Charles Chace, Stephen Birch and Peter Deadman, as well as the many clinicians with whom I studied in China. I am very grateful to my great friend Dr Liu Ying who worked at my clinic for many years, and who helped with the translation of source material. Sabine Wilms kindly commented on my coverage of Sun Si-miao. I would also like to express my appreciation to Jessica Kingsley and everyone at Singing Dragon who helped to get this work into print.

Finally, I wish to thank my wife Marianne for allowing me the time in our relationship as well as the space in our house to indulge my passion for this medicine. Without your support and encouragement this work would never have been completed. Thank you, love of my life.

DYNASTIES OUTLINE

Note: For simplicity I have chosen to use Joseph Needham's system for dates. Where a positive date is self-evident the + is omitted.

Xia	−2100 to −1600
Shang	−1600 to −1060
Zhou	−1060 to −256
Western Zhou	−1060 to −771
Eastern Zhou	−771 to −256
Chunqiu (Spring and Autumn)	−770 to −476
Zhanguo (Warring States)	−475 to −221
Qin	−221 to −206
Han	−206 to +221
Western Han (Xian)	−206 to +8
Xin	+8 to 23
Eastern Han (Lo Yang)	+23 to 221
Three Kingdoms	+221 to 280
Jin	+265 to 479
Northern and Southern Dynasties	+479 to 581
Northern	+479 to 502
Southern	+502 to 581
Liang	+552 to 587
Sui	+581 to 618
Tang	+618 to 907
Five Dynasties	+907 to 960
Song	+960 to 1279
Northern Song	+960 to 1127
Southern Song	+1127 to 1279
Jin	+1115 to 1234
Yuan	+1260 to 1368
Ming	+1368 to 1644
Qing	+1644 to 1911
Republican	+1912 to 1949
People's Republic of China	+1949 onwards

1

INTRODUCTION

Chinese people are proud of their long and distinguished culture, and for most, that sentiment includes some acknowledgement of the value of their traditional medicine; such pride has continued despite the recent romance with all things Western. Many are aware that Chinese medicine deserves its place as the world's pre-eminent pre-modern medical system, and that it still has a significant contribution to make to healthcare today, despite all the advances in scientific biomedicine. Having hit a nadir a century ago as a consequence of social and political conditions, Chinese medicine (encompassing Chinese herbal medicine, acupuncture, moxibustion, *tui na* massage, traditional dietetics and its associated explanatory models) has recovered to a point where it is now fully institutionalised into state-controlled healthcare in the universities and hospitals of modern China. For most Chinese people, however, Western biomedicine currently holds a higher status as a profession as it appears more modern and connected to technological industries and to Western-style corporate branding by which so many are beguiled. When asked about healthcare choices, most Chinese people will say they prefer to rely on modern medicine, although in practice, their actions may be different. Those polled often report that their culture's traditional medicine is the choice of old people and those living in the countryside, although this belies the fact that numerous large, traditional hospitals are also located in the cities, and of the millions who spend time in their waiting rooms each year, many are neither peasants nor elderly. In fact, demand for traditional medicine is kept alive by all sectors of Chinese society. Just as people in today's China often wear formal Western business suits as well as traditionally tailored silk outfits, the educated middle classes as well as the upper echelons of Chinese society tend to play safe by backing both horses, so to speak – consulting Western medicine specialists when it seems appropriate, as well as maintaining relations with traditional medicine hospitals or the new and more exclusive private Chinese medicine clinics, where well-heeled patients can consult with renowned physicians. Ever pragmatic, the educated classes tend to follow the healthcare policy of the old communist era that aimed to integrate the two medical systems, an approach informally referred to by a doctor I met in China in 1990 as the 'walking on two legs policy'.

In the West, acupuncture and Chinese medicine has often been categorised as 'fringe therapy' in the minds of many, and so it may be useful to contextualise, by sketching its dimensions in China today. In China's current state healthcare system, approximately 350,000 full-time doctors of Chinese medicine enter professional practice after graduation from a medical college training that is taken full time over five or more years. The requirements for entry into a career in Chinese medicine match those expected for medical school entry in the West. Roughly half of the taught component is Western biomedicine, which ensures that biomedical diagnoses can be understood and tests interpreted, and so communication with colleagues in biomedicine departments can function properly. Working alongside these Chinese medicine physicians are degree-level health professionals with somewhat lesser training: nurses, physical therapists and professional acupuncturists trained in acumoxa, but without the rigours of a full Chinese medicine doctoral training. One estimate puts the total number able to provide acumoxa treatment in China's health service at just over one million. A vestige of Chairman Mao's desire to integrate the best of Eastern and Western medicine remains in the inclusion of some study of Chinese medicine theory and practice in the Western medical school curriculum, although I gather that the sport for students of biomedicine is to sleep through these classes.

China has over 2800 regional traditional medicine hospitals that are roughly the size of the largest teaching hospitals in the West. In addition, 68,000 smaller hospitals and clinics that are able to offer Chinese medicine serve the healthcare needs of those in towns and rural areas. Chinese government statistics say that these medicine hospitals and clinics treat 230 million patients each year. As well as professionally delivered Chinese medicine, there is also a large market for traditional treatments available as over-the-counter preparations of famous herb prescriptions, called *chengyao* (ready-made medicines). Just as Westerners know some remedies for common ailments, so most Chinese people know that they can take *gan mao ling* or *yin qiao san* (honeysuckle and forsythia powder) if they are coming down with a cold. They know to take *shi Quan da bu wan* (all-inclusive great tonifying decoction) for fatigue or to help recovery from illness; they know to take *bao he wan* (preserve harmony pill) for indigestion. The list of classic prescriptions known to the public is long, and the origins of this can be traced back to the benevolent efforts of governments in the Song, Jin and Yuan dynasties (+960–1368) in setting up pharmacies for the benefit of the public (see Chapter 5). There is also a widespread public understanding of the techniques and application of acupuncture; many Chinese people will self-treat, using moxibustion in particular for maintaining health. I came across an example of this after asking two young office workers for directions in Shanghai in 1990. Hearing of my profession, they pointed to an acupuncture point, challenging me to name it. '*Zu san li!*' I said. They became visibly excited and pointed to another – '*Da zhui!*' I said, and they laughed some more. I expected this game to end after a couple more points, but it continued on for another 20 minutes or so! Ordinary young office workers knew dozens of acupuncture points.

Later, when I employed a Chinese doctor as an assistant at my clinic, we had a lunchtime discussion of *yang sheng*, the long-standing Chinese obsession with personal health maintenance. We watched as Dr Liu Ying flashed back to her primary school days. Taking on a shrill and bossy primary school teacher voice, she simultaneously recited and performed the eye care massage regime that her class had been taught and that was a standard part of education in her childhood. This included a chant of the Chinese names of each of the acupuncture points around the eyes whilst massaging them, an example of one of the many ways that ordinary Chinese people come to understand their bodies and how to look after them according to a deep-rooted medical tradition. A Confucian ethic is the sense that your body is not entirely your own but has been handed down to you by your ancestors, a viewpoint which brings with it a heavy responsibility to take good care of it. As Dr Ted Kaptchuk, one of my Chinese herb tutors, said, 'the Chinese make the Jewish race look like they don't care about their health!' (Ted is classic New York Jewish). Chinese medicine remains strongly rooted in everyday culture in China and across much of Southeast Asia.

Westerners have become used to the word 'acupuncture', but in this book I often use the term 'acumoxa', which needs some explanation. *Zhen jiu ke* (针灸科) are the characters you will see above the entrance to a hospital acupuncture department; they mean the '*needles* and *moxibustion* department'. Moxibustion is a heat treatment that mainly uses the downy hairs refined from mugwort leaves to heat or cauterise the body surface; it is often used when deemed appropriate in addition to needles or sometimes instead of them. Even the term *zhen jiu* (acumoxa) should really be seen as shorthand for a wider range of physical stimulation techniques including the use of suction cups (*ba huo guan*), massage (*an mo*), channel massage (*tui na*), scraping (*gua sha*) and other methods in the acumoxa therapeutic armoury. Working alongside clinical specialists in the traditional medicine healthcare sector are large numbers of ancillary specialists such as herbal pharmacists who have to take specialist university degrees in order to be employed as traditional pharmacists. They learn herb identification, quality control, pharmacy management and skills such as preparing creams, pills and herb prescriptions for decoction. Again, this has existed as a formally trained profession for many hundreds of years.

Also serving the traditional medicine sector is an army of growers, producers and processors across China, with different regions and provinces specialising in the cultivation and supply of particular herbs. The People's Republic of China (PRC) government figures for 2008 say that, in addition to medicinal herbs collected from the wild, over 300,000 metric tons of herbs were cultivated, and about 12 million kilos of a single herb, the blood-nourishing herb *dang gui* (Angelica sinensis), are cultivated annually. These are distributed through wholesale markets, one of the largest of which is in Bozhou in Anhui province, where 6000 tons of herbs are sold daily to roughly 50,000 wholesalers – a trade that amounts to roughly US$1.5 billion. This industry is regulated by law and by teams of government inspectors who ensure that national medicine quality standards are upheld. One example of this is in the licensing of centres that process the herb *shu fu zi*, an aconite product that is dangerously toxic until it is rendered safe and effective by these factories. Historically, of course, these medicines were all organically grown or gathered from the wild. In the last few decades, with the introduction of modern farming methods, the Chinese government is now fighting to curb the use of pesticides and other contaminants by growers, and so regulation itself has become a significant industry.

As well as those professionals engaged in clinical medical practice, there is a profession of specialist scientists who follow careers researching into acumoxa and Chinese medicine. These include scientists studying the pharmacology of herbal medicines, chemists and biochemists investigating active components, those researching agricultural methods for herb production and those engaged in laboratory research into acupuncture and moxibustion. The last five decades of such work has created a significant scientific body of research to support clinical practice. All the 300 or so commonly used herbs have been researched for their effects, screened for toxicity and had their active constituents chemically identified. Recently, with China's adoption of a more Western mindset, we have seen a move from a pure science approach to realisation of this work's potential for bringing novel pharmaceuticals to market, a change that has introduced ideas of intellectual property ownership that did not previously play much part. This provides a difficult mix of gains and losses for Chinese medicine – more research and more funding, but more secrecy and a proprietorial approach to knowledge.

The Chinese medicine clinical profession has its own research agenda that disseminates its findings through more than a hundred professional journals. By any standards this is a significant body of medical literature as these are among the world's largest medical journals. *Zhongguo Zhenjiu* (Chinese Acupuncture and Moxibustion), for example, reports a circulation of 300,000 (for comparison, *The Lancet* in the UK has a circulation of 18,000). Traditional doctors in the state healthcare system engage in some form of research, as this is a contractual pre-requisite to promotion and career advancement. This policy has led to the publication of tens of thousands of clinical studies, although the great majority of these should be classified as clinical audits rather than high-grade explanatory trials. Surveys of this literature find that roughly 5 per cent warrant a score of three or more on the Jadad scale (or the Oxford trial quality scoring system), which indicates a moderate trial quality and gives an approximate guide to reliability. A significant amount of research work is now being carried out in the West that is often good quality, and so there is a drive to further improve standards in China. As well as clinical trials, basic laboratory research has explored the mechanisms of acumoxa, and has delved into the pharmacology of Chinese herbal medicine; much of this work has been repeated in the West. A drug discovered by Chinese herb pharmacologists in a herb that was traditionally used to treat malarial fevers is currently saving about 200,000 lives a year in Africa.

Taken altogether, there is sufficient high quality evidence for traditional Chinese medicine to be taken seriously in modern healthcare. Given the size of the Chinese medicine academic world, it is surprising that it is taking so long for awareness of the scale and value of this medicine to reach the Western world. As the prejudices born out of ignorance weaken, and as patient interests begin to override the hegemony of big pharma, a new respect is beginning to appear outside the confines of Chinese medicine enthusiasts in the West, initially for acumoxa, and latterly for Chinese herbal medicine. Chinese medicine has a past, and it certainly has a future.

Ironically, an indicator of success, of the increased acceptance of Chinese medicine in the West, is seen in the way that it is being increasingly challenged by those whose interests are threatened. Evidential standards are demanded for Chinese medicine that are so high that they are met by only a small minority of currently accepted biomedical treatments – most prescribed drugs do not meet the evidence standards that sceptics demand of Chinese medicine. Although current medico-political issues are beyond the scope of this text, some of the other hindrances and misunderstandings that Chinese medicine has faced do warrant some attention.

Active opposition aside, Chinese medicine has long suffered as a consequence of the East–West language and culture gap. A satisfyingly succinct expression of the way that misapprehensions arise came from Eugène Ionesco who said, 'The French for London is Paris.' When we lack actual knowledge of something we tend to assume that the unknown is essentially the same as something we are already familiar with. In terms of medicine, we are familiar in the West with folk herbalism, faith healing and the vitalist-spiritualist ideas of the 19th century. And it is easy to jump to the conclusion that China's medical tradition is similar.

Given a better understanding of the roots of Chinese medicine we can gain a more reliable sense of what the tradition contains and what it has been about; this serves to counter some of the false assumptions that continue to exist. In particular, there is an urgent need to rise beyond notions of this medicine as a quaint, folksy and primitive play medicine that one might turn to in desperation. Indeed, the evidence is increasingly showing that it can help patients who cannot be treated safely or effectively with current biomedicine.

Misapprehensions exist amongst advocates in the West; these include the idea that classical Chinese medicine came into being 5000 years ago, and that what it is today is essentially what it was in its earliest times. Many suffer from the delusion that it is primarily based on spirituality and metaphysics, and I have heard exasperated Chinese doctors plead, 'This is not a religion – it's just a way of doing medicine!' There is also a perception that acupuncture and Chinese medicine ignores the study of disease in favour of balancing *qi*, *yin-yang* and *jing-luo* channels, and that those who developed it cared little for anatomy, physiology or pathology. Again, a different picture should emerge on reading this book. Although only presenting a tiny sample of the whole story, it chronicles Chinese medicine more correctly, showing it as a relatively successful quest by serious, educated and rational people to create a system of medicine able to maintain health, reverse suffering and stop disease.

As a consequence of recognition by the Chinese state in the 1950s and its widespread incorporation into the university system, the historical medical tradition was trimmed and modernised so as to be more in accord with curriculum requirements and the need for greater congruency with modern biomedicine. This sanitised version of Chinese medicine appeared a decade or two before the growth of interest in the West, and so strongly influenced understanding outside China.

Providing helpful clarification at first, it has led, in the last decade or so, to realisation of a need to map the historical tradition more thoroughly. A new generation has appeared armed with the skills to re-examine the historical literature, to check for the 'babies that have been thrown out with the bathwater'. This scholarly work has been facilitated by improved communications that have allowed much easier access to ancient source texts, helped, too, by levels of scholarship in the West that have improved spectacularly, and by the new ease of travel to East Asian countries.

Better-informed debate comes as a result of this exploration of the wider classical medical tradition, but it also feeds factionalisation as gurus establish their own fiefdoms and proclaim their way as the one true way. One successful movement emphasises interpretations of the Eastern Han dynasty classic, the *Shang Han Zhabing Lun*, and a subset of herbal medicine practitioners are choosing to emphasise this methodology in their clinical practice. As we will see later in Chapter 7, this represents a re-run of history when, for centuries, various different styles contended for primacy. A deeper appreciation of the *Shang Han Lun* is valuable, but I hope that my work will help us appreciate some of the other ideas and provide a wider perspective on what the tradition offers.

Classical and folk medicine

Since my focus here is on 'classical Chinese medicine' I need to highlight the distinction between what we can rightfully call a 'classical' medical tradition and 'folk' medicine. Folk medicine exists today, and has always existed throughout the world, as a relatively informal attempt to deal with health matters. It is based on the use of lore that is shared by a population and perhaps understood in greater detail by particular individuals. In folk medicine the base theories are simple and tend to posit a one-to-one correlation between a symptom and a treatment – say, a herb or a chanted prayer. Little or no diagnosis or theory sits between noting the main symptom and the therapeutic response, and there is little perceived need for a systematic or rational explanatory model. Interestingly, studies of primates and other animals have shown that they use folk medicine – they seek out specific plant materials when they have digestive upsets, and on occasions these have been found to be exactly the same substances taken by local people for similar complaints. Even some lower vertebrates seem to have folk medicine traditions. Chickens, for example, are known to educate their chicks to avoid toxic grains, and many animals seek out substances with medicinal properties when they are unwell. Generally, folk medicines are communicated from generation to generation, gradually becoming refined or degraded over time, depending on the fidelity of the process by which folk medical knowledge is transmitted between individuals and from generation to generation.

Classical medical traditions are distinctive in using a more systematic approach – an explanatory model that can be tested by experience, which seeks to understand causality and is concerned to see that this knowledge base is subject to cycles of critical evaluation. A classical tradition aims to reach beyond the presenting symptom to a deeper and more specific understanding of what has gone wrong that can be labelled and described systematically. Modern biomedicine does this largely by using technology to discern physical or chemical changes underlying ill health. Chinese medicine had more limited technology, and so aimed to extract more information about underlying processes by meticulous observation with the senses, codified experience of previous generations and a systematic logic. China has always had folk medical traditions alongside classical medicine; indeed, the vast majority of medical practice through Chinese history has been folk medicine. The folk tradition barely gets a mention in this book, however, except for mention of its value to the literate physician classes as a handy resource from which to borrow.

The Victorian medical grandee Sir William Osler (1849–1919) is famed for saying to his medical students, 'By the time you are in practice half of what we are teaching you will be known to be wrong – the problem is that we do not yet know which half.' Modern medicine continues to evolve by abandoning obsolete beliefs – in theory, if not always in actuality. Only a decade or so ago most doctors believed that cardiovascular disease resulted from fat depositing itself on the wall of arteries – a picture now known to be inaccurate. Throughout its history, acupuncture and Chinese medicine has focused on finding ways to label, model and influence function. For the most part this process has continued by simply piling new ideas and discoveries on top of the old. Critical appraisal has not always been characteristic of this medicine, but when it has occurred at the hands of innovative thinkers, the medical tradition has benefited greatly. If Chinese medicine was a house, it would be like one belonging to a compulsive hoarder – packed to the rafters with a mixture of junk, antiques and precious artefacts. When we ourselves survey its contents, a discerning clarity of mind is needed to distinguish the two as well as some understanding about the way that situations change through time. The treatment of leg oedema in modern Westerners today might not be usefully informed by ancient writings when we realise that, historically, the most common cause of this condition was beriberi. Nevertheless, most of the great physicians of Chinese medicine have carefully examined the historical medical legacy.

The study of the history of medical science contributes almost nothing to a modern biomedical clinician's education or medical understanding – old notions are by default obsolete and outdated, to be confined to the curiosities cabinet. In general it provides an opportunity to be amused by the quaint ignorance of the past and to celebrate how clever we are now. Even more amusement is to be derived from examining past folk medical customs from Europe and around the world – ye olde herbals, the leeches, the bloodletting and the strange beliefs. So it may be difficult for some to conceive how the study of the ideas of long-deceased physicians might be to practitioners today. The belief is that many of the tenets of traditional Chinese medicine are as valid today as they were a thousand or more years ago, but many will be baffled as to how this can be the case. Although this is not an explicit theme of this book, it may be that readers will finish their reading with a sense of how this might be possible – how a different approach to the acquisition of knowledge might produce a different and perhaps robust knowledge set. For example, a fundamental dichotomy present at the start of classical Chinese medicine was the distinction between *xu* (deficiency) and *shi* (excess). This is the realisation that we can divide most patients' ills into those that arise because some essential part of function has been weakened (*xu*) versus those that are due to the presence of something in the body that should not be there (*shi*) that is interfering with proper function. This remains as helpful clinically today as it was when introduced well over two millennia ago; the idea has not become obsolete and contains the potential to be polished and made more clinically relevant through repeated application. This is not to say that we therefore uncritically accept everything that has been handed down, but simply that we might aim to distinguish those truths that are immutable from those that are more subject to becoming obsolete.

So, Chinese medicine's cluttered house is actually a repository of useful knowledge, as well as perhaps some junk. Recent findings in genetics suggest that much of what science once considered to be 'junk DNA' turns out be a record of our adaptation to, and our protection from, past diseases. The discovery that our DNA still contains genetic records of our ability to fight viruses that affected us when we were a type of shrew 100 million years ago is a startling example of the potential inherent in what once may have seemed like junk. Similarly, Chinese physicians have faced innumerable different illnesses at different times in history, and we still have the written records of the solutions they found; this may be 'junk information' now, but we may just need it again. More important, perhaps, is the opportunity the study of ancient thinkers gives to gain insights into the thinking processes that allowed them to find solutions to the health problems they faced. How was it that the Tang dynasty physician Sun Si-miao was able to work out that people suffering goitre in highland regions could be cured by bringing them seaweed thousands of miles from coastal regions? We can learn from Sherlock Holmes and we can learn from the principles established by Sun Si-miao, Zhang Zhong-jing and Ye Tian-shi. In addition, by studying what has gone before, practitioners will be better placed to appreciate our own position in the wider scheme of this great medical tradition.

Chinese culture is traditionally envisaged as a fabric woven from the weft of each generation, intertwined with the constants that are provided by the warp threads that are the ancient precepts lying at the root of Chinese medicine. We will see that classical Chinese medicine is not really a single tradition but the constant re-interpretation and adjustment of classical doctrine to meet the changing clinical challenges of different times, and yet supported by the structure that the ancient truisms gave. In my experience as a clinician, these truisms remain inherently holistic, rational and wise in modern times. When we understand the historical legacy, a shift begins in the relationship we have with what was learned in our basic training. An understanding of the historical styles opens up avenues of clinical investigation to which we might otherwise be oblivious. We learn that there are many more tools in the box than can be squeezed into undergraduate training. We learn that China's medical tradition is complex, multifaceted and always ready to adapt to current circumstances. Also, we learn more about the mindset of the great physicians of the past – in particular, the way that so many of them rooted their thinking in observation, rationality and pragmatism, with an equal measure of creativity and wisdom.

How this book came about

Having subscribed to Beijing's English language *Journal of Traditional Chinese Medicine* since its founding in 1979, I read its articles on traditional Chinese medicine history and used these as a means of adding depth to my teaching work. Then, through the work of pioneering publishers such as Blue Poppy Press and Paradigm Publications, it became possible to piece together a clearer understanding of the contributions of individual scholar physicians and their styles of practice. This way I learned about Huang Fu-mi, Li Gao, Wang Shu-hu and many others. I gained sufficient knowledge of Chinese to allow investigation into areas that I wished to clarify and that were poorly covered in the existing literature. Realising, for example, that my practice perhaps over-emphasised the use of supplementation methods, I was frustrated to find the existing texts only devoted a few lines to the work of the Jin-Yuan dynasty expert on pathogen expulsion, Zhang Cong-zheng, and so I spent some time translating some of his ideas. In 1990 I obtained Fu Wei-kang's *Zhongguo Yixue Shi* (History of Chinese Medicine), for me a Rosetta Stone offering more detailed access to the historical tradition and which provided a means of filling in the blind spots left from study of other sources. I also gleaned information by a wide reading of the Western academic literature, notably the texts written by authorities on Chinese medical history and anthropology such as Paul Unschuld, Donald Harper, Elisabeth Hsu, Nathan Sivin, Judith Farquhar and others. Some useful and informative input came from academic theses by authors such as Asaf Moshe Goldschmidt and Peter Nigel Daly. I consulted existing texts on Chinese medicine history, many of which I found had not quite satisfied my desire to really understand things. Worth mentioning, too, are writings on the borderlines of the field, works on early philosophical warfare and political theory, in addition to the many authors on the Yijing, Laozi, Zhuangzi, Sunzu and Han dynasty thought; I was especially taken by the insightful work of François Jullien and Shigehisa Kuriyama. A fuller account of the main sources accessed is provided in the Bibliography at the end of the book.

Reading the sources on Chinese medicine history has its frustrations. Some texts devote half of their content to discussions on political and social background, and many are hard to read. High quality sources tend to be written from academic standpoints, arguing for particular academic positions rather than discussing the issues that are of interest to clinicians. Sinologists like to make the case for a thesis that they are trying to prove, and this too often distracts from the content by adopting a scholarly style that obfuscates more than it illuminates. Naturally, historians emphasise issues of interest to historians and anthropologists discuss what interests anthropologists, but my reading suggests that the perspectives of these specialists rarely match the interests of practitioners, who are more interested in issues such as how knowledge was acquired, who developed it, what it actually means and what aspects might be relevant in clinical practice today. Instead, we find emphasis on the socio-political context or writings that highlight the differences in medical practices amongst different social strata, and that place information in relation to changing cultural beliefs and practices. Practitioners are less interested in counting changes in the numbers of herbs or acupoints listed in texts at different times in history – this does not contribute to the business of gaining insight into the thinking, ideas and practice of the ancient architects of this medicine. Even great scholars appear to have significant blind spots when it comes to Chinese medicine, and some even appear actively prejudiced against its clinical application.

At times I have sensed a seemingly wilful lack of a hermeneutic, insider perspective. Paul Unschuld's *History of Pharmaceutics* charted the development of China's *bencao* (*materia medica*) literature from its origins to modern times. The thematic thread that was applied tracked the discussions on one specific medicinal – *ba dou* (croton seeds) – in the various *bencao* editions through history. This is a substance with violent effects that induces massive fluid loss through the bowels, and might only be appropriate in the pre-terminal ascites stages of severe liver disease. The choice to focus on a drastic purgative like this, a substance that is almost never appropriate in the Western clinical setting, seems almost specifically designed to alienate practitioners who would be far more interested in following a thread about medicinal substances they actually prescribe on a daily basis and might wish to understand more fully.

Unhelpful distortions also arise in the way that aspects are included or excluded in some of the academic writings. So, in a quest for completeness in studies of 'medicine in China', some academics seek to encompass all of the practices carried out in the name of medicine, and then evaluate them as if they were all part of the same thing and so deserve the same attention. Few Chinese medicine practitioners will be wishing to help patients by burning pieces of paper on which they have written special characters, asking them to swallow burned lice combs or the dust swept from beneath a hangman's gibbet. Along with academic processes of conjoining the literate and scholastic tradition with shamanistic medicine, folk traditions, magic and ritualistic healing, there comes a dilution of the real achievements made by the literate traditions. The tarred brush of populist superstition too easily paints over the achievements of the real scholars of history.

Some writers may seek to demonstrate something in relation to the current discourse of another field. Some feminist scholars focus on the place of women in healthcare or seek to demonstrate how women have been subjugated by medical practices; some anthropologists aim to show how current traditional Chinese medicine should be considered an 'invented tradition'. Sometimes the consequences of such scholarship are completely absurd, for instance, by allowing those with little knowledge to suggest that the history of classical Chinese medicine is entirely non-existent. Baffling, perhaps, but not quite on target for insiders and clinicians who simply want to gain a better understanding of the root ideas and key historical influencers of this medicine. So, my intention is to skip much of the off-message stuff and to highlight instead the intellectual strands of actual medical thought and practice, to be more relevant to the task of enriching a practitioner's sense of connection with this medicine by focusing on the evolution and refinement of the medicine itself. This is not intended to be high-level academic sinology, but it is a challenging task, and one that will, no doubt, be completed by others to a degree that I can only aspire to. I hope my work succeeds to some extent in outlining where Chinese medicine's teachings come from and what their relevance is to modern practice. Readers will hopefully gain a sense of this medicine as an evolving tradition of professional medicine, developed largely by intelligent and rational thinkers who have responded well to changing times and conditions.

Themes, style and structure

Anticipating that my readership values accessibility and interest over strict academic rigour, this work does not formally propose new ideas or critique the work of others. For me, over-referencing hinders readability, and can even become an unnecessary affectation, and so I have chosen to provide my sources as an appendix. I have tried to ensure that my personal interpretations and speculations are flagged as such, using the usual un-academic 'weasel words' such as 'probably', 'in my view', 'it may be that', and so on. All the rest, of course, is derivative of the numerous sources drawn on, and I would like to express my gratitude to the many who have given me shoulders on which to stand. My skill has resided mainly in deciding which parts to borrow and in the ways that the information can be interpreted and represented, although these conclusions may not always be the same as those given by my sources.

I have also chosen to defy some other conventions in order to de-clutter the text and keep it compact. With this in mind I have been sparing with my use of Chinese characters, as putting these in on every occasion would hinder readability. Similarly with the Latin names of medicinals – these have been included mainly where the substance mentioned is less commonly used. For dates I have chosen to follow Joseph Needham by using – or + to stand for BC or AD, except where the context makes it self-evident. The temptation to pepper the work with footnote statements has also been resisted, and so the main concession to the general reader has been to provide a glossary of terms likely to confuse outsiders to the field (see Appendix 1). Academic conventions are important in high-level scholarly work but can be considered affectations when simply presenting, as faithfully as ability allows, a relatively uncontentious record of the received narrative of history. The slippery nature of truth becomes evident when we take different perspectives or when we chunk up or down to different levels of analysis. Sometimes, for clarity, a complex situation has to be covered with a generality. A British Prime Minister once asked the Russian Head of State, 'How are things in Russia?' 'Good!' came the reply. Hoping for a little more detail, the Prime Minister asked, 'Could you expand on that a little?' 'Not good!' came the more detailed reply. For so many aspects of human affairs truth is a slippery and possibly even mythical beast, and this is especially true of history. If ever there was an endeavour where the maxim 'an ounce of lie saves a ton of explanation', it is in the presentation of Chinese medicine history.

So, in writing this book, the aim was to draw on reliable sources in English and Chinese, and to offer plain and readable content covering the ideas of Chinese medicine – what they were, when they appeared and why. In telling this story I inevitably pluck information selectively or omit some information and so distort a little, but I have come to realise that even the most academically rigorous include distortions and even some misapprehensions. Anticipating that my readership values accessibility and interest over the strictest academic rigour, I also give little space to referencing individual statements.

The text is structured chronologically, and there are some themes that run loosely through the chapters. These include the issue of physician education and approaches to febrile epidemics. A central aim is to outline the most well-known texts from each era, and to sketch out what is known about the most famous thinkers and clinicians, as well as presenting the particular contributions made. Readers may notice that some of the major historical classics, such as the *Neijing* and *Shang Han Zhabing Lun*, do not quite get the coverage they deserve. These were downplayed somewhat because I realised that it was impractical to do justice to these complex texts in just a few pages. I think it is also true to say that others have already given sufficient detail on their meaning and content. Space has instead been devoted to the presentation of information that is less accessible, some of which has been specially translated by myself and by my friend and colleague, Dr Ying Liu. Inevitably some readers will spot glaring omissions; indeed, it is my spotting more and more of these that has contributed to years and years of delay in getting this into print – work was started about 15 years ago!

An early draft included much more recent history as well as an outline of the spread of Chinese medicine to the West in the 20th century. Better coverage on this has now appeared at the hands of others, and eventually I came to the conclusion that this material was a distraction that could safely be edited out. In addition, my writings give little attention to the way that Chinese medicine was adopted and adapted by countries such as Japan, Vietnam and Korea, and the way that it influenced medicine in India. My own studies have neglected these countries – my library is weak in this area and so my understanding here is weaker. Also only touched on are discussions of folk medical practices and *yang sheng* practices such as *qigong*, dietetics and religious and sexual health practices. Inclusion of all these would make for an unwieldy project; the omissions have also helped to keep a tighter focus on the medicine's core roots in mainland China. Apart from these gaps, knowledgeable readers will certainly be able to spot many other aspects that have been neglected, either because of the limits of my knowledge and abilities, or because I simply forgot to include them.

...if you want to change history, become a historian.

2

MEDICINE IN CHINA PRIOR TO THE HAN DYNASTY

For convenience, we can call the medical style that was systematised by scholars in the Han dynasty 'classical Chinese medicine'. Having labelled this strand of medical practice, and distinguished it from the many other medical styles practised in China, we can follow a continuous narrative of its progress, from the metaphysical ideas, investigations and fragmentary medical writings in the millennium prior to the start of the Han dynasty in −206, through a flowering due to the work of medical scholars in the Han dynasty itself, on through all the dynasties leading up to modern times. This story is a remarkable one, so vast, diverse and profound that all writers struggle to meet the challenge to accurately encompass its contents and its value.

Given the diversity of styles, practice and therapeutic traditions that have existed in China and its satellite cultures, it is possible to trace numerous other narratives that differ from those covered in this text. These might examine folk herbal medicine, shamanic healing, Daoist magical traditions, Buddhist chanting and prayer, the use of talismans and spells and the many other approaches to healthcare that deviate from what we choose to delineate as the classical style. Many of these other traditions survive today. Folk traditions, for instance, continue to exist in China and East Asia and across the world. These apply simple remedies that are cheap and accessible to everyone; they encompass sense and nonsense, they differ in degrees of simplicity and sophistication and often provide effective first aid measures for day-to-day ailments. Every rural province, for example, will have its local folk methods for the treatment of dysentery, the majority of which I think are effective. Daoist, Buddhist, magical, shamanic or superstitious traditions that might be characterised by the use of chanting, the performance of rituals, wearing lucky talismans or burning paper on which special characters have been written – all of these have formed part of the spectrum of medical care through China's history, and are mentioned here mainly to acknowledge the fact that there has always been an interchange between vernacular therapies and the classical tradition. Silk-clad classical physicians have often looked to folk medicine for inspiration, and conversely, folk practitioners have often sought to aggrandise their position by adopting the terminology and mannerisms of those higher up the social and intellectual ladder. The main focus of this book

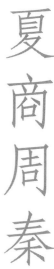

is the classical medical tradition in China as represented by a relatively restricted collection of famous figures and their ideas. Although emphasising the ideas of a particular social elite, this medicine nevertheless created a literature that runs to tens of thousands of texts and drew on the work of vast numbers of clinicians.

The Han dynasty scholars who laid down the foundations for classical Chinese medicine, nearly all anonymous, detailed their ideas in a handful of texts, some of which have survived reasonably intact to the present day. Textual analysis of Chinese medicine's most famous founding canonical text, the *Huangdi Neijing* (Yellow Emperor's Inner Classic), indicates that the core content was the work of roughly 30 different scholars, a handful of whom are named. The medical style they defined and set down was aggregated from the ideas and medical practice that had been current in the preceding century or two, so it makes sense to set the context by first picking up some of these early threads. These tributary medical lineages were themselves rooted in the various philosophical, metaphysical and pre-scientific beliefs that existed in the millennium before the Han dynasty. Very few writings on healthcare survive from these pre-Han times and so, inevitably, this chapter includes a certain amount of author speculation and interpolation – which has hopefully been adequately highlighted as such where it occurs.

Prehistory

Legend tells us that the history of medicine in China begins with Shen Nong, the 'Divine Farmer', who is said to have lived around −2750. He is credited with introducing agriculture to the Chinese people and is reputed to have selflessly poisoned himself many times whilst testing plants and other potential medicinal substances for their effects on the body. Tradition also claims that his medical experiments were recorded in the *Shennong Bencao* (Divine Farmer's *Materia Medica*). It is certain that herbal medicine was practised in prehistory. Residues of medicinal plants such as yarrow and camomile have been identified in the tartar of Neanderthal teeth found in northern Spain, providing direct evidence of medicinal herb use. However, modern scholarship of the *Shennong Bencao* tells us that the text that has been passed through to modern times could not conceivably have been compiled before the first century; for instance, the place names mentioned in the text were those in use during the Eastern Han (+23–221). This helps date authorship to that period even if, as seems likely, its content was derived from writings circulating in the previous centuries amongst those providing medical care.

Shen Nong, a legendary healer

Said to have lived prior to the Xia dynasty, Shen Nong is traditionally credited with inventing the plough and introducing crop planting. His selfless medical experiments are legendary. Having such an iconic hero invites emulation by later generations, and so his story probably contributed much to the development of medicine in China,

夏
商
周
秦

inspiring similar investigations and, ultimately, almost every substance in the environment that was accessible in China was studied and its qualities recorded for future generations.

If a historical figure named Shen Nong actually existed five millennia ago, as many contemporary medical historians in China believe, he may actually have been a notable tribal leader or a charismatic healer. It is also possible that the name may have referred not to a specific individual, but to a clan, perhaps part of the Neolithic Yang Shao culture that was active across today's Henan, Shaanxi and Shanxi provinces around −2600. Various Neolithic cultures in ancient China have been investigated in recent years, but the Yang Shao is especially celebrated by archaeologists and ceramic connoisseurs for their finely crafted pottery decorated with intricate chocolate-brown patterns and swirling motifs. Some hints of the thoughts and beliefs of these people can be discerned from their ceramic decorations. For example, swastika-like motifs (卍), that are said to represent the rotatory movement of the heavens, point to man's early fascination with observation of the night sky. These constant, reliable and reassuring cyclic movements seem to have symbolised to Neolithic peoples that all was well with the universe, and that the spirits of their deceased were content in the afterlife. The forces that manage such regularity needed to be encouraged – the darkest fear was that the stability and regularity might fail or even be plunged into reverse, the sun and moon might fail to rise, or the seasons may lose their regularity, leading to catastrophic consequences. (That in the 20th century the Nazis chose to reverse this ancient emblem of peace to symbolise their activities perhaps should have been taken as a warning of their intent.) It seems likely that these ancient people had a cultural memory of a time of prolonged wintery darkness, perhaps as a result of a volcanic catastrophe, instilling fear that this might be repeated if the ancestral spirits were displeased. Indeed, modern genetic analysis suggests that in prehistory mankind suffered a population hiatus during which the world population was reduced from many millions down to roughly 30,000 due to the 'nuclear winter' following a large meteor strike. Cultural memories of this catastrophic event may have driven a need in ancient times to enact rites conducted at sacred sites at the winter solstice intended to ensure continued cosmic regularity and the return of longer days rather than a continued retreat into darkness, illness and death. Beyond such speculations, a near complete absence of textual evidence from these Neolithic times means that we can say little about the earliest medical beliefs and practices.

PRE-HAN DYNASTIES

Xia −2100 to −1600

Shang −1600 to −1060

Zhou −1060 to −256

　　Western Zhou −1060 to −771

　　Eastern Zhou −771 to −256

　　Spring and Autumn −771 to −476

Warring States −475 to −221

Qin to −221 to −206

夏
商
周
秦

Fu Xi and Huangdi

Another legendary founding father of Chinese culture and medicine from prehistory is Fu Xi, who is credited with introducing agriculture, fishing with nets, the first written characters and, almost certainly incorrectly, with the eight-trigram symbols (*ba gua*) used in the *Yijing* (Classic of Changes), a text discussed later in this chapter. Traditionally considered to have lived around −2500, Fu Xi is also said to have devised the system that was used for most of China's history to track cycles of time and that formed the basis of the traditional calendar. This consisted of the successive paired interaction of a cycle of ten heavenly time periods, called stems, with twelve earthly attributes, called branches. The cyclic interaction of these resulted in a 60-part cycle where stems and branches paired successively to create a calendar that charted seasonal changes, information that was useful in an agrarian environment. It also served to model the moment-by-moment environmental and climatic qualities and their effect on the affairs of mankind. Much later, in the Tang and Song dynasties, this system was incorporated into a cosmology-based medical style. Various other contributions to civilisation are attributed to Fu Xi, but it is impossible to verify any of these.

Completing a triad of ancient heroes is Huangdi, who is said to have lived around −2680 and to have founded the Daoist healing arts. Because the *Huangdi Neijing* summarised earlier material on medical practice, it was respectfully attributed to him, even though we can be certain that none of the content came from such early times.

Whether or not any of these three named legendary rulers represent actual individuals, we know that charismatic clan leaders existed in these ancient times and exerted their rule, in part at least by virtue of their ability to convince others of a personal and influential connection with the spirits of the ancestors in the heavens. The rulers' professed power to mediate the will of heaven, earth and the destiny of mankind is reflected in an early character for chieftain that shows the three levels of heaven, earth and mankind connected and unified by a vertical line (*wang*, 王).

The three powers: heaven, earth, mankind

The three powers (*san cai*, 三才) idea, a fundamental theme of the *Yijing*, was a theory derived from Neolithic cosmology that described the relationship between heaven, the earth and mankind. In the heavens only three external energetic influences were seen to reach the earth from above – the sun, the stars and the moon. The sun was plainly associated with daylight, warmth and so on, influencing day length and the changes over the course of a year. With its changing elevation in the sky, the sun was seen to have a profoundly *yang* influence on the changing seasons and growth and development on earth. Even in ordinary modern Chinese usage the word for sun is *taiyang*, extreme *yang*. The moon was also considered to influence the earth,

夏
商
周
秦

in a darker and subtler way, in the tides and in the menstrual cycles of women. Representing the souls of departed clansmen, the stars, and especially those that form the Milky Way, were also considered to influence events on earth and the affairs of mankind.

Heaven, represented by the character 天 (*tian*), was seen to be the epitome of reliable regularity in its behaviour and its cycles. Ordered and boundless, it was the abode of the ancestors and the source of the natural order of things. Its pristine influence descended to earth, normally working to ensure that man and nature did not deviate from their proper order. Those occasions where the heavens were seen to deviate from their exact regularity were therefore significant. Their long-standing obsession with sky watching means that ancient Chinese records are a useful resource for modern astronomers studying past cosmic events, such as supernovae.

In heaven–earth–man cosmology the energies of heaven and earth meet and react together to create life on earth and, in a sense, this is true from a scientific standpoint. Lacking the *yang*, the warming and transforming influence of the sun, the earth would be dark, cold and lifeless – *yin*, in other words. The heavens do indeed influence life on earth. Science would disagree about the extent to which events on earth can influence the heavens, although unarguably heaven and earth react together to create all the complexities of life. By understanding and describing these forces, including their movement and changing qualities, the ancient Chinese believed they would have the key to understanding what benefited and what hindered mankind. Man stood in the middle, with the bright, energetic, stimulating, non-material clear-sky influence from above, energising, warming, transforming, ordering and clarifying. Below was the earth, with its dense, dark, muddy and turbid qualities, providing material existence and sustenance. In this conception it was the interaction of the two that would allow man, and indeed life on earth, to flourish.

Use of medicinal herbs in prehistory

There can be no doubt that plant materials and other natural substances were used as medicines in China at around the alleged time of Shen Nong. Well-preserved desiccated bodies dated to the second and third millennia before Christ have been found in desert areas bordering modern China; one was found to be carrying a belt pouch containing the herb *ma huang* (Ephedra sinensis), a medicinal that remains important in Chinese medicine today to treat respiratory disorders. A main active component of this herb is ephedrine, an effective bronchodilator that was adopted into Western medical practice early in the 20th century when it became established as the first effective pharmaceutical drug for asthma. With the introduction of newer bronchodilators, it has since been relegated to use as a nasal decongestant; nevertheless, it is interesting to reflect on the fact that a pharmaceutical drug commonly used in modern medicine was first introduced into healthcare by people living around the end of the Neolithic period.

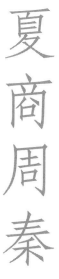

夏
商
周
秦

Other medical therapeutics in prehistory

In addition to herbal medicine, there is evidence of various other therapeutic procedures employed in prehistoric China, although acupuncture does not seem to have been in existence at this time. A skull with a carefully executed 3cm round hole dating from the Shang dynasty (roughly −1600 to −1060) has been unearthed in China. Scientific examination of the degree of local bone healing indicates that the subject lived for at least two months after the operation was carried out, and the procedure must have almost certainly required some form of anaesthesia. Most scholars in China consider that the area was probably numbed using ice prior to incision.

Apart from a few archaeological traces that have been found in China dating from roughly −3000 to −1500, the earliest documentary evidence available in relation to medicine and health practice dates from the Shang (c. −1600 to −1060) and Western Zhou (−1060 to −771) dynasties. Unfortunately, these are also too fragmentary to construct a clear idea of the standard health practices of this early time, although there is sufficient evidence for a rough picture to emerge of shamanic practices that often attributed ill health to ancestor displeasure.

SHAMANIC MEDICINE

Illness, along with most other calamities, was often blamed on displeasure of the ancestor spirits meting out retribution to the living who had failed in some way to satisfy their needs and desires, for example, by not carrying out the appropriate rites of appeasement at the proper times, rites that may well have been devised by those in the community with schizotypal and obsessive personality disorders. The shamanic diagnostic process was similar to that used for any other problem facing the clan – it consisted of divining which particular ancestral figure was responsible for the difficulty, and identifying what placatory actions the living could take to help restore normality. Typically this consisted of an offering and conducting a ritual, a prayer or a sacrifice. This early conception of the underlying meaning of disease differed from our modern sense of the word because an individual's illness carried with it implications beyond the concerns of an individual or family; it could imply ancestral displeasure that carried with it ramifications for the larger social group – a person's illness might be a harbinger for medical catastrophe on a wider scale. In cases of epidemic illness, of course, the effects of ancestor displeasure could quickly spread to affect many people, and so suitable appeasement measures were crucial for the well-being of everyone. So the fact that one individual had been targeted for retribution did not rule out the possibility of others becoming affected too, and things were especially ominous if the person affected was a high-status individual. Rapid appeasement was important before deeper trouble set in.

Further, beyond the medical consequences for the individual or the potential for epidemic disease, unresolved ancestor displeasure might entail an even wider package of associated adverse events – perhaps impacting on the whole clan, such as

夏
商
周
秦

infertility of livestock, floods or losing battles with neighbouring clans, and so on. With such ramifications to consider, the appropriate response sometimes required remedial measures that were targeted not only at the sick individual, but the social group as a whole, for instance, by performing rituals that were evident to the whole community.

Given that the ruler and his clan were responsible for the maintenance of harmonious relationships between the ancestors in the Milky Way, the earthly climate and its numerous ghosts and the affairs of the living, it was especially incumbent on them to employ the most powerful shamans available to ensure proper regulation of ancestral relations. In prehistory, tribal rulers may themselves have been shamans, but later kings could simply employ them to assist in state administration. This relationship, based on respect and fear, meant that for much of China's early history a degree of tension existed between the shamans, with their schizotypal personalities, and the rulers. In the Warring States period (−475 to −221) the influence of the shamans declined and they lost some of their influence to the then burgeoning scholar classes, but tensions between advisers and the ruling aristocracy continued. Such advisers, shamanic or scholarly, were a necessary part of government, but were also prone to overreach themselves, plot and scheme for their own advantage and generally bicker and cause trouble. Later, court eunuchs also became renowned for joining in the intrigue and profiteering game.

An important way that the power and legitimacy of early rulers was demonstrated to those around them was by effective divinatory activity. If rulers could accurately predict, and thereby appear to be in control of, eclipses and other events in the heavens, catastrophes, changes in climate and so on, then their credibility and position was more assured. Repeated crop failures, famines, disease epidemics and so on were tangible evidence for both ministers and the populace that the heavens' support for the current ruler was waning. The shamans and court scholars were therefore an important part of this aspect of government, and when predictions came to pass, the veracity of the claimed links between the rulers and the spirits of the ancestors was confirmed. The use of clan folk beliefs and superstitions, hallucinatory trance states and magic provided an extra dimension to the more mundane aspects of statecraft, such as punishing wrongdoers, ensuring grain supplies and defending against marauders. Of course, a skilful court mystic could predict a catastrophe, enact a solution and then be celebrated for his power when the disaster failed to occur.

Individual shamans probably achieved their credibility and hence their influence and position by having learned to perform a set of convincing, perhaps awe-inspiring, tricks and illusions that combined magic, chanting, acoustics, hyperventilation and hallucinogenic drugs. This was a trade that gave access to influence. At the very least these specialists needed a demonstrable track record in summoning ancestral spirits and ways of proving to everyone that they had done so. Being privy to secret knowledge of astronomy enabled some to make predictions of heavenly events such as eclipses, comets and retrograde planetary motions. The diurnal rotation of the

夏
商
周
秦

heavens was the most universal constant imaginable. Its frequency could be calculated and then represented as a musical note. This understanding allowed sacred rites on earth to be tuned by the emperor and his advisers to resonate with, and therefore communicate with, the heavens – the abode of the ancestors. The geometry of the Ming dynasty Temple of Heaven in Beijing appears to reflect this, as do many much more ancient structures across the world, such as Stonehenge in England. Speculating for a moment, with their roughly 32-metre diameter, the Temple of Heaven and Stonehenge are resonant with overtones of the frequency of the apparent rotation of the universe which approximates to the note F. Clan voices singing a low F note two octaves below middle C would resonate with the structure, and so, in theory, with the universe itself. With the structure roofed and the walls closed up, the acoustic standing wave from this chanting would likely create impressive effects, such as swirling dust and smoke along the entrance tunnel and the 'spirit path' that leads up to it. There is archaeological evidence of cremated remains here in Neolithic ritual sites such as Stonehenge, a site that also has the inside stones slightly hollowed in a way that would enhance their response to chanting. With this acoustic trick, dust from the cremated remains of recently deceased tribal leaders, lit by the rising sun on the winter solstice, along with chanting and the use of hallucinogens, such effects would serve quite well as convincing demonstrations of awe-inspiring shamanic supernatural power and influence. Resonate with this overtone of the fundamental note of the universe and, as a shaman, you could feel quite sure you were getting through to those in the heavens and the ancestral spirits, themselves revolving around the pole star. And sure enough, from that moment on, the days would get longer and lighter, and the rejuvenation of spring would appear. These prehistoric notions of a resonant connection between the heavens, the natural world on earth and the affairs of mankind persisted from prehistory into the beginnings of documented history in China in the Shang and Zhou dynasties. The power of the mandate of heaven could be demonstrated annually by ritual and magic.

Understanding the great potential of resonance to ancient peoples is an important aspect of understanding some of the thinking behind early medical practices.

Shang and Zhou cultures

Thriving roughly from –1600 to –1050, the Shang civilisation was located on the plains of the Yellow River in northeastern China. Their capital was called Yin, a place that corresponds to the city of Anyang today. Towards the end of this period the Zhou clan, who were confined to territories further to the west, referred to their neighbours as the Yin Shang, or simply the Yin, a term that is often used by historians today. The Yin Shang people are remembered today for their iconic and skilfully cast bronze ritual vessels. They ruled with the aid of military force and, like many civilisations of this time, ancestor worship was at the centre of their belief system.

The people of the Shang dynasty, in common with most cultures ancient and modern, were keenly interested in the effects of ingested substances on mind and body. They made beer (*chang*) out of the fermented tubers of the mild intoxicant *yujin* (Curcuma longa), a relative of the ginger plant that remains a commonly used medicinal in Chinese medicine today. Grapes, together with medicinal herbs such as *shan zha* (hawthorn berries), have also been identified from fermenting vessels from Neolithic times, which may indicate a crossover between medicinal and recreational use. It is certain that many other plants and substances were employed in prehistoric times for their therapeutic properties, although substantive understanding of the way that medicine was practised at this time is virtually absent, and so we have to hunt carefully for clues.

Components of the character 醫 (*yi*), the Shang and Zhou word for healer, give hints about the tools that medicine used at the boundaries of history and prehistory. One part of the character suggests the sticks clattered together by shamans to drive away malevolent spirits. Another part shows a quiver full of arrows said to represent the lances, or perhaps stone arrowheads, used to drain abscesses, boils and other pustular swellings. The lower part suggests medicinal wines and decoctions made from herbs and other substances used to treat illness or to strengthen an ailing patient. *Yi* can therefore be interpreted as summarising some of the main activities inherent in medical practices of the Shang era.

In contrast to the classical medicine of the literati that was to develop roughly a millennium later, herbal medicine was almost certainly practised in a folk medicine style – meaning, single medicinal substances applied symptomatically, with little by way of systematic diagnostic or theoretical foundation. Folk medicine differs from the more systematic literate medical traditions by the relative paucity of its written corpus, by the limited formal training of its practitioners and by the simple matching of symptom to treatment. Incidentally, the term 'herbal medicine' is used here as a convenient label despite the fact that therapeutic usage was not confined to plant materials. Throughout the history of Chinese medicine, physicians went to the trouble of systematically investigating the therapeutic properties of pretty much every imaginable substance found in nature – plants, insects, rocks, animal droppings and beyond. Moss scraped from the north wall of a house, the oviduct of a particular frog, flying squirrel droppings, dandruff and dust swept up from below a hangman's gibbet, the quest was to investigate the properties of everything. This work was driven by curiosity and by the medical imperative. In addition, during times of famine there was a survivalist imperative to distinguish substances that could serve as food sources from substances that were inedible or poisonous.

The great majority of substances listed in the historical *bencao* (herbal pharmacopias) are not in common use today in medicine, although the vast database of possibilities remains. Demand for substances whose properties were explored historically, such as rhino horn, bear bile and tiger bone, comes today not from mainstream professional Chinese medicine practice but from the whims and desires of the wealthy keen to possess expensive rarities.

夏
商
周
秦

Founding of the Zhou dynasty

Towards the end of their dynastic domination the Shang rulers became increasingly cruel and autocratic, behaviour that left them increasingly vulnerable both to internal rebellion and to invasion. The breakdown eventually happened somewhere between −1060 and −1050, when the Zhou people crossed the Yellow River, invading eastwards to overthrow the Yin Shang and to establish more civilised rule. The new regime gained control by installing their own princes widely across the region, and by appointing fiefdoms that were beholden to, and generally related to, the Zhou rulership. In contrast to the Yin Shang who had claimed that their rule was an enactment of the will of ancestral spirits, the Zhou introduced the concept of rule by the more impersonal concept of the mandate of heaven – the emperor ruled because the heavens willed it, and less so because of the actions of individual ancestral spirits. This mincing of words and concepts may have been a necessary expedient to win over the Yin Shang population to the new rulers – whose ancestral spirits were obviously not the same as those of the indigenous population. So, despite the word changes, the idea of the influence of the ancestors on the people remained an important part of the cultural belief system, and liaison with them continued.

The Zhou clan introduced a new, more efficient bureaucratic style to government, something that is evident in the extensive divinatory and other court records from this time that have been unearthed, inscribed on animal scapula bones and tortoise shells. Tortoise shells were an especially auspicious medium because they normally had a long lifespan (and so had virtue); their shape was auspicious as it was itself a microcosm of the universe itself, embodying the connection between the heavens above (dome shaped) and the earth below (flat). This shape suggested that it was able to resonate with the affairs of both heaven and earth. Being very resistant to rot, tortoise carapaces were also very useful for record keeping – indeed, so good that many survive today. A high bureaucracy such as that of the Zhou people consumed a lot of writing materials, so when tortoises subsequently became scarce, the scapular bones of domestic animals were used instead. The records on bones and carapaces that have been unearthed numbered in their hundreds of thousands, together with writings on bronze ritual vessels, and similar inscriptions from the Shang dynasty have provided us with a few fragmentary medical writings and some glimpses of the medical beliefs and practices of the time.

Jiagu wen, shell and bone writings

In 1899 the first of the *jiagu wen* writings were found in a village near Anyang in Henan province. The initial discovery was made when an archaeologist noticed that the 'dragon bones' (*long gu*) dispensed by the local herb pharmacy were inscribed with a mysterious and almost indecipherable script that was clearly related to subsequent Chinese writing. In 1928 a full excavation of the source of this cache of bones and carapaces was carried out, and since this initial find, more than 150,000 *jiagu wen* have been excavated and studied as textual sources providing insight into the Yin Shang and Zhou dynasty cultures. Some 4500 different characters have been identified, and a few thousand of these early 20th-century texts have been interpreted. More recently, various other *jiagu wen* of the Western Zhou period (–1060 to –771) have been discovered in Shanxi province, and these have provided further glimpses into medical theory and court health practices during the Shang and Zhou dynasties.

The vast majority of the *jiagu wen* writings are court and government administrative records, and records of the divinatory activities of the shaman advisers to the ruling elite. Relatively few provide information about medical matters, but they do help inform us of the way these ancient people thought. Typically, the texts ask questions such as 'Is now a good time for the prince to go hunting?' and other such routine dilemmas of the ruling classes. Brief questions were first inscribed, and then a hot metal implement was pressed into the bone or tortoise carapace so that the expert could divine the answer following inspection of the pattern of cracks. The answers usually came in the form of a 'yes' or 'no', and the outcome of the consultation was then also inscribed on the bones and shells. In the minds of these ancient seers the actual process of the formation of cracks was itself emblematic of the predictive process. Cracks symbolised the idea that subtle changes in the fabric of the world, when viewed alongside a knowing observation of present circumstances and conditions, could be predictive of developments in the future. As modern householders living in areas prone to subsidence know, tiny cracks presage future change. They are emblematic of the earliest stages of change. This is something that is depicted in the character ⼘ (*bu*), which means to divine. In terms of the crucial life-and-death issues facing mankind, such as warfare and sickness, the principle was that early recognition of change allowed timely, and therefore minimal, intervention – a stitch in time saves nine. This is relevant to medicine because later down the historical line similar thinking was transferred to medicine – subliminal changes, subtle diagnostic 'cracks' observable in the bodily landscape, could be interpreted as portents for future progress into illness.

In the Shang and Zhou dynasties a skilled seer was one who was especially adept at being able to read revealing prophetic signs in the environment, such as the behaviour of particular birds or even maggots in rotting meat, and to be able to sense the likely path of future events. The seers felt that these events were pregnant with meaning – that these were communications from the ancestral spirit world.

Such ideas might appear nonsensical to the modern mind, although sometimes signs in the environment are indeed significant – but because of our different experience of the world, our sense of dread is triggered in different ways. Most of us today would experience a real sense of dread if the tide suddenly went out as we lay on a tropical beach, for example – we have acquired a learned association that might save our lives. And changes in bird behaviour have even been known to precede earthquakes and tsunamis. One problem with this portent method, apart from most of them being rather unreliable, was that many of the signs presupposed

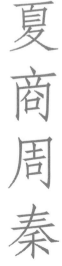

'being out there', connected to the natural environment, with one's portent antennae adjusted to full sensitivity. Not so good if you are confined to a palace. There was also the practical difficulty that one had to wait patiently for the meaningful cracks to appear – not so convenient for a busy court seer under pressure to be productive. What was needed was divination on demand, hence the development of the *jiagu wen* system based on the interpretation of cracks inflicted on turtle shells and animal scapulas that offered instant prediction without the inconvenience of waiting for environmental portents.

As the Zhou dynasty progressed into the Warring States period, some questioned the use of mystical prognostication methods. How reliable was it, when life-and-death issues or the survival of the state were at stake, to put your trust in patterns of cracks interpreted by intoxicated epileptic seers? So, in –5th century Kongfuzi (Confucius) proposed that government and the ordering of society should be based on clear social rules, and over the following centuries, a new class of educated rational gentlemen, the *shi* scholars, grew to have ever-increasing political influence. Another pragmatist was the famed military strategist Sun Zi, who specifically urged that divination methods should be abandoned in favour of insightful strategy, deep cunning and military skill. Later, in the decades before the Qin and Han dynasties, other figures also advocated abandonment of superstitious beliefs.

Yijing, invention of a mathematical model of change

As discussed, predictions provided by the early shamans, mystics and seers were based on the supposed meaning of portents observed in the environment that were perceived as pregnant with significance. It may have been a skylark that inspired one such signal from nature: *the bird that sings in flight – don't ascend – descent will be fortuitous!* These passed from generation to generation as simple *aides memoirs* for these signs, some of which survive in the oldest parts of the *Yijing* (Classic of Changes). The Zhou clan collected these aphorisms together to help bureaucratise the business of prognostication and decision-making; they then formulated a mathematical means to access the portents and to model change and transformation through time that bypassed the need for direct observation of nature.

Authorship of the *Yijing* is traditionally attributed to the clan chiefs the Duke of Zhou and King Wen at the start of the Zhou dynasty, but in reality the text we have today evolved through subsequent centuries. The mathematics that formed its structure is so lucid and symmetrical that it bears the hallmarks of the involvement of at least one mathematical genius savant. With the addition of archetypal symbols and a form of binary digital mathematics later in the Zhou dynasty, it offered a model for understanding and predicting change and transformation, and provided philosophical ideas for contemplation as well as a map of the thought structures of the unconscious mind. Known also as the *Zhou Yi* (Changes of the Zhou Clan), it

夏
商
周
秦

claimed to provide a systematised symbolic representation of the manner in which events unfold through time, the implication being that such contemplations facilitated timely action before events had progressed to beyond rescue. The *Yijing* offered a way of joining together an understanding of the evolution of events through time in a satisfying framework that mixed the beliefs of the seer with the lucidity of a seemingly rational mathematical schema.

Centuries later, the *Yijing* and its underlying ideas and mathematics had a profound influence on early medical thought as well as on Chinese and indeed East Asian thought as a whole. Its beauty and its claim to model processes of change and transformation have made it an eternal object of veneration. (We return to it later in this chapter.)

Yijing origins

The people who devised this system believed that the key to understanding change through time lay in the relationship between the sky above and the earth below, and the effects these had on the affairs of mankind. This is summarised in a passage in the *Yijing* that says:

> Looking upwards we can contemplate the manifestations [of change] in the sky, looking down we examine the patterns [of change] on earth. In this way we can understand the characteristic [changes] of the dark and the light [*yin* and *yang*]. ('Da-juan', *Yijing*)

Seemingly abstruse and metaphysical, these ideas are rooted in basic truisms that describe links between the cyclic changes in day length, position of the sun, moon and stars with climate cycles, and therefore life itself. Questionable to the modern mind is the extent to which the modelling of such things could be extrapolated to things such as the relationships between people; nonetheless, it provided a framework and an impetus for the detailed study and classification of natural phenomena for which the Chinese are renowned.

Looking upwards, the stars of the Milky Way were believed to be the place where the ancestral spirits were concentrated. The pole star, the still and central pivot of the night sky, was felt to be crucial as it held pride of position as the axis of the movement of the entire universe. One ancient Daoist *qi* cultivation technique involved forming a mental connection between this point and the acupoint Du 23 (*shang xing*, highest star) with the intention of drawing personal strength from this pivot of the universe – a powerful mental image that may well induce psychosomatic effects. From this central reference point the sky was divided into four quadrants that, together with the central pole position, allowed a five-part division of space. The Chinese character for the number five (五) shows this map, with the pole and its four quadrants shown as 十, the sense of the connectedness between 'heaven and

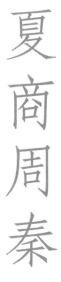

夏
商
周
秦

earth' indicated by the two horizontals (二) and the vertical (l). The short vertical line then suggested rotational movement and change.

Modelling the intermingling of heaven and earth, the creators of the *Yijing* codified the relationship into a hierarchy of gradations of *yang* and *yin* (light and dark). This scheme progressed from the simple two-part *yin-yang* distinction, through a four-part division, then an eight-part and on to a 64-part model of patterns of change. Its originators considered that it could be extended to encompass the complexity seen in the 'ten thousand things' – shorthand for the entire world.

The character *yi* (易) in *Yijing* means 'change' and also 'easy', perhaps suggesting that this was a simplified model of the way things transform, or the apparent effortlessness by which the natural world transforms itself through time. Use of the word 'easy' may also have been an expression of the Daoist belief that the most effective and effortless form of action was a form of prescient minimal action based on careful reflection rather than brute imposition of will.

The word 'easy' also suggests the idea that one could get to grips with the extreme complexity of the natural world by subjecting it to an analysis using a series of binary distinctions, that the analogue world could be represented and interpreted using a digital thinking schema. The factors underlying and influencing change and transformation were multifactorial, obscure and subtle, only discernible by very careful observation; the belief was that these complex interactions behind the unfolding of events could be modelled by simple binary mathematics. The simplest logical tool, a product of a basic way that the mind operates to interpret sensory information, is the idea of binary contrast: *yin-yang*, light-dark, hot-cold, above-below, inside-outside, solid-hollow, hard-soft, and so on. By means of ever more detailed refinements of this binary logic tree, the gentlemen scholars of the Warring States period believed that all phenomena could be encompassed and understood.

The extent to which the Zhou court scholars were able to make this scheme work as an effective tool for state administrative affairs is debatable, but in the process of trying, they hit upon an interesting and powerful logical tool, one that in modern times has been adopted as the mathematical basis of computing and digital communications. The flexibility of this thinking model meant that it could be applied either to pragmatic real-world problem-solving, at one end of human endeavour, or to esoteric metaphysical speculation, at the other. Nevertheless, it was later to become central to classical medicine.

Yin and *yang* (阴阳) originally meant the shady and sunny slopes of a mountain respectively, and early forms of these characters predate the Shang dynasty (–1600). The words, which have no English equivalent, accumulated more shades of meaning (see below) to broadly represent all the dualities observable in the universe and the affairs of mankind.

YING-YANG BINARY HIERARCHY

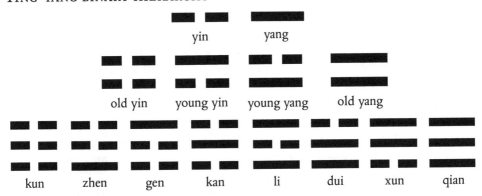

The use of six lines allowed 64 basic states of change to be mathematically represented by the hexagrams of the *Yijing*. The text suggests that this scheme may be extended infinitely to represent 'ten thousand things', or everything in existence; it provided a framework in which to fit observations about the patterns of change and transformation seen in nature. These observations led to a set of axiomatic generalisations and beliefs about the application of this explanatory and predictive model to the world.

Over 2000 years after these Chinese scholars created their binary system, a Jesuit missionary living in China became fascinated by its possibilities, and described it in letters he wrote to his mathematician friend in Germany, Gottfried Leibniz (1646–1716), describing his study of the *Yijing* and its novel mathematical system. Leibniz himself is credited with the invention of binary mathematics that was later to become a fundamental basis of computing and digital communications that we use today to model the analogue world digitally. What we see as a very modern way of managing information has its origins in the ruminations of scholars working in ancient times.

> **SOME AXIOMS OF THE *YIN-YANG* DOCTRINE**
>
> - Everything can be classified using these attributes.
> - The attributes are relative rather than absolute.
> - Nothing is entirely either *yin* or *yang*.
> - Nothing remains unchanging; there is always transformation and change through time.
> - When one situation reaches a peak, it already contains subtle indicators of its transformation into its opposite.

Yin-yang interpenetration

The *yin-yang* relationship between the sky above and the earth below is an idea that probably extends back to prehistory and was viewed as analogous to sexual interplay. When these two fundamental aspects of the universe and nature worked together properly, were fully intertwined with each other, then there could be life. Under these conditions things were generated and there was thriving health and

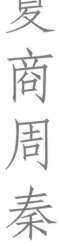

vitality. Harmonious *qi* was created by this interplay of *yin* and *yang* whilst, at the same time, this *qi* itself helped maintain the interpenetration of and connection between these opposites. Dissolution and death implied a separation of *yin* and *yang* – when *yin* substance is no longer animated by the presence of *yang* activity, they are no longer unified together. Both at an individual and universal consciousness or spirit, *shen* (神) was considered to be one product of this healthy interplay of *yin* and *yang*.

The relationship between *yin* and *yang* was also compared to the transformational relationship between fire (*yang*) and water (*yin*). The action of fire when placed below water generates steam, which is *qi*-like in its insubstantial qualities, but an enduring excess of one or the other is not sustainable. The Mawangdui manuscripts suggest this happens in mankind, too, proposing, for example, that in health man has a cool head but warm feet – that his *yang* fire activities are properly placed below so as to generate *qi*. In this context we might understand *qi* as akin to the modern idea of metabolism. We should, however, bear in mind that the actual meaning of *qi* is very context-dependent. Seemingly alchemical in nature, this scheme is not especially metaphysical; it is true that life on earth depends fundamentally on the interaction of the *yang* energetic influence of the sun and the *yin* material nature of the earth, and that life is an interpenetration of activity (*yang*) animating substance (*yin*). When decoupled, life is no longer sustained, and so the idea behind many health-maintaining practices was to enhance integration of *yin* and *yang*.

Hexagram 63 of the *Yijing* represents this near-ideal state of *yin-yang* inter-penetration in man by alternating *yang* (unbroken) lines with *yin* (broken) lines. The bottom group of three lines represents warmth, *yang* and activity; the top trigram represents coolness, water and *yin*. The balanced interaction of the two is emblematic of health. This hexagram is called *jiji* and was often used historically in medical scholarship to denote a state of health balance.

Early surface anatomy

By the end of the Shang dynasty numerous written characters existed to describe surface anatomy. According to the eminent contemporary medical historian Fu Wei-kang, some parts were named with reference to their physiological function, for example, in relation to pregnancy – birth, breasts, urine, blood and so on. Apart from the character for heart, the *jiagu wen* (shell and bone writings) only rarely mentioned the internal organs. It is hard to imagine, though, that no knowledge of the internal organs existed in these early times – the slaughter of animals inevitably involves exposure to their inner

Basic anatomical characters found on Shang dynasty divinatory bones include: head, face, eyes, mouth, tongue, nose, eyebrow, ears, teeth, hands, elbows, humerus, feet, shin, knees, toes, neck, back, abdomen and hip.

夏
商
周
秦

workings, and given the human propensity to engage in combat and war, people must have noticed that they, too, possessed similar inner workings. Examining Shang dynasty writings on bronze, bones and tortoiseshell, we find many of the very early anatomical terms used have survived into modern Chinese, although the actual form of the characters has mutated through time.

In traditional cultures, medical knowledge usually accumulates as oral folklore, and such traditions are known to have evolved in China amongst midwives, sores specialists and bonesetters who, in the course of their work, inevitably acquired anatomical knowledge and other medical insights. In the Shang and Zhou dynasties the progress to the professionalisation of medicine was hindered by the weakness of the communication systems available and low literacy rates of the time. The adoption of this medical folklore into systematic medicine had to wait until the Han dynasty, when conditions were more favourable. For example, prior to the Han dynasty, the need to write on carapace, bone and bamboo slats precluded any detailed discussion of medicine, much less the processes of discovery that led to the conclusions. Even with the much-increased literacy in the Han dynasty, and when paper became available, detailed discussion was difficult. The important thing was the actual knowledge itself and its coding in compact form. Because the epistemology underlying much of early Chinese medicine's 'facts' is obscured due to these factors today, we are forced to choose, according to our mindset, to interpret any particular 'fact' from Chinese medicine's ancient history, either as groundless speculation or as the result of an actual investigative process. It is clear, though, that much of the information that formed the basis of the early classical medical tradition could only have been the result of formal investigative processes.

Basic examples of this include anatomical information described later. Even seemingly esoteric statements of fact are probably rooted in real-world observations. For instance, one traditional fact that survives into modern Chinese medicine is the statement 'spirit consciousness travels with blood'. Often seen as a rather speculative metaphysical statement, this idea may actually come from the more mundane observation that animals or humans quickly lose consciousness as a consequence of haemorrhage. Other aspects of traditional medical doctrine are vulnerable to a similar disconnect from their epistemological origins whilst others have become indecipherable as a result of the language, temporal and cultural distance between us and ancient scholars. In general, the early medical texts may be seen as a mosaic of innumerable observations and experiments mixed together with folklore and speculation, and bound together with an ever-evolving explanatory model incorporating the ideas of the intellectual classes of the time, such as *yin-yang* and *wu xing* ('five phase') theory.

Alongside the inherent tendency for ancient people to seek to acquire useful skills and condense these into compact aphorisms and pithy written texts, there was also a need for those in possession of such knowledge to keep the information secret and to resist pressure from outsiders to access that knowledge for their own advancement. The possession of secret and valuable knowledge and skills provided

夏
商
周
秦

income, mystique and power that would be diminished by free dissemination. For this reason, proprietary knowledge of medicine, longevity practices, philosophy and statecraft was often encoded in obscure language with the deliberate intention of excluding non-initiates. This has long been one function of technical languages in the West, too. This imperative to exclude non-initiates makes the interpretation of early medical texts especially problematic, because generally they were not *meant* to be easily understood by outsiders, even in their own time. Medical and other scholarly texts were manuals to be used alongside the explanations and practical input from a mentor following vows of secrecy.

Early knowledge of diseases

Study of the *jiagu wen* (shell and bone writings) from the Shang and Zhou dynasties allowed some illnesses to be identified. Most often these were named using the format of 'body part' character as well as a character for 'illness'. Examples included illnesses affecting the head, eye, ear, mouth, teeth, tongue, nose, neck, limbs, abdomen, urinary tract, feet, hands, hips and knees. Obstetric and children's diseases were also found named in this way. Other diseases were labelled according to the main characteristic of the illness, such as *ji yan* (speech disease), most likely referring either to hoarseness or post-stroke aphasia. Medical historian Fu Wei-kang discusses another term seen in the *jiagu wen* writings that appeared in relation to pathology, namely *ji nian* (disease year). This term is believed to refer to years when epidemic diseases were rife. A further example is a *jiagu wen* character that consists of a part meaning worm or insect and a part meaning 'bowl'. This is the ancient form of the modern character *gu* (蛊), and may originally have referred to a specific parasitical disease or a group of such diseases.

夏商周秦

An interesting connection that spans the last 3000 years is seen when we look at the modern characters for tooth decay, *qu chi* (齲齒). *Chi* means teeth, and the ancient bone script form of the character for *qu* is assembled from parts signifying teeth, worms and holes – suggesting wormholes in the teeth. These examples, and the ones mentioned earlier, highlight the fact that specific diseases were recognised and named in the Shang and Zhou dynasties, and that modern scholars perhaps over-emphasise ancestor displeasure to the exclusion of real-world aetiologies.

The term *gu* was used through much of subsequent history in China to refer to an intractable poisonous curse administered by those with malevolent intent. *Gu* poison was created by collecting one each of the 'five poisonous animals' (venomous snake, scorpion, centipede, bufo bufo toad and spider), putting them in a container with the intent that one would consume all the others, and thereby accumulate all the poisons together. The surviving creature is then killed, ground into a powder and covertly administered to somebody with harmful intent.

Treatment methods in the Shang and Zhou dynasties

Study of the *jiagu wen* offered a glimpse of some treatment methods used in the Shang and Zhou dynasties, which included surgical lancing, massage, bonesetting, teeth extraction and herbal medicine. Fu Wei-kang uses the modern word 'acupuncture' (*zhen ci*, 针刺) rather than 'lancing', but this is misleading as there is no evidence from the Shang and Western Zhou dynasties to support the idea that needles were used in any way akin to the energetic system of medicine that was later to appear in the Han dynasty, implied by the term 'acupuncture'. Finely crafted stone needles have been unearthed from Shang and Zhou tombs, but these were almost certainly used for surgical lancing procedures rather than the wider therapeutic intent suggested by the word 'acupuncture'.

Other evidence that is sometimes offered to support the idea that acupuncture was practised in the Shang and Zhou dynasties comes from two characters on inscriptions from these times. Some *jiagu wen* inscriptions use the characters *qi yin* to mean 'sick person'. *Qi* (其) means 'him', and *yin* (殷) combines representations of a person lying on a sickbed paired with character components representing sharp tools or weapons, so this character might be taken to imply 'lancing therapy' and has sometimes been interpreted as evidence for early acupuncture. More likely, though, it refers to minor surgical procedures such as the debridement of wounds. On oracle inscriptions the expression *qi yin* often appears in divinatory questions asking whether or not to treat a patient with this form of therapy.

Such routine references to divine authorities before giving treatment may well have served as much to protect the physicians themselves as to gain high-level advice. It was quite important to be in a position to sidestep responsibility if things went wrong.

There is also evidence of an understanding of hygiene practices in Shang times – bone inscriptions mentioning the routine washing and bathing habits of the Yin Shang people indicate that they practised basic personal hygiene. In 1935 archaeologists unearthed a complete sanitary set from a Yin Shang tomb in Henan province, including a kettle for warming bathing water, a water container, a ladle and a washbowl. Clean water was obtained from wells, and excavations have even found underground drains serving Shang dynasty townships. This suggests that there was a good understanding of the links between clean water, disposal of waste water, personal hygiene and the maintenance of health.

> Other *jiagu wen* divinatory inscriptions ask:
>
> - The Yin Emperor has elbow dislocation disease – should we treat using elbow manipulation?
> - Emperor Wu Ding has a teeth sickness – should we extract?
> - Yin Emperor Wu Ding is ill – should we treat this with *da zao* (medicinal dates)?

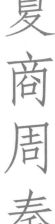

Medical specialists to the Zhou court

Members of the Zhou dynasty court were served by personal physicians who were probably appointed to official service after gaining repute as medical experts in the community. This idea is supported by the official record of the Zhou dynasty activities (*Zhouli*, Rites of the Zhou), where three types of medical specialist at the imperial court are described. There were two dietary specialists, who were classed as upper masters (*shangshi*, 上师), eight general physicians or middle masters (*zhong shi*, 中师) and eight surgeons or lower masters (*xia shi*, 下师). Veterinary specialists were also classed as *xia shi*. This statement is taken to indicate that the Zhou courts included a range of medical specialists, although we should bear in mind that the term *shi* was also used at this time as a general term to mean an educated literate scholar. Later in this chapter we find further clues as to the types of medical thinking used at court in the Warring States period.

Beyond what can be understood from the sparse references discussed so far, the medical beliefs and practices of Shang and Western Zhou times can only be guessed at. Basic herbal medicine was used, but probably in a folk medicine or symptomatic style admixed with rites, lore, magic and superstition. One folk belief that still survives in the Chinese popular imagination today claims that carrying the aromatic herb *wu zhu yu* (fructus evodia) in a pocket protects against malevolent spirits; this may be an example of the kind of belief current in the early era of medicine. Through much of China's history shamans and diviners were influential, and rulers and the population were in awe of their professed powers, although they were also viewed with suspicion, and not all disease causality was directly associated with moody ancestors. As we see in the next section, mundane factors such as falls and injuries, as well as climatic and lifestyle factors, were also understood to cause disease.

Medicine in the Spring and Autumn period

By −771 the Western Zhou dynasty rule was floundering due to increasing difficulties with rebellious fiefdoms and declining relations with neighbouring states. This heralded the start of the Chunqiu, the Spring and Autumn period (−771 to −476) of the Eastern Zhou dynasty, characterised by a flourish of intellectual and cultural activity alongside a fragmentation into about 170 squabbling small states. Coincidentally, whilst early Greek thinkers were reflecting, debating and writing on philosophy, statecraft and the organisation of society, some notable thinkers in China were doing the same. Indeed, based on the similarities between these cultures, some have claimed that there must have been extensive East–West exchange in these early times. These suggestions seem inconclusive, but I was interested to see a cast bronze head from −8th-century China in the collection of the Shanghai Museum that is not ethnically Chinese and clearly portrays a person of African descent. This supports the idea that, even in ancient times, adventurers travelled across continents, presumably bringing a cross-fertilisation of ideas and beliefs.

夏 商 周 秦

The Chunqiu period was the time when Confucius (–551 to –479) was setting down his ideas on the way that civilisation could be harmoniously organised by following his model of social order between individuals, ideas that would be adopted by the state a few centuries after his death. Also, at around this time, the reputed founder of philosophical Daoism, Lao Zi (real name Li Dan, c. –550 to –480), in his *Dao De Jing* (Path of Virtue Classic), was espousing his profound and poetic reflections on the links between the ways of man and nature as a philosophical guide to life, thought and wise governance. Alongside the *Yijing*, these and a few other great writings helped set the warp threads on which the coming millennia of Chinese civilisation was to use to weave its cultural fabric. A true understanding of China's culture and medicine begins with study of these works.

Whilst good writings on philosophy, culture and statecraft survive, there are few specific textual sources on medicine from this time. A text called *Lushi Chunqiu* (Lu's Spring and Autumn Annals) includes the statement, 'Throughout life the new replaces the old and so the *jing-luo* are unobstructed, *qi* is gained and pathogens are expelled.' However, although this text has Spring and Autumn in the title, it was actually written much later, around –240, by a man who was to become the first prime minister of the Qin dynasty, and it can only be taken as indicative of ideas of that later time. Another key record, which was probably written around –450, at the end of the Spring and Autumn period, is the *Chunqiu* (Spring and Autumn Annals). This includes some important early discussions of two 'pre-classical' professional physicians, Yi Yuan and Yi He. This text is also likely to have been written some time after the events described, but is considered to have been derived from other more contemporaneous records that are now lost. These brief passages offer rare insights into the minds of two prominent physicians working in the centuries before the founding of the classical medical tradition and before its basic ideas had been fully defined.

Yi Yuan, the physician

His true family name is unknown, but the physician Yi Yuan is said to have lived in the state of Qin during the Spring and Autumn period. According to records in the *Zuo Zhuan* (Chronicles of Zuo Qiu-ming), in –581 the ruler of the Jin state, Jin Jing-gong (ruled –599 to –581), fell ill. Initially a shaman from the Mulberry Fields (Sang Tian, now Lingbao in Henan province) was summoned to attend. Using divination methods, he concluded that Jin Jing-gong's illness had been inflicted on him by the spirits of Zhao Tong and Zhao Kuo, two doctors whom the ruler had previously ordered to be executed. The shaman predicted that the ruler would die before collection of the wheat harvest and, sure enough, Jin's condition continued to decline. Knowing the high repute of doctors of the neighbouring state of Qin, an official request was issued for a doctor to attend and, in response, the Qin ruler dispatched his physician Yi Yuan. After his clinical examination he, too, pronounced that Jin Jing-gong's illness was incurable. Yi declared:

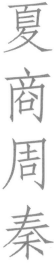

This disease is located above the *huang* and below the *gao* [inaccessible internal anatomical locations]; puncturing this place is impractical and medicines are also unable to reach it. For this reason it cannot be cured.

Jin Jing-gong is said to have listened closely to Yi Yuan's prognosis and to have exclaimed, 'What an excellent doctor!' Yi was awarded valuable gifts in payment, and was returned safely to his home, in the state of Qin.

This story suggests that during the Spring and Autumn period the ruling elite could access various types of healer besides the usual artisan healers specialising in wounds, midwifery and so on. These were shaman healers with their professed skills in influencing malevolent spirits, and an emerging class of professional physicians who had learned to diagnose internal illness by clinical examination followed by treatment using either herbal medicines or some form of puncturing therapy. One reason this specific incident was deemed worthy of recording for posterity may have been because it highlighted the contrast between these two styles of medical practice, with the imperial endorsement being given to the more modern style of physician. In other words, this may be an indication that shaman healers were beginning to lose ground with the ruling elite who were beginning to favour a new style of more pragmatic and methodical physician, using clinical examination rather than divination. It is also possible, given Emperor Jin Jing-gong's propensity for executing doctors, that the court advisers may have suggested summoning help from a neighbouring state to reduce the likelihood of further needless waste of local medical expertise. Rulers might wish to avoid souring relations with neighbouring states by refraining from executing their ruler's favourite physicians, and the story may have been recorded to suggest this strategy to future generations of court advisers.

Over the next few centuries it became increasingly common for the burgeoning class of *shi* scholars, possessing all kinds of useful skills besides medicine, to peddle their services to competing states, creating some confusion over loyalties. So, on another level of statecraft, requests for the attendance of a physician from a neighbouring ruler might also have been a handy ploy to test neighbourly relations – a ruler intending to wage war might be much less keen to dispatch his physicians to serve another ruler. This story also tells us that at this time the doctors of the state of Qin were known for their skills. For me, the most important subtext is that those in high places were beginning to attach more credence to trained scholar physicians than to the shaman classes.

Yi He, the physician

The other medical practitioner to have been recorded in the *Spring and Autumn Annals* is Yi He, another professional physician practising in the state of Qin. The *Zuo Zhuan* tells us that Jin Ping-gong (ruled –557 to –532), emperor of the Jin state, fell ill and

夏
商
周
秦

summoned the medical assistance of doctors from the Qin state. The emperor of Qin dispatched the physician Yi He who, after the consultation, is reported to have said:

> This illness is incurable. It is called *jin nu shi* [being too close to the women's room]. This illness is similar to *gu*; it is not attributable to ghosts and is not due to food, but it is lustfulness that has made you lose your spirit. Your majesty will die and [even] heaven will be unable to save you.

Yi He further explained that Jin Ping-gong's insatiable lust had made his spirit confused and obsessive. In a unique exposition of pre-classical medical theory, he then proceeded to outline his general understanding of the causes of disease:

> There are six heavenly [i.e. environmental] *qi* that generate the five flavours [and these] manifest in the five colours and the five sounds. Disease is caused by excess [of these so] there are six disease types. The six *qi* are *yin*, *yang*, wind, rain, mistiness and brightness that appear in the progression of the four seasons and the five festivals (*jie*). When these become excessive they cause problems. *Yin* types of *yin* [environmental excess] cause cold diseases, *yang* types of *yin* cause heat diseases, wind *yin* causes diseases of the extremities (*mo*), rain *yin* causes abdominal diseases, dull *yin* causes diseases of confusion, bright *yin* causes heart diseases. Women are *yin* [and so] relate to cloudiness and mist; excessive contact with them causes internal heat which ends in *gu* disease. Your highness is intemperate, so how can you possibly avoid contracting an illness such as this?

In this brief explanation of his medical doctrine, Yi He gives us the earliest known mention of the concept of the 'six adverse environmental factors' (*liu yin*) which seemed to its authors to provide a more rational and real-world explanation for aetiology than the ghosts and spirits aetiology offered by the shamans. Furthermore, this new model offered the possibility of finding ways to avoid and treat medical problems beyond simple appeasement of the spirits by the faithful. This new idea can be seen as a prototype of the six factors that, by the time of the *Neijing*, had been refined into the six *yin* of the subsequent classical medical tradition: wind, cold, summer heat, dampness, dryness and fire. Also notable in this passage is Yi He's identification of pathogenesis resulting from emotional and lifestyle indulgences. This early identification of untrammelled emotional states as internal factors in disease causality re-appeared later in a more evolved form in the more developed theories that were set down centuries later in the Han dynasty. Furthermore, in this brief text we see the early hints of the application *yin-yang*, five-flavour, five-colour and five-sound correspondences that were later to develop into much more detailed *yin-yang* and *wu xing* (five phases) correspondence theories. At this time, however, although some five-part classifications of nature existed, actual *wu xing* theory had to wait another couple of centuries before its introduction, probably by Zou Yan in the −3rd century, discussed in the next chapter.

夏商周秦

Contribution of Zhanguo (Warring States) statecraft to classical medicine

After the country's fragmentation into about 170 small states in −771, and throughout the subsequent 250-year Spring and Autumn period, warlords contended with each other for power and territorial control until, eventually, four main states predominated, Qin, Jin, Qi and Chu. By −475, the beginning of the Zhanguo (Warring States) period, the typical ruler was no longer a warlord but an educated nobleman which, ironically, meant that warfare activity escalated. Such a state of constant strife and political intrigue created an increased demand for scholars − people of high ability required for the administration and survival of the state. Armies were professional, large and well equipped, often numbering 50,000 to 150,000 men clad in thick rhino hide armour, on horseback and riding in chariots, armed with razor-sharp iron weapons and powerful, deadly accurate crossbows. The Warring States period is a time that is celebrated in Chinese culture for the positive effects it had on strategic thinking, and many of the cautionary tales and aphorisms that have been learned by Chinese children for millennia originate from this time. The strategic thinking that was the fruit of this two-century period of turmoil also contributed to medical thinking.

The continual strife meant that life-and-death survival depended on bringing to bear every available tactic to avoid defeat; for instance, farmers in the border regions were instructed to plough their fields in the direction that offered the bumpiest ride to invading chariots. Rulers who recruited the most skilled military tacticians, technologists and sages to their court were more likely to see their state and its population survive. It is hard to envisage a more powerful impetus to develop high-level skills than the constant, centuries-long threat of annihilation at the hands of neighbouring regimes, and so ingenuity was nurtured to the maximum possible extent. Later we discuss some of these ingenious ideas, such as methods of detecting invading armies from afar using drums or examining atmospheric effects. Diplomatic and military strategies of bluff and counterbluff motivated the development of cunning spycraft, strategic thinking and resourcefulness. Ministers and envoys who were skilled at face reading, body language interpretation and spotting deceptive voice 'tells' were invaluable not only in negotiating with neighbouring courts, but in divining their intentions. Court

WARRING STATES TACTICS PRESERVED IN SHORT SAYINGS THAT SURVIVE TODAY

- The expression 'blocking the retreat to redouble the fight' refers to a Warring States general who forced his troops to fight to the death by blocking their retreat path.

- 'Watching the fire from the other side of the river' refers to a general whose tactic was to allow his enemies to fight each other to exhaustion before stepping in later to snatch an easy victory from the weakened survivors.

Even today, most Chinese know these sayings, and sometimes apply the principles in their lives.

夏商周秦

scholars competed to refine such abilities so as to win power, wealth and influence for themselves. Eventually, collateral benefits appeared when it was realised that some of these scholars' skills were also applicable to medicine.

Under conditions of such strife a pragmatic approach to problem-solving that was based on meticulous observation and strategic thinking made more sense to the educated classes than mystical divination using shamans and cracks in bones. With the survival of the state at stake, the old divinatory practices came under question. Among those calling for rationality was the renowned military strategist Sun Zi, whose *Art of War* ridiculed the use of mystics. Another proponent of hard-nosed reality in the −3rd century was Han Fei-zi, the prominent political thinker and proponent of the legalist style of government, who famously proclaimed, 'It is stupid to claim certainly without corroborating evidence.' So, at the end of the Zhanguo period, just as the first texts and ideas of the classical medical tradition were being created, a desire for rationality had become widespread in intellectual circles. This, too, informed the spirit of the nascent new medicine that would serve the literate classes.

Like chess masters, the elite scholars who ascended to court service aimed to take account of every subtle nuance of a military or political situation, such as the advantageousness or otherwise of the terrain of the landscape as well as the *shi* (strength) or *xu* (weakness) of the enemy, so as to weigh up all relevant factors to arrive at the perfect move. They would 'gaze' (*guan*) on the totality of a situation to apprehend all its nuances, using the same mindset as later classical physicians 'gazing' upon the clues to be observed in their patients. The same thinking styles, terminology and tactics that had been developed by Warring States scholars were later applied to creating the new style of medicine. When, for instance, early Han dynasty medical scholars turned their attention to medicine, their first instinct was to map the bodily terrain in detail as if it were a military terrain. So, although only a few Warring States medical writings survive, wider reflection on the ideas in common currency at this time helps inform our understanding of Chinese medicine.

Dawn of the classical medicine tradition in the Warring States

So, various key contextual factors help our understanding of the birth of the classical medical tradition through the Warring States period; these include the political state of the country, discussed above, and the rise of the *shi* (gentleman) scholar.

Confucius was the archetypal example of a *shi* scholar (士). He tried to develop his career by seeking influence with individual rulers, offering them his own blueprint for statecraft and governance; these advances were generally rejected, although he did eventually gain some respect by becoming a minister for the state of Lu. His personal qualities as a teacher and scholar inspired many followers who continued his work after his death. The *shi* class that burgeoned over the following

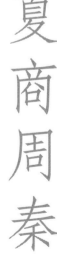

centuries encompassed gentlemen scholars, intellectuals, philosophers, natural scientists, physicians, warriors and military strategists. These were literate men, often distantly related to the nobility, who existed for generations as an aspirational sub-elite operating on the margins of power and influence. As the Zhanguo period progressed, they increasingly crept into government circles, often filling the vacancies in official posts that had been created by the ongoing wars and that had previously been occupied by the aristocracy. As their influence and numbers grew, so did their sense of entitlement and self-esteem. Increasingly intoxicated with their own success, they then made themselves indispensable to the running of the state and to military security matters. Operating both within the corridors of power and networking with their educated peers spread through the community, they began to see themselves as the intellectual superiors to, and the natural teachers of, the ruling classes. They strived to persuade everyone that they were a superior race, the natural holders of wisdom, the inheritors of the Dao and indeed the whole spectrum of intellectual and professional skill. The *shi* would have happily subscribed to the maxim 'knowledge is power'.

Most educated and literate gentleman preferred to study philosophy, statecraft and the art of warfare as a key to advancement, but increasingly, through the Warring States period, scholars became attracted to the secret medical knowledge contained in the private texts passed from master to pupil on medicine and in secret lore, such as alchemy. They sought to accumulate expertise, appropriating the secrets of the Daoist mystics, hermits and sages; they borrowed wisdom from secret mystical societies, specialist tradespersons, from artisans in various fields including medicine, and perhaps even from the shamans. Literati scholars gathered their informational wealth in personal libraries that were, in the decades leading up to the Han dynasty, seen as so threatening to the rulers that mass book burnings were ordered.

The *shi* scholars laid claim to ownership of the wisdom they had gained, and positioned themselves as the inheritors of the philosophical and mystical traditions of China – the *Yijing, Laozi,* the investigation of nature, Daoist yoga and so on. As well as borrowing the Daoist adept's breathing and contemplation techniques, they also explored ways of using sexual activity and dietary regulation to maintain health. Towards the end of the Warring States, the maintenance of health became fashionable in elite society, and people began to collect and study healthcare texts; a subset of *shi* scholars began to formulate theories of health preservation and personal spiritual development based on their conceptions of the relationship between mankind and nature, cycles of change and ideas that they took from the *Yijing* and from seers in the community.

> The sages of old emphasised disease prevention just as good government prevents war. Giving treatment when illness is established is like trying to suppress revolt when it has already broken out. It is like digging a well when you are already thirsty or casting weapons when fighting has already broken out. We have to ask, are these actions not already too late? (*Neijing, Suwen*, Ch 2)

夏
商
周
秦

Seeking to maintain health, the upper classes became interested in the health cultivation methods that had been developed by Daoist sages such as breathing techniques, exercises, diet regulation and sexual alchemy (the use of sexual practices for health). We see this in the *Daoyin* exercise instructions that survived as illustrations and texts in the Mawangdui manuscripts (–168) that were retrieved from the tomb of an upper-class family, and that probably functioned as a home help guide to the special exercises considered useful for maintaining good health.

As we saw when discussing the physicians He and Huan, intellectuals tended to value scholarship over shamanism. They claimed ownership of the ancient wisdom and high culture passed on from earlier times in texts such as the *Yijing*, the *Shijing* (Book of Songs) and the Confucian classics. To the ancient ideas taken from such ancient writings, they added an element of rational enquiry, enquiry into the outer world of nature and the inner world of man, in the vaguely scientific manner of educated gentlemen. They believed that insights into the nature of heaven, mankind and earth could be accessed through *neigong* (inner alchemy training and secret longevity practices) and *Daoyin* (the leading and guiding of *qi* in the body by breathing techniques and mental effort). They were also practical experimenters – they could see the dividends that had come from the study of, for example, metallurgy and the management

> Texts on Daoist breath cultivation instructed the practitioner to send their breath down to 'the moving *qi* between the kidneys' that is generally taken to mean the middle of the pelvis. Given that the testicles were also referred to as the kidneys, I suspect that, to the early Daoists, this was code for the perineal area, where the prostate is located. Elusive language was used to make it harder for non-initiates to make sense of Daoist secrets. The seemingly poetic names used formed a special kind of technical language.

of watercourses, and wanted to study and record the way things worked and the way they could be made to work better. They explored change and transformation, including the changes that could be explored by alchemy, and were fascinated by, for example, the way that heat applied to cinnabar created a liquid metal – mercury. The desire was to create a universal rational science that encompassed the resonating network of everything in the universe, in nature and in mankind, in a grand scheme.

The *shi* classes included political thinkers who sought better ways to administer the state; they included diplomats to negotiate with neighbouring states, warfare strategists as well as spies and educated people of skill and guile. This explains why so many of the writings that survive from the Spring and Autumn and Warring States periods are about statecraft and warfare – even seemingly philosophical Daoist texts, such as Laozi's *Dao De Jing* and the philosopher Zhuangzi's writings, have a distinctive, and often overlooked, undercurrent of politics and statecraft. The *shi* were as much concerned with the survival and health of the state as intellectual nicety. As the Warring States period progressed, the numbers of scholars proliferated, both in state service and in the general community; competition for power and position was strong, which meant that professional secrets needed to be guarded.

夏
商
周
秦

Such protection was achieved by the exclusion of outsiders, initiation rites, secret oaths and by surrounding the teachings with obfuscation and secret terminology. Even in ancient China the professions conspired against outsiders. The *shi* scholar classes realised that their ownership of these theories, beliefs and practices gave them opportunities; they represented a way of making a living, advancing socially and gaining power and influence, and so the teachings were kept within families or social groups or transmitted as secret lineages taught to others for profit. An important characteristic of these ideas was the sense that man was linked to and analogous to the natural environment, and that he reflected the cycles and activities found in heaven and earth, especially the movement and cycles of water, wind and growth and decay.

By the −4th century the *shi* scholars had become well established as a bureaucratic class, making a crucial contribution to society, and they succeeded in gaining ever-increasing official utilisation of their skills. The most famous early academic group of *shi* scholar officials was the Jixia Academy (*Jixia Xuegong*), which was founded in the state capital Linzi in −315. This was sponsored by the rulers of the state of Qi (the area of today's Shandong), and was an elite academic institution made up of the leading academicians of the time. Its luminaries debated politics, statecraft and philosophy, and were employed as advisers to the ruling nobility of the Qi state for about three decades. The Jixia Academy was specifically intended to attract the very best scholars from distant states, and the Qi rulers succeeded in this by offering the highest prestige and showering their scholars with material finery. This tactic worked too well, however − loss of their most talented officials soon became a concern for the rulers of the other states.

Most intellectuals emphasised the study of statecraft, political theory and philosophy, as these were the pressing difficulties of the time; medicine was less attractive as a profession. In terms of medicine and health, the influence of the Jixia Academy scholars is seen in their discussions of meditative *qi* cultivation methods that were set down in the *Nei-yeh* (Inner Cultivation) text that was added to an earlier text, the *Guanzi*. The Jixia Academy also indirectly influenced the development of medicine through the ideas of some of its leading lights, such as Zou Yan, who popularised *yin-yang* and *wu xing* (five phase) theory, and the rationalist Han Fei-zi, who was a pupil of the top Jixia scholar Xunzi. Having such an accumulation of the best *shi* scholars of the era was threatening to the rulers of other states, and, in −284, the city of Linzi was stormed by armies from the powerful state of Yan to the north, and the Academy was destroyed. By −250 the largest gathering of scholars, numbering over 1000, had moved, and was now under the patronage of the state of Qin.

One particular skill that came to the fore amongst scholars in the Warring States period was face reading or, more generally, person reading, because ultimately it involved the ability to sense personality types and to read thoughts by using a cultivated acuity of the senses. Subtle signals such as a change in voice tone, a facial

夏
商
周
秦

flush, a fleeting expression or a change in posture were all considered to be 'tells', able to reveal when a person was lying or to divine their true intentions. The character *se* (色), although translated as 'complexion', also carries the sense of the face's complete information readout – as one saying had it, 'Facial expressions reflect the feelings of the heart as a seal reflects its impression.' Such beliefs were transferred to medical practice and remain part of Chinese medicine diagnostics today.

The modern Japanese scholar Shigehisa Kuriyama recounts how Duke Huan of the state of Qi plotted secretly with his chief minister to attack the state of Lu, but somehow the secret plan became known. The *shi* scholar Dongguo Ya confessed that it was he who had leaked the information. When asked how he had found out about the secret, he explained that he knew the plan was afoot simply by reading the minister's face. Dongguo Ya said that he had learned to tell when the minister was joyful or reflective or hyped up for battle. 'By observing his expression and connecting it with the current political situation I was able to sense what was being planned,' he explained. The emphasis placed on visual diagnosis by the classical medical writings that appeared a century or two later is almost certain to be rooted in these endeavours. Legendary physicians would later claim to be able to diagnose illness by applying a knowing gaze on the subtleties of the facial complexion, and even to predict future illness sometimes years in advance using this method. Various systems of face reading and physique reading seem to have been devised by the Warring States *shi* for personality typing, and some of these were

> **LINGSHU 72**
>
> Huangdi: I am told there are different types of people who can be distinguished by *yin-yang* theory; tell me about this.
>
> Shaoshi (少师, little master): Yes, and all things can also be approximated using *wu xing* theory. By means of the ever-greater subdivisions of *yin-yang* we can distinguish complexity that reaches beyond what can be expressed in words.
>
> Huangdi: Tell me about the way that sages maintain *yin-yang* balance.
>
> Shaoshi: Physiques can be classified as *taiyang*, *taiyin*, *shaoyang* or *shaoyin* or evenly balanced. They look different, their tendons and bones differ and the *shi* and *xu* of their *qi* and *xue* (blood) differ too.
>
> Huangdi: Explain the difference.
>
> Shaoshi: The *taiyin* type lacks benevolence, is insincere and ungenerous. He takes but dislikes giving, the harmony of his heart is not expressed on the outside and he shows little interest in doing good or caring for others. *Shaoyin* people like to gain petty advantage over others, sometimes even plotting to harm them. They feel gain at the misfortune of others and become jealous and irritated when others are honoured. They have no sympathy for their fellow man. The *taiyang* type is smug. Although lacking in competence, does not hesitate to discuss grandiose projects. He ignores ethical niceties and feels he is always right, then, when he fails, he feels no remorse. The *shaoyang* man is cautious in his dealings but, thinking himself remarkable, likes to boast of and broadcast his prestige even when his position is lowly. He enjoys social networking but neglects the one he should love most. The *yin-yang* balanced person is calm with neither fright nor excessive joy and is content in his work. He does not strive for advantage but adapts to changing circumstances. In high position he is modest and in lowly position he is not subservient.

夏商周秦

adapted for medical diagnosis. The boxed example on the previous page, from the *Lingshu*, seems to have been cut and pasted from the earlier face reading tradition with little attempt to add a medical gloss; it seems more of a guide to understanding people in the court circles than to medical diagnosis.

So, towards the end of the Zhanguo period, the *shi* scholar classes had grown both in numbers and in political influence, and the point was eventually reached where the knowledge and power they held was a threat. With an ever-mounting and increasingly plainly expressed disdain for the court and for the ruling aristocracy, they often proclaimed an arrogant sense of their own superiority over the rulers. The fact that they had made themselves and their skills indispensable to the rulers gave the *shi* considerable power and influence, creating rising levels of suspicion and intrigue. In a sense, their indispensability and continued power was built on the continued state of disharmony, so they had an investment in the ongoing tensions between states.

Medical education

There are no records of any formal medical academies in the Warring States period and before; we see from the stories of early physicians, however, such as the aforementioned Yi Yuan in −571, Yi He in −532 and Chunyu Yi (discussed in the next chapter) in about −200, that a class of professional and educated physicians existed plying their trade amongst the higher sectors of society. From the case records of Chunyu Yi we can surmise that these physicians often apprenticed under a relative or a mentor paid to reveal his secrets. A medical apprenticeship began with the taking of a ritualised oath of secrecy, sometimes sworn in blood, with restrictions on the further transmission of the material. One or more of the mentor's lineage texts was then provided for hand copying and memorisation by the disciple. To help ensure that the medical secrets did not easily fall into the wrong hands, the texts were written in obscure language, often using metaphysical code or employing vernacular words with new specialist meanings in the context of medicine. This is akin to the use of Latin by European professionals such as physicians, lawyers and priests that functions to create mystique, enhance the sense of value of the knowledge and to maintain exclusivity of access to insider information.

After the text had been received in this way, the master would, over a period of months or perhaps years, proceed to decipher and explain its meaning and demonstrate to the initiate the practical clinical skills required for clinical application. The main Han dynasty medical classic, the *Huangdi Neijing*, is largely a later compilation and annotated re-editing of such early texts. One measure of a medical master's expertise and position in the hierarchy was the number of texts he himself had been made privy to, and so some early physicians progressed from one mentor to another, gathering their transmitted teachings and acquiring a repertoire of styles. Wealth and family connections thus gave access to wider knowledge and better training.

夏
商
周
秦

Practical instruction was crucial. Although none have survived into modern times, herbal medicine writings from this time almost certainly lacked illustrations, so they would have had limited value without guidance from a mentor able to provide identification of the plants and substances used and the methods of harvesting, preparation and use. Similarly, acumoxa study relied on practical tuition in finding the acupoints and applying the correct needling and moxibustion methods. The mentor–disciple relationship is often represented as one-to-one tuition; there are indications that this may be mistaken, as, in records from subsequent centuries, we find teachers running mini-academies teaching dozens of students.

The writing of texts and the academic networking of the new class of scholar physicians represented the start of a bid to compile and re-evaluate the existing medical knowledge, to collect and decipher the written traditions and to make the information acquired congruent with the elite rational thinking of the time. Such thinking included the *yin-yang* and *wu xing* models combined with the strategic wisdom derived from statecraft and military tactics. In short, they were working to develop a new coherent and systematic form of medicine, derived from but also distinct from the previous anarchic mix of medical practices that had evolved through various previous medical lineages. The *shi* scholars interested in medicine worked to reconcile the information and so lay the foundations of a new classical medical tradition, unified and codified to fit with the dominant intellectual beliefs of the time, to create a medicine more suitable for the elite than shamanism. Given that the traditional medical lineage involved the passing on of arcane written texts accompanied by oral explanations, this may explain why so much of the *Neijing* consisted of question-and-answer sessions between the Yellow Emperor and his physicians. Its commentaries in dialogue form may represent an attempt to get around the exclusivity of the master–disciple relationship, allowing the know-how to be revealed in written explanations.

Chinese medicine at the end of the Zhanguo period

At the end of the Zhanguo period seven states existed: Qin, Zhao, Wei, Yan, Qi, Han and Chu. These were conquered in quick succession by Qin Shi Huang, who declared himself the first emperor of this newly unified China in –221. The founding of the Qin dynasty completely changed the position of the *shi* scholars, many of whom were now humbled, vulnerable and facing the possibility of redundancy under the new regime. At a stroke, their indispensable role in games of interstate intrigue was taken away. Emperor Qin seems to have wanted to 'put them in their place' and, in the infamous book burning episode of –213, he singled out scholar groups in the wider community in an attack aimed at removing some of their power by destroying their knowledge base. On pain of death, all privately held books were, with a few exceptions, to be destroyed. The fact that the new court itself kept reference copies of the books seized in this way in the imperial library tells us that he was not averse to the actual knowledge itself – just to it remaining in the hands of the inner circle

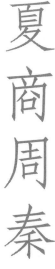

of the *shi* scholar classes. He may also have wanted to remove writings that could threaten the stability of his new state. A little later, in −214, Qin Shi Huang is alleged to have taught the *shi* scholars a lesson by disposing of over 400 of them in a live burial – although some say that this was Han dynasty propaganda against the memory of the Qin rule.

Like all new regimes, Qin Shi Huang needed to consolidate his position; it made sense to rid the state of those whose instincts and training might lead them to continue in intrigue and warmongering, and thereby threaten his hard-won termination of centuries of military strife. Although criticised for tyranny, the new emperor was skilful in his ideas for unifying the country, and seemed dedicated to bringing centuries of turmoil to an end. Indeed, we might ask if his famous burial of the Terracotta Army may have been intended more to symbolise an end to militarism than to function as a resource for continued warfare in the afterlife – he probably did not expect to die quite so soon after his founding of China. Qin Shi Huang's governance emphasised cultural unification – for example, he standardised weights and measures and the written language across the empire. Now, with militarism off the agenda, and with the overbearing *shi* scholars suitably put in their place, the path was open for the next generation of scholars to turn their attention away from warfare and to focus instead on the next most pressing threat to life and limb – disease. The strategic military skills, and theories gained through centuries of statecraft and military cunning, turned to the problem of medicine and, more generally, to more peaceable pursuits – the Han dynasty search for knowledge, its version of scientific investigation.

Clues to the military roots of this emerging new medicine are seen in the way that many of the ideas and terminology that had previously been applied to warfare were now transferred to the medical domain. We saw earlier how the mapping of the body territory was conducted using the approach of a military strategist, and how the strength or weakness of an enemy's forces described in Sun Zi's *Art of War*, in terms of *shi* (replete) and *xu* (weakened), had parallels in medicine. Further military metaphors and terminology were applied to the relationship between a pathogenic invader and the body's normal constituents. In the past, one's home state was referred to as *nei* (inner) and foreign territories as *wai* (outer); this same idea was now applied to the politics of the relationship between the body and its environment, and between the exterior of the body and its interior. On a smaller scale the court was *nei* and the country was *wai* – which, incidentally, allows us to explain the naming of the *Neijing* (Inner Classic) as the 'court medicine classic' rather than the 'classic of internal medicine'. Much of this book was about the physiology and pathology of the body exterior; crucially important in the new medicine was the guarding of the body's boundaries between exterior and interior. Military analogies are here, too – the exterior boundaries guarded by *wei qi* (defensive *qi*) linked to the recognition that armies cannot function without nutrition, and so the *wei qi* function is inextricably linked to the provision of *ying qi* (nutrient *qi*).

夏

商

周

秦

So, military scholars developed methods to detect military threats from afar, an idea that was itself rooted in the *Yijing* belief that 'what is distant can be discerned from that which is nearby'. One interesting group of *shi* scholars perhaps worth our attention are the so-called 'cloud watchers', who were said to have specialised in interpreting cloud formations with a view to guiding battle strategy. Although this may seem like an absurd idea, it does conceivably have some rational basis.

> If dust rises up high in a clearly-defined column then chariots are coming. If it is low and broad then infantry are advancing. If it is dispersed and rises in thin shafts they are gathering firewood. If it is sparse and intermittent it indicates an encampment. (Sun Zi, *Art of War*)

Military historians describe court cloud watchers as mystical diviners, and some of the writings do indeed appear nonsensical. It is likely, though, that an army of tens of thousands would indeed generate dust clouds when on the move, and it is feasible that the size of an army and its movements could be discerned from a long distance. Heat from fires and cooking would likely be sufficient to disturb overlying clouds, and so observation of atmospheric disturbances above an enemy encampment may well provide useful information. The size of an enemy encampment and the adequacy of its food supplies could probably be estimated in this way. An army that was not cooking food at mealtimes was an army whose food supplies were exhausted and whose generals were facing a choice, either to retreat or to imminently invade. An army running short of food and with deteriorating morale may show little cloud disturbance, as may an army that was very small or more vulnerable to attack. It may have been expedient for cloud watchers and other experts to represent what they were doing in hard-to-fathom or mystical terms so as to conceal their real methods – especially when asked to write their methods down. They may also have wished to keep their options open to defect to the service of a rival court, which they commonly did, and so would prefer to obfuscate.

Cloud watchers not only observed clouds, but also discerned coloured atmospheric hazes, mist, smoke, dust and subtle vapour effects such as might be seen over a lake on a warm day. In other words, the object of their attention lay on a spectrum, from the relatively tangible to the very subtle, and they were one of the first groups to routinely use the word *qi*, often in the compound term *cloud qi*, and it may well be this *shi* scholar profession that introduced the *qi* concept that was later borrowed for medical use. Indeed, the *qi* character first appeared around the end of the Spring and Autumn period and entered common usage in the Warring States period. The earliest character to represent *qi* was a graphic of clouds and later the *mi* (rice radical) was added to suggest the aroma rising from cooking rice.

Another early warning system devised by court scholars near the end of the Zhanguo period appears in the political writings of the renowned Jixia Academy philosopher, Mozi (Mencius). This was designed to detect the rumble of the horses and chariots of an approaching enemy from afar by listening to a bamboo pole

夏商周秦

resting on the skin of large drums buried in the ground. This is an idea that is akin to pulse diagnosis that aims to detect the hidden rumblings of disharmonious *zangfu* organs from convenient locations on the limbs.

Many other concepts of military strategy and intelligence seem to have been carried over into medicine. As we have seen, surface anatomy was mapped topographically and examined by palpation and by visual inspection; its signs could be interpreted and the internal dysfunction underlying illness symptoms could be categorised. 'Know the territory' was a cornerstone of military strategy described in Sun Zi's *Art of War*. Transferred to medicine and health, this meant naming every mountain, marsh, pond, valley and stream of the body topography, something that survives today in the *jing-luo* system and the names of acumoxa points. In a wonderfully direct connection between our minds and those of ancient scholars, their work survives today in many of the acumoxa point names.

> **SOME TYPICAL ACUPUNCTURE POINT NAMES**
>
> *Qu chi* (curved pond) (LI 11)
> *He gu* (joining valleys) (LI 4)
> *Tai yuan* (great abyss) (Lu 9)
> *Jing qu* (across the ditch) (Lu 8)
> *Qu ze* (curved marsh) (PC 3)
> *Kun lun* (Kun Lun mountains) (Bl 60)

Other core ideas of early classical medicine

Other basic precepts underpinned the new medicine, dozens of which can be identified as themes in the Han dynasty medical literature, and which represent a synthesis of earlier medical styles, the prevailing philosophies and metaphysics together with ideas derived from military strategy. We now survey some of these.

Zang xiang theory

By the end of the Warring States period it appears that palpation of the body surface, including the arterial pulses, along with visual observation of the body exterior, emerged as a prime means of diagnosing and making clinical assessments. Early evidence for this comes from the records of the elite physician Chunyu Yi, who was working near the start of the Han dynasty, and who is discussed in detail in the next chapter. He repeatedly refers to his routine diagnostic process as 'examining the vessels', which is taken to mean palpation and visual assessment. Later, the *Neijing* articulated this approach to diagnosis in the maxim 'the state of the deepest roots is reflected in the highest branches', a way of expressing the belief that the condition of interior organ function is reflected on the exterior. This was the start of *zang xiang* (organ manifestation) theory.

The *zang xiang* idea became a central hypothesis of the classical medical tradition, one that has remained one of its defining characteristics up until the present day. It holds that the body-interior and body-exterior are intimately connected and mirror each other; in a sense the *zangfu* organs are believed to be visible from the outside,

夏
商
周
秦

especially on the face, and the arterial and *jing-luo* systems. In some ways this is self-evidently true. In people under chronic stress we can usually palpate increased tension and tenderness in the trapezius that is usually centred round the acupoint *jian wang* (GB 21). This is one part of the way that stress patterns of activity in our brain and spinal cord are expressed externally. No doubt we could list many other external manifestations of internal stress states. Stimulation of the point *jian wang* by massage or needling not only helps relax the muscle locally, but can also have a more general soothing effect on the internal neurology. This suggests a reciprocal relationship between this point and our neurological mechanisms linked to the stress response. Recognition of this two-way communication appears to have been one of the key discoveries of the first acupuncturists who, having identified this as a hypothesis, embarked on investigations intended to create a detailed map of these reciprocal interior–exterior links. This principle is quite explicit in early medical writings; it is clear that at the end of the Warring States period scholar physicians considered that important diagnostic data were available from the arterial pulses, the complexion, palpable changes along the channel tract system, strength of voice, bodily appearance and other bodily manifestations.

LINGSHU 45, ON EXTERIOR ASSESSMENT

Huangdi: I've learned some acupuncture but I still don't quite get it. I know it is based on understanding the complex changes of heaven, man and the seasons but can you sum things up concisely for me?

Qibo: Great question your majesty! In your work of ruling the country, despite its complexities, you employ some overarching principles. Similarly there are principles at work with acupuncture practice too.

Huangdi: OK, tell me!

Qibo: Like the shadows of the sun and moon, or water and its reflections, or a drum and its sound – physical form and activity are inextricably linked; stimulus and response connect and resonate with each other.

Huangdi: That's great! A brilliant insight into *yin-yang*! Now I understand how we can examine the patient's overall condition, check our conclusions by palpation, then determine the specific patterns by inspection, and in this way reach an accurate diagnosis. The *zangfu* are manifested in the voice and complexion; when the voice lacks resonance and the five colours are indistinct we know the *zangfu* are faltering. This exemplifies the mutual connection between interior and exterior, a link that is as inextricable as a drum and its sound or the body and its shadow. This is the way we can discern *zangfu* disease patterns from the outside and, given prior knowledge of *zangfu* disease, it is how we can teach ourselves the associated manifestations. This is the basic principle that allows us to diagnose conditions of the *zangfu*; it is an example of the idea that things at opposite poles from each other have mutual linkages.

The explorations were not limited simply to the links between the interior and exterior of the patient; the grand plan was to map the characteristics of the wider web that connects our health with all things in nature in an overarching cosmology.

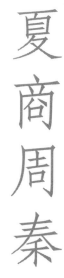

Xie–zheng

Besides the interior–exterior dialectic, another important distinction that contributed to the founding of classical medicine in the Han dynasty was the one posited between the normal tissues of the body: blood, bodily organs, fluids and *qi* (collectively known as upright *qi* – *zheng qi*, 正气), and pathological influences called *xie qi* (pathogenic *qi*, 邪气). The origins of the idea of *xie qi* can be traced back to the Shang and Zhou dynasties; for example, one of the *jiagu wen* divinatory writings mentioned by Unschuld asks, 'Has Princess Hao been afflicted by *xie*?' So, the existence of malign 'stuff' having an adverse effect on health had long existed. Later, as we saw from the Warring States case involving physician Yi He with his hypothetical disease-causing agents such as 'wind', 'rain' and 'mistiness', medical scholars came to distinguish specific types of *xie qi*. As the medicine progressed, the different forms of pathogen were standardised and defined in more detail. With further experience and study, their associated symptoms, signs and effects on the body could be elaborated more fully, leading to clinical guidelines such as 'coldness stagnates and contracts', 'dampness sinks', 'wind moves', etc. The effects of these factors on the various organs and tissues of the body became an important area for investigation in the run-up to the compilation of the Han medical classics.

Reference to the diagnosis and quarantining of lepers is found on Qin dynasty (–221 to –206) writings on bamboo slats, and these tell us that there was also a basic conception of illness factors that were transmissible from person to person. Strangely, though, this knowledge of transmissible disease appears to have been ignored by the writers of the *Neijing*. Pathogenic *qi* could also be formed from normal body tissues that had become diseased, for example, when *qi*, blood or fluids failed to circulate properly, leading to bruising, haematoma, pain, swelling, oedema or phlegm accumulation. For example, midwives' experiences of post-partum fatalities due to retained lochia will have highlighted the potentially pathogenic nature of retained stagnating tissues.

A significant part of the development of classical Chinese medicine over the subsequent millennia involved ever more refined empirical elaborations of the relationship between the various types of *zheng qi* and the various forms of *xie qi*. This has led to the complex map of energetic aetiology and pathology used in modern clinical practice, where even discussions of what can happen after a sneeze can run to thousands of pages of technicalities.

Movement and stasis

Another important distinction that appeared in the centuries prior to the founding of classical medicine was the idea that health involved maintaining a proper movement of substances in the body. The proper flows of *qi*, blood, food and fluids became central to classical medicine's conceptions of health, and it became axiomatic that hindered movement was, by definition, pathological. With the importance of irrigation and water management in Chinese civilisation, the issue of movement

夏
商
周
秦

and stasis had long been a matter for investigation; the conclusion was that lack of movement had adverse consequences. An early reference to this idea in relation to health appears in −239 in Master Lu Bu-wei's *Lushi Chunqiu* (Spring and Autumn Annals), in an essay called 'On Reaching our Allotted Years':

> …the reason flowing water does not become putrid and the pivots of a door are not eaten by insects is because they move. The physical body and its *qi* are like this too. If the body does not move then the essential *qi* does not flow. If this does not flow then the *qi* clogs up.

Some disease states were self-evidently linked to stasis of normal substances in the body: oedema, often a sign of significant pathology, was clearly a failure of fluid transportation. Blood stagnation, evidenced by cyanosis, menstrual blood clots, venous congestion or pain with purple discolouration locally or on the tongue, lips or nose, indicated the urgent need to invigorate the circulation of blood. Failure to do this led to increasingly adverse effects on health.

Like the cloud watchers' fascination with the finest subtleties that could be perceived in the atmosphere, or the seer's study of the environment at the very limits of perceptual acuity, the concept of *qi* stasis described a subtler dysfunction in the movement and transformation processes in the body, requiring careful observation of the bodily landscape. Sometimes, inhibited *qi* movement was visible to the trained eye or could be surmised from subjective physical sensations such as distension or bloating. Alternatively, poorly circulating *qi* could manifest as alterations in emotional state. Movement and exercise tend to help people feel more energetic, invigorated and psychologically balanced, and this may have also given the hint that inactivity and stagnation was unhealthy. Subtle *qi* stasis could also be assessed, and its locality defined, by palpation, and its significance could be interpreted in terms of the *jing-luo* channel model. Tenderness or pain along the *qi* pathway of the *xin* heart channel, for instance, could be taken to reflect dysfunction in the heart *zang* itself.

The idea of stagnation of *xue* blood, *qi* and *jinye* fluid was therefore central to the emerging explanatory model of the emerging new medicine. Early writings from the Warring States period mentioned *mai* vessels and their function in circulating blood, and there was no mention of the idea of *qi* circulation or the *jing-luo* paths that the *qi* was later said to travel in. In other words, blood circulation was understood first, but the search for greater subtlety of observation led to the identification of *qi* and the *jing-luo*. Knowledge of blood vessels comes naturally, both from butchery of animals and, very much in the Warring States period, of people. With the introduction of the idea of a more subtle circulation involving *qi*, health cultivation practices began to include ideas that emphasised activity. Health advisers to the nobility prescribed physical exercise to counter the tendency to stasis, along with the use of *qi* guiding (*Daoyin*) that employed breathing and mental concentration that had been devised by the body-mind alchemy of the Daoists. Secret Daoist lore taught that inhaled *qi* could be stored internally as increased personal power – just as alchemists used bellows to create extreme heat to transform and forge metals, the lungs were the

夏
商
周
秦

bellows of *qi* that strengthened the ability to move and transform in the body as well as the wider world.

The observation that the stimulation of acupuncture points and the use of some herbal medicines eased pain and made the body feel invigorated indicated that these worked because they removed stagnation. In clinical practice, when applying acupuncture to an area where the skin appears dull, it is common to see a colour change to a healthier pink, which today we would attribute to a local vasodilation response. Given that it was axiomatic that actions in one place also have effects distantly, stimulating one part of the body can exert beneficial effects further away. For example, systemic and distant responses to acupuncture have some support in modern neuro-physiological research that has tracked localised cranial vasodilation in response to needling of points on the foot.

Rebellion and chaos

In addition to the free flow of *qi*, blood and fluids, the proper direction of flow of these was also seen as important to health – any reversal of the appropriate direction of movement was, by definition, pathogenic. The character *ni* (逆) describes this form of pathology, and has the sense of rebellion and adversity, or to go against the proper flow. Doctrinal statements on the subject of adverse flow fall strangely on modern medical ears, but this idea was probably derived from ordinary clinical realities. Vomiting is one example of adverse *qi* movement, and it is reasonable to characterise vomiting as an abnormal flow of the *qi* of the stomach, stuff not moving in the direction it is supposed to. Closely associated with vomiting, nausea is also categorised as an aspect of the energetic dysfunction label, rebellious stomach *qi*. The icy limbs of a person in end-stage febrile disease was seen as a sign of *qi* and blood retreating away from the extremities rather than extending to the fingertips. With coughing and dyspnoea, the *qi* of the lungs, instead of descending, is rebelling upwards. The red-faced plethoric appearance of a patient heading for a heart attack or stroke plainly, in the eyes of ancient medical thinkers, implied an inappropriate and unregulated movement of hot *yang qi* upwards to the head. These are all examples of the energetic disease category *qi ni* (气逆), the rebellious or abnormal flow of *qi*. The diagnostic label itself points directly to the appropriate treatment principles – countering the adverse movement and re-establishing correct flow. In the case of vomiting, this means normalising the direction of oesophageal and gastric peristalsis. Fresh ginger has this effect, and so the *bencao* literature records that it is able to 'descend stomach *qi* and harmonise the *qi* of the stomach'.

Other contrasting pairs

Early medical thinkers applied many other contrasting pairs to labelling physiology and pathology. These included distinctions such as movement-stillness (*dong-jing*), tip-root (*biao-ben*), clear-turbid (*qing-zhuo*) and above-below (*shang-xia*). Those that

夏
商
周
秦

came to be seen as the most important ones are what in modern times have been labelled the 'eight principal patterns' – yin-yang, empty-full (*xu-shi*), cold-hot (*han-re*), internal-external (*nei-wai*) – although skilled physicians understand and apply most of the other distinctions when the context demands.

Floating-sinking and expansion-contraction are interesting ones to consider. Spending time in meditative breath watching the Daoist scholars had a sense of tidal changes of expansion and contraction, of tension and release, and the cycles of nature were seen in similar terms, with spring being seen as a time of expansion and winter as a contraction. A sense of these activities cycling naturally, spontaneously and in an appropriate manner in nature and in the body was seen as indicative of proper order. Disruptions to orderly cycles were taken as indicative of unhealthy states, and a sense of these dynamics informs study of classical medicine. We see examples in the discussions of coordinating breathing with acupuncture needling which are based on the idea that on the in-breath the body's *qi* retreats inwards slightly from the exterior, and on the out-breath the *qi* tide moves outwards. Forcefully breath holding forces *qi* excess to the exterior so strongly that it brings extra blood with it and we go red. In winter, in response to cold, our *qi* moves more deeply, and in summer our *qi* lies more on the surface.

So, one aim of diagnosis was to identify, characterise and label dysfunction in these dynamic terms. Confident of the reliability and rational nature of this approach, the route to its refinement was considered to be to seek greater and greater subtlety. A single hiccup might presage a more significant rebellion of stomach *qi* to come. A greenish cast to the nose might indicate future respiratory problems. A renowned physician might predict illness months, years or decades ahead to demonstrate his penetrating medical vision. Logical at its root, if the system had a fault, it was in this tendency for romance with the intangible and esoteric subtleties that attracted the *shi* scholars, a fascination with the limits of perception.

On the treatment side, the aim of needling, moxibustion or treatment by medicinals could be pitched at correcting and harmonising such aberrations so as to restore normal functioning. Pungent-tasting *yang* herbs and *yang* forms of acumoxa would be expansionary in nature whilst, for example, sour-tasting *yin* medicinals and *yin* physical stimulation would contract and astringe things where appropriate. Where the need was for health preservation, then diet, exercise, regulated sexual activities and self-discipline would be recommended.

Health cultivation, yang sheng

An important aspect of the background theory of health cultivation for the elite in the years around the start of the Han dynasty was to engage in activities believed to promote the continued close integration of *yin* and *yang*. Health meant cultivating a firm interpenetration of *yin* and *yang*, *qi* and substance, whilst death was the separation of *yin* and *yang*, body and soul. Real life existed between these extremes. Activities included using the mind and breathing techniques to circulate *qi*, blood

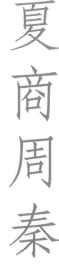

夏
商
周
秦

and fluids, and to encourage their union and interactions. The lungs were conceived as *qi* bellows, and inhaled air directed as if it were stoking up a metabolic fire in the lower parts of the body, the *dan tian* (丹田, cinnabar field). Numerous breathing methods and meditative techniques were devised with the intention of exploring the body landscape and its possibilities. In the centuries leading up to the Han dynasty some medical ideas came out of these introspections to provide ideas about the circulation of blood in the *mai* vessels, of *qi* in the *jing-luo*, of *xue* (blood) in the arteries and of acupoint *xue* 'caves', where *qi* could be affected. These experiments provided one tributary of ideas to classical medicine – in particular, descriptions of the eight extraordinary channels (*qi jing ba mai*) theories probably came from this work.

Sexual activities were also seen by the educated and aristocratic classes as holding the potential for *yang sheng* or health preservation and, more specifically, as a means of consolidating one's own internal *yin-yang* relationship. Loss of semen was viewed as potentially weakening, and so ejaculation was deliberately limited. Intercourse could be combined with breathing exercises and mental control of the *qi* and *jing-luo* circulations.

Much attention was also devoted to the study of diet, and this was recognised for its influence, either for good or for harm. Health could be regulated by appropriately matching the intake of warm *yang* substances, such as meat spices and ginger, with *yin* nourishing foods, such as fruit and root vegetables, based on knowledge of one's own current state and the state of the climate. The ideal norm used in *yang sheng* health cultivation was the *Dao*, the natural way of the universe. Through the Warring States period a prime intellectual endeavour of the scholar gentlemen classes was to investigate the *Dao* of nature and to encapsulate it in the overarching explanatory model that was to be more formally structured in Han dynasty medicine. So successful were these ideas that, even today, most Chinese people, and people across East Asia as a whole, have an inbuilt sense of them, for instance, in their approach in harmonising diet and lifestyle in a manner that accords with the seasons, nature and the *Dao*.

Daoist alchemical experiments with mercury

From the Warring States period onwards the Daoists had a particular fascination with alchemical experimentation and were especially intrigued to discover the properties of cinnabar – mercuric sulphide ore. When freshly mined and powdered, cinnabar looks like dried blood, *yin*, dry and dead looking, but when some *yang* is introduced in the form of heat, a wonderful transformation takes place – liquid mercury metal runs out. This appeared to be magical proof of the way that when *yin* and *yang* (heat and substance) are brought together, an *essence* is created, heavy (*yin*), but able to flow (*yang*), and able to reflect images in a manner akin to the conscious mind. This epitomised the truth of the transformational properties of the meeting of *yin* and *yang* and echoed the belief that the essence of longevity could be cultivated by the

夏
商
周
秦

action of the *qi* of breath on *jing* essence to create an enhanced and everlasting *shen* consciousness. In the culture of the time, those who purported to understand these things would have been held in awe by most people, so many of the intelligentsia were beguiled into alchemical study. Their ideas gained a momentum that carried the ideas for thousands of years – even in the face of opposition of those who could see a harmful side. When influential people suggested that mercuric substances were the basis of immortality, most would believe them. Although they brought death to many, the alchemists also brought a hands-on experimental approach to the investigation of chemical transformations.

More than a millennium later garbled information on alchemy reached Europe, triggering the fascination of Western alchemists and their own occult yearnings for the secrets of the universe. The origins of the science of chemistry were in mediaeval European alchemy, but in turn, its origins can be traced to China's alchemists. The fascination with alchemy continued long after the Warring States period, and led to the development of many of the fundamental techniques of basic chemistry, such as distillation, filtration and sublimation, and the study of transformations happening during chemical reactions.

Gan ying, resonant causalities

Intending to understand the way the world functioned, Warring States scholars considered various types of causality. At a mundane level simple cause–effect relationships were self-evident – you fall from a tree and your leg breaks – but for things where the chain of causality was less evident, or if everything seemed to be going wrong, intangible mechanisms such as ancestor displeasure might need to be invoked. Studying the networks of relationships found in nature led to the conclusion that some types of causality were subtler; things happen in concert with each other where the connection is obscure. Something else often seems to be going on other than physical causality. Nature appears to orchestrate itself. The moon and the tides change in concert, spring arrives and everything everywhere just seems to know what to do. Early thinkers believed that all the things around them in nature existed in a web of relationships whereby one thing affected another by a resonant connection, with each other and, ultimately, in response to changes in the cycles of the skies. Things that connected most strongly were things that had similar qualities in their nature; it was the similarities that created a response in each other. Evidence for such invisible links between things could be identified in the real world. One famous observation concerning this influence of one thing on another comes from Dong Zhong-shu (−179 to −104), who said:

> The…kung note struck upon one lute will be answered by the…kung notes from other stringed instruments. They sound by themselves in complementary resonance. This is a case of comparable things being affected according to the classes to which they belong.

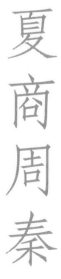

In other words, when the strings were tuned to exactly the same pitch, there was an invisible resonant connection between them. So, an important quest of the 'science' of the time was to understand, label and map these qualities, something that was done using *yin-yang*, the calendric emblems (*wu yun liu qi* – five movements and six *qi*), and with colours, textures, tastes and so on that could be grouped using the *wu xing* (five transitions, or 'five elements') doctrine. The current view, however, is that Dong Zhong-shu's writings on *wu xing* were later additions.

For understanding medical pathology, this *gan ying* (感应, resonant influence) idea served to explain the relationship between the environment and health. According to this hypothesis, the various *jing-luo* channels and *zangfu* organs could resonate either harmoniously or adversely with the climate, with the cosmos, with foods or with emotional disturbances. In terms of treatment it meant that therapies could work because they had some quality that evoked a beneficial resonant response in the channel or organ that was disturbed. In this conception acumoxa stimulation at the surface of the body, if it had an appropriate quality, could induce beneficial responses deep inside. Medicinal herbs worked less by pharmacology and more by inducing a *gan ying* response. Therapeutic causality was seen as being a consequence of things having a similar nature; herbs were able to change activity in the body because they had a *qi* quality that was related to that function in the body. This idea might seem quite esoteric until we reflect on the fact that this is a fundamental basis of modern telecommunications – it is resonance that enables a tiny current transmitted from a mobile phone to communicate afar to equipment that is tuned to exactly the same frequency.

The *gan ying* idea was a method of understanding the more subtle connections and influence between things: the way that nature orchestrated its activities as if a guiding force were at work – in spring, plants and animals were all stimulated to growth and development whereas in the autumn they began a coordinated retreat in readiness for winter – and the way that man's physiology also danced to this tune without evident instruction. I think that it is important to realise that the *gan ying* model served to characterise the mysterious dance of nature but it did not replace or preclude more mundane and obvious causality – a skull fractured by a lump of wood or a burn-induced blister. The belief was that the mapping of all nature's concordances would give understanding and the power to influence change. In medicine this meant labelling the body's anatomy and physiology in health and disease using the same terms that were used to map nature so that interventions could be applied that resonated in a beneficial way to restore health.

Essence of the clinical gaze

The French sinologist François Jullien has described the high esteem that early Chinese thinkers attached to those who had developed the ability to sense from the myriad details of a situation its essential possibilities for development through time. This idea is expressed by the character *shi* (势), meaning the possibilities inherent in

夏商周秦

any configuration of things or events, something that is key to timely and pragmatic action. This was the skill that was most valued in military strategists and court political advisers since the Warring States period. The realisation was that those who are prescient enough to discern the crux of a complex situation at its earliest germinal stages then have the greatest degree of control over their fate because they are in a position to make subtle but perfectly pitched interventions, actions that require minimal expenditure of effort and create minimal disturbance. This fine ability to discern and interpret subtleties and then act before others were even aware of a disturbance was what was meant by 'sagely action'. It is the true sense behind the Daoist ideal of *wu wei* – something that has sometimes been misconstrued as an inactive *laissez-faire* approach rather than a perfectly judged and prescient 'stitch in time'. This idea was popular in the Warring States period, and by the beginning of the Han dynasty is an idea that was seen as pertinent to medicine as it was to warfare. In warfare military intelligence could be gathered by spycraft, but in the case of medicine, this involved seeking out and appropriating medical knowledge from the community – midwives, herbal practitioners, battlefield trauma specialists and even butchers. In clinical medicine 'sagely' practice meant applying subtle observation of changes in the patient's bodily landscape using all the senses to understand the configuration that underlies their malaise.

In much the same way that the mind of a chess master functions, *shi* referred to the ability to gaze knowingly on a complex situation and fully apprehend all the nuances and interrelations and be able to sense its pivotal point such that the perfect, most elegant and economic intervention could be made. In the Han dynasty it was realised that this mindset was just as applicable to the complexities of medicine as it was to warfare.

Origins of acupuncture

Finely crafted stone needles dating from the Shang dynasty have been excavated from archaeological sites, and these *bian* stones have been offered as evidence of prehistoric acupuncture practice. The *Dong Shan Jing* section of the *Shan Hai Jing* (Classic of Mountains and Seas) mentions Mount Gaoshi, in Eastern China, as a prime source of these *bian* stones. Such implements are believed to have been used for medical treatment as they do not have the eye needed for sewing; this view is also supported by an entry in a Han dynasty dictionary that defines *bian shi* as 'a type of stone used to treat illness by pricking the body'. The manuscripts unearthed at Mawangdui (dated exactly to −168) mention the use of *bian* stones as a treatment for haemorrhoids. Given that the ideas in the Mawangdui texts were those current in the decades prior to their burial, *bian* stones were used to treat haemorrhoids at least as early as the −3rd century. However, this information is not sufficient for us to say that any therapy resembling energetic acupuncture was being practised at this time. The Shang and Western Zhou dynasty stone needles were almost certainly used for lancing boils, for puncturing haemorrhoids and perhaps for other surgical therapies,

夏
商
周
秦

but not for the more complex energetic-based system of general medical therapy that was to characterise acumoxa practice from the Han dynasty onward.

We also have no documentary evidence of the existence of the acumoxa meridian tract (*jing-luo*) system in the Shang and Zhou dynasties, or the identification of acupuncture points. These ideas almost certainly emerged through the course of the −3rd and −2nd centuries. The Mawangdui tomb finds are one of the best sources of information we have providing a snapshot of medicine at around the start of the −2nd century. This find contained medical texts owned by a noble family together with a model that crudely outlined 11 of the acumoxa tracts. As this model included no acupoints, it has been taken to indicate that channel theories predated the identification of acumoxa points. The context of this find, though, seems more suggestive of a wealthy elite hobby interest in health preservation than of professional medical practice, so it is not necessarily representative of cutting-edge professional medical knowledge at that date. The elite classes of the time were especially interested in *yang sheng* (health preservation practices), some of which involved stretching exercises where basic knowledge of the acumoxa tracts would be helpful. What was sealed in this tomb was perhaps more *Readers' Digest* than *Gray's Anatomy*.

Unromantic as it may seem to acupuncturists today, it is likely that boil lancing, sore draining and bloodletting medical practices were the key fortuitous points of departure for the invention of acupuncture, fortuitous because its originators seem to have stumbled on the observation that stimulation of specific places on the body surface evoked a wider range of body responses than might be expected from the simple removal of local pus or clots.

Trauma specialists flourished with the conditions of continual warfare that existed in the Warring States period, and these artisan practitioners were given plenty of opportunity to develop their skills. They used medicated dressings based on substances such as cinnabar, arsenic and alum to stop infection and to aid healing.

> Before or after pus draining and debridement medicines are applied externally to treat sores, swellings, wounds, injuries and ulcerations, before or after draining of pus…all external illnesses can be treated using *dan*, an externally applied medicine made from the five poisonous mineral drugs shi dan, dan sha, xiong huang, fan shi, ci shi. ('Tian Guan Zhong Zai', *Zhouli*)

Patients presenting an abscess or pustulant wound to an early healer or *yang yi* (sores specialist) might expect to be lanced by a *bian* stone and the pus drained away. Pain relief would follow such debridement, together with relief from feelings of malaise accompanying the infection. A common side effect of acupoint stimulation is mild euphoria, understood today as a mild 'kick' resulting from endorphin and other neurotransmitter changes. Current practice also shows that needling can trigger other subjective responses such as an aching or tingling sensation that propagates along the limbs from the puncture site. Physicians and patients alike will have noted the visible evidence of *xie qi* (pathogenic *qi*; in this case, pus) associated with tissue

夏
商
周
秦

infection – the presence of something in the body that, in health, should not be there. Bacterial infection that enters lymph vessels on the limbs leads to visible red lines of inflammation that spread proximally, and this probably contributed to the development of *jing-luo* theory. The *jing-luo* were viewed as another near-invisible subtlety that lies behind what is visibly manifested on the body surface as colour, movement, lively well-nourished tissue, relaxed musculature and so on. Physicians studied the visible and the palpable to assess the invisible and the hidden.

So, besides visual evidence of illness, the unwelcome presence of pathological foreign material was considered to be evident from local tenderness to pressure. With the success of surgical therapies that aimed to drain pus and debride necrotic tissue, the hypothesis then arises that besides local pain, heat and swelling, many other illnesses might also result from the presence of foreign material. Pathogenic *xie qi* might sometimes be less visible, stealthily not revealing itself by local swelling and pain, but detectable only by tenderness on pressure. My view is that this led some of these early healers to a new hypothesis, that disease was often caused by the presence of a pathogenic foreign substance that had gained access to the body, one that was more subtle than pus and whose location could be revealed by palpation of tell-tale tender spots, and that indicated to the perceptive healer the best place to drain away this less tangible form of *xie qi*. Tenderness indicated both the presence and location of *xie qi*, and highlighted palpation as a key diagnostic and investigative procedure that allowed the identification of disease loci and eventually the naming and classification of acupoints. At the same time, it gave a simple research methodology that led practitioners to investigate and map the body's responses to health imbalance. Systematic palpation allowed the creation of an experiential map of the places where reactive spots were most often found in ill health – the *xue* (acupuncture points or 'caves'). These are indeed the *ahshi* ('that's it!', tender) places on the body that often become very tender to pressure in patients seen today in the modern clinic.

One piece of evidence that supports this transition from pus draining to piercing intended to remove less substantial *xie qi* (pathogenic *qi*) is found in the observation that some sections of the Han dynasty classic, the *Neijing*, are near-identical to earlier writings, except that the word pus (*nong*, 膿) has been replaced by the term *xie qi*. This seems to indicate a conceptual shift of intent from removing a tangible pathogenic substance from the body, pus, to removing a subtler and more intangible one, pathogenic *qi*. Part of the success that spurred these pioneers on was the happy accident that needling tender spots did indeed often evoke a rapid and tangible response, such as relief of pain or mild endorphin euphoria. Such a response would encourage further hypothesis generation and investigation, leading to the emergence of a new explanatory model of disease. Had the first experiments with therapeutic lancing failed to provide any response, the method would most likely have petered out.

The modern experience of acupuncture practice suggests that the *ahshi* hypothesis is also applicable in the absence of *xie qi*, for example, when tender points appear

夏
商
周
秦

in skeleto-muscular injury or even in response to emotional changes. This could not have gone unnoticed by the Bian Que healers, and probably also contributed to the new brand of medical knowledge becoming mainstream in the century before the start of the Han dynasty. The large numbers of literate doctors who began to adopt *qi*-based acupuncture themselves began to investigate the acupuncture phenomena, which they explained using the 'science', metaphysics and beliefs in vogue at the time, such as *yin-yang, wu xing* and the other concepts discussed earlier. From the end of the Warring States period to the end of the Han dynasty, greatly increased numbers of acupuncture points were described, and ever more detailed explanatory and diagnostic models came into being amongst the medical literati.

The dawn of energetic acupuncture in the Warring States period

The pre-eminent medical figure said to have been working a century or so before the founding of Han dynasty medicine was Bian Que, who is seen as a pioneering new style of healer. His clan are the most likely innovators behind the invention of acupuncture.

Bian Que

Bian Que (aka Qin Yue-ren) is a semi-legendary figure considered to be the first recorded physician to combine folk shamanism with theoretical doctrine. He is said to have lived between −407 and −310 and, according to Unschuld, he epitomises the combined attributes of shaman, folk physician and classical physician. Writing a few centuries later (around −75), historian Si Ma-qian wrote that Bian Que ran a boarding house that was visited by an elderly sage called Chang Sang. Nearing the end of his life, the old physician chose to pass on his secret knowledge to Bian Que, and as a part of the process he is said to have given him a medicinal decoction saying, 'Drink this with fresh dew for 30 days and you will gain special sight.' The legend has it that this enabled Bian Que to see into people's bodies and also through walls. Plainly an exaggerated account, we might re-read the story as: 'Drink this decoction and learn my teachings and you will enhance your acuity and your ability to assess people medically.' As we have seen, the culture of the time admired those possessing sensory acuity and a strategist's gaze, people skilled at reading subtle clues and able to deeply assess a situation to ensure that the most beneficial outcome can be gained. The real understanding conveyed by Chang Sang to Bian Que may have been an understanding of *zang xiang* – the view that the body's hidden internal workings are readable by knowing observation of the exterior.

Tradition credits Bian Que with three important contributions to medical practice. He is said to have founded the systematic *sizhen* (四诊, four diagnostic methods) approach to diagnosis, namely looking, listening-smelling, questioning

夏 商 周 秦

and palpation, which remains a foundation of clinical examination today. Because different medical lineages of his time probably emphasised different diagnostic and theoretical methods, the references to the four methods may be taken as code to imply that Bian Que had studied and drawn widely from various traditions, and so had a more complete grasp than most other physicians of his time.

Tradition also claims that Bian Que contributed to the writing of the *Nanjing*, although current scholarship suggests that it was largely compiled in the +1st century, but it may have included later versions of texts from Bian Que's time. He is also credited with what is claimed to be the first documented use of acupuncture, the treatment of the Prince of Qin in −501. Some have wondered how it could be possible for the Prince of Qin to be treated by a physician who was not due to be born for another century. Indeed, when all the fables about Bian Que are put together, we find him working not only across an implausible time span, but also sometimes simultaneously in places very far apart from each other. So although there may well have been an historical Bian Que, the name is likely to also have become a generic label applied to a particular clan of medical shaman physicians with a similar medical style and practising an early form of acupuncture. They appear to have originated in today's Shandong province and to have plied their medical trades mostly across Eastern China, perhaps dressed ceremonially as birds, their clan emblem. The character *que* (鹊) in the label Bian Que means magpie, and it is possible that their choice of tribal emblem may relate to Shang dynasty mythology which held that it was bird spirits who controlled the wind that was said to have originated from 'caves' (*xue*, 穴). *Xue* is the character used in both the *Neijing* and today for acupuncture loci.

Bian Que should perhaps not be seen as an individual person but as a charismatic medical brand synonymous with an innovative style of medical practice. The Bian Que healers synthesised existing knowledge and made new discoveries to create a new class of healer that would be the template for a new scholar physician class which developed rapidly over the coming few centuries. The notable medical sinologist Paul Unschuld positions the Bian Que healers as representative of the transition from folk healer to the more investigative scholar physician. Championing acupuncture treatment, they introduced important innovations to the lancing therapies that had previously been limited largely to pus draining and wound care.

In the absence of reliable documentary evidence, we can tentatively suppose that it was the Bian Que tribe who made the conceptual leap from surgical lancing to the use of physical stimulation of the body surface as a more complex energetic therapy able to treat a wider range of illnesses. They seem to have hit on the idea that low-level physical injury could evoke therapeutic responses and, in the process, appear to have made the innovative leap from simple surgical treatment to a *qi*-based 'energetic' reflexive therapy. Such transitional healers, who were neither simple folk artisans nor high-level classical scholars, prepared the ground for the Han dynasty literati by pioneering the palpatory investigation of the bodily landscape and its responses to physical stimulation. They began the process of mapping the tender

夏
商
周
秦

points that can appear on the bodily terrain, and began to name the special places where the invisible disease-causing *qi* could be drained away.

A famous Han dynasty stone relief is said to depict Bian Que as a shaman dressed as a bird giving acupuncture treatment to finely dressed ladies. Dating from a time when shaman healers were under suspicion for their mystical outlook and yet somewhat feared for their professed powers, I personally interpret this relief as a satire on the unsatisfactory state of affairs faced by the upper classes – your silk-clad wife having to seek the help of people such as Bian Que for medical help because they had stumbled on more effective treatments than those used by the court physicians. What aristocrat wants to see his family seeking healthcare from the lower orders? What better motivation could there be for finding ways of appropriating their knowledge and sanitising it for the benefit of the elite? Indeed, legend has it that a court physician called Li Hai murdered Bian Que as he was jealous of his skills.

The Bian Que tribe emphasised acupuncture as distinct from its sister therapy, moxibustion. The use of smouldering moxa as a medical therapy almost certainly predates the introduction of energetic acupuncture, and was probably initially used as a localised method for soothing pain and skeleto-muscular injury. It seems likely that, just as the *Neijing* claims, needling and moxibustion were developed in different parts of China and by different groups of healers. The Mawangdui manuscripts reflect this other healing tradition; they describe moxibustion but not needling, and *jing-luo* channels rather than points, which suggests that the date −168 roughly marks the time when these aspects of treatment merged to form Han dynasty acumoxa therapy.

Besides Bian Que, the other most notable early physician whose activities were documented by the historian Si Ma-qian is Chunyu Yi, discussed in the next chapter.

Jing–luo conduits

Modern practice confirms that stimulating the body surface using needles or strong heat frequently causes aching and tingling sensations to propagate along the limbs, head or, to a lesser extent, the trunk of the body. The course and speed of these responses has been investigated, and even the way that the sensation can be hindered by pressure or by cold ambient temperatures. The ancient physicians labelled these phenomena as movement of *qi*, and meticulously mapped their apparent trajectories, an effect that was almost certainly a key factor in the development of the *jing-luo* explanatory model of the living body that continues to inform current acumoxa practice. An acupuncturist asked to treat menstrual pain might palpate the acupoint *sanyinjiao* (Sp 6) area above the medial anklebone to locate the most actively tender location. Needling this point can send a dull ache or numb feeling radiating up the leg that, when it reaches the abdomen, often relieves acute pain. Early healers seem to have concluded that pricking such places was effective to expel *xie qi*, clearing away bruising, swelling and the associated stagnation. Also, disease was considered to respond because the needling was able to send the body's healthy *qi* along the

夏
商
周
秦

limb to correct the dysfunction and pain. The fact that the sensation followed a predictable course suggested that the movement was akin to blood circulation in that it progressed along some kind of communication tract or channel.

Besides palpation, visual inspection also seems to have contributed to early channel theories, much of this based on the imperative of the time to create a detailed map of the body's anatomical terrain. Blood vessels were considered to be part of the circulatory network, and previous identification of the function of blood vessels was probably the inspiration for the concept of substances moving and circulating in the body. Fleeting mention of blood vessels is found in Warring States texts that predate any mention of acupuncture or the *jing-luo* tracts. These arteries and veins were referred to as the *mai* vessels, and it is clear that they were clearly understood as a transport system for a tangible material substance – blood. Later on, medical scholars moved their attention from obvious anatomy to greater subtleties and, with the observation of *qi* propagation sensations along the limbs, the need arose to map the less tangible currents in the body. So, as well as a *mai* vessel system circulating blood, the *jing-luo* system was conceptualised based on investigation of sensations elicited by acupuncture and moxibustion. In modern terms this less obvious circulation might be seen as reflecting lymph circulation or electrochemical propagation through excitable tissues such as nerve, muscle and possibly arterial smooth muscle and even connective tissue.

Interruption to the flow of blood by arterial or venous occlusion from pressure results in colour changes, and highlights the importance of blood circulation. This is a simple observation to make and is especially evident when we cut the blood supply off to the head. Pressure at other places where there are no major blood vessels also results in changes that are not related to interruption of blood circulation, and it appears that these were interpreted as interruptions to the circulation of a more subtle substance – *qi*. Pressure at the acupoint SI 8 (*xiao hao*), where the ulnar nerve passes, results in numbness and tingling along the limb, but none of the rapid colour changes seen on blood vessel occlusion. A similar response is seen when pressure is applied to the sciatic nerve near the acupoint *huan tiao* (GB 30). So, besides the responses to actual stimulation with needling or moxibustion mentioned earlier in this chapter, simple palpation of the body surface probably contributed to the idea of a circulation that was parallel to but subtler than blood circulation. Investigations of this kind are likely to have contributed to the *qi* circulation and *jing-luo* theories that appeared towards the end of the Warring States period, and offered tangible evidence to early physicians of the existence of more subtle conduits apart from the blood vessels through which healthy *qi* circulated and through which *xie qi* could progress proximally, as could be seen in bacterial lymphangitis. Such an observation was important because experience would show that contamination of the *jing-luo* system by pathogens represented a significant risk to the patient's health, from septicaemia, for instance. Exposure to cold or to simple pressure on the skin causes blanching, and it seems that this too was considered to be evidence of tiny vessels

夏
商
周
秦

that were referred to as *luo mai* (network vessels) or *sun luo* (grandson networks), that we would recognise as capillaries today.

In all, we can reasonably suppose that the points of acupuncture, its *jing* channel and *luo* capillary vessel ideas, probably developed as a mix of observation and experiment of the manner in which the body responded to different stimuli. The conclusions of these investigations were fitted into the mix of rational and fanciful proto-science ideas current in the few centuries before the Han dynasty.

Qin and han dynasty strip writings

In 1975, extensive writings on bamboo (笺, *jian*), dating from between −250 and −201, were excavated from graves in Yun Meng county in Hubei province. Most of these recorded Qin dynasty (−221 to −206) legal decrees, but a few described medical practices of the time and, in particular, their relation to forensic medicine in these early times. In 1972, in Gansu province, wooden strips describing Han medical practices were also found, and other texts written on bamboo slips were excavated from Han dynasty graves in Hubei's Zhang Jia Shan in 1983. The latter writings contained more medical discussions than earlier writings, including material on Chinese herbs, formulae and other therapies, and mentioned treatment principles and early Chinese medicine pattern diagnosis.

Qin dynasty jian and crime investigation

The Qin dynasty writings on bamboo *jian* slips from Yun Meng county included details of forensic practices of the time. These were in the form of official directives on crime investigation stipulating the methods to be used by officials when examining assault victims, crime scenes and corpses that had been discovered; they indicate that a systematic approach to traumatology was in place in these early times. When examining assault victims, investigators were instructed to formally identify and classify the type and degree of injury – the term *da yi*, for example, was used to label an injured person who was either without limb fracture or in recovery from a leg fracture at the stage where support was needed in order to walk. The procedures to be used in inspecting crime scenes involving suspected murder, presumed suicide by hanging and in examining corpses that had been unearthed by grave robbers were clearly stipulated. The texts described the way that, during investigation of a suspected murder, attention should be paid to recording details of the scene, the position of the body and other clues at the crime scene such as blood marks, hand prints, foot prints, knee prints, marks on the body left by weapons and any other evidence found at the scene.

When examining corpses the initial focus was to identify whether there were any obvious indications of murder, and whether the death was caused by hanging or strangulation. Those investigating murder were instructed to systematically collect evidence by noting the location, direction and size of any injuries, the pattern of

夏商周秦

bloodstains on clothes and the condition of damaged clothing. The height of the body, style and length of hair, skin colour and old scars was also to be noted. When investigating hangings, detailed evidence was recorded that was intended to distinguish murder from suicide based on the condition of the rope, the path it takes from the body to its anchorage point, whether or not the victim's tongue was protruding, the presence or absence of incontinence of urine or stool, and whether the mouth and nose were agape. The precise nature of tissue injury and of the rope imprint on the neck was considered especially valuable. Dark purple skin bruising was a key sign of hanging occurring prior to death as distinct from hanging that occurred subsequent to death in an attempt by a murderer to give the appearance of suicide. It was also noted that when rope marks were seen to extend right across the back of the neck, this indicated prior strangulation, whereas death due to hanging left tissue undamaged at this place. The writings advise, 'If the tongue is not protruding, if the mouth and nose are not open, if the rope imprint does not show bruising and the end of the rope shows no signs of attempted escape, then we should hesitate before concluding that hanging was actually the cause of death.' In this manner, Qin dynasty law applied some surprisingly perceptive and rational forensic methods.

Qin dynasty law also provided measures in relation to leprosy, stipulating that people infected with it must be quarantined at an infectious disease centre, suggesting that the contagious nature of this illness was recognised. These texts also specified that doctors who diagnosed lepers should be specialists in forensic medicine. The signs of leprosy were described in detail and included loss of eyebrow hair, sunken nasal cavity, absence of a sneeze reflex, deflection of the nasal bone when subjected to pressure, deformation of the feet, ulcers on the soles of the feet, lack of hair on the hands and hoarseness of voice. These descriptions of leprosy are far more detailed than other medical literature so far discovered from the Qin dynasty, and can be seen as evidence of a rational and systematic approach to medical matters as part of the establishment of a new unified and more peaceful civilisation in the decades leading up to the Han dynasty.

Early moxibustion and heat treatments

Heat has obvious therapeutic potential, sometimes offering quick relief from pain, for example, in soothing menstrual pain, or for soothing pain due to arthritis or from trauma, so it is likely that this modality has been in use at least from Neolithic times. Throughout history we see mentions of 'baking' and 'scorching' treatments which amount simply to warming an affected part near to a fire, sometimes in conjunction with the application of herbal compresses. In classical moxibustion treatment heat stimulation is given either by burning the substance directly on the skin or applied at a short distance, as a form of radiant heat.

In the centuries before the Han dynasty various smouldering plant materials were in use as therapeutic heat sources, including charcoal, grass, feathers, herbs,

夏
商
周
秦

firewood and the pith extracted from juncus grass. Strictly speaking, then, the term 'moxibustion' is an inaccurate translation because the term *jiu* refers to a variety of different heat treatments. The Mawangdui manuscripts (−168) suggest that, from the Qin and the beginning of the Han dynasty, moxa, the woolly material sifted from the dried leaves of artemesia vulgaris and burnt as a fragrant heat source, became the main heat source used therapeutically. We know, however, that moxa was also in use in the centuries before the Qin and Han dynasties because a passing mention of it is found in the Warring States philosophical treatise, *Mengzi*, where it says that people should 'use three-year-old moxa to treat a seven-year-old illness'. Moxa is the preferred heat source for *jiu* treatment because it smoulders reliably to provide a convenient,

> Moxa 'punk' comes from the leaf of artemesia argii, a weed that is found worldwide. The best quality is produced in Qizhou, where the late spring leaves are sun-dried and coarsely powdered. Leaf and twig debris are sifted out, leaving downy wool from the underside of the leaf. Sun drying and sifting is repeated until soft, pale moxa wool is obtained. High-grade moxa is spongy, pale brown, has no twigs or coarse leaf material, and burns with a light and fragrant smoke.

strong, even and prolonged heat. The character *jiu* (灸) consists of a part meaning fire (火) combined with a part meaning prolonged heat (久). With characteristic inventiveness, numerous different ways of applying therapeutic heat stimulation have been developed through Chinese medicine history, most of which are still in use today. In addition to the use of smouldering plant materials various irritant substances, such as mustard paste, garlic, ginger (*xi xin*), aconite, euphorbia root (*gan sui*) and cloves, are sometimes used to provide a burning stimulation, a process called 'heavenly moxibustion'.

Earliest textual references to herbal medicine

The earliest written references to medicinal herbs are found in the *Shijing* (Book of Songs), a chronicle of social history written at the end of the Spring and Autumn period (−770 to −476). Although this text is mainly a collection of folk songs from previous centuries, and was not specifically a medical work, its verses include some poetic descriptions of the collection of medicinal herbs such as *yi mu cao* (motherwort), *ze xie* (alisma), *bei mu* (fritillaria bulb), *ai ye* (moxa) and *deng xin cao* (juncus grass), which, as mentioned, were also sometimes used in heat treatments. The inclusion of these discussions helps to confirm that many medicinals that are still current in today's *materia medica* were in use in about the −5th century.

Another text that was written in the era prior to the dawn of classical medicine is the *Shan Hai Jing* (Classic of Mountains and Seas), believed to date from the Warring States period, also including a few scattered references to medicinal substances. Consisting of two parts, a *shan* (mountains) section and a *hai* (seas) section, this is essentially a work that discusses geography. The *hai* part of the text has been dated to about −250 and makes no mention of medicinal herbs. The *shan* section dates

夏
商
周
秦

from about −400 and mentions various commonly used medicinals such as *rou gui* (cinnamon bark), *chuan xiong* (ligusticum or Chinese lovage), *dang gui* (Angelica), *sang bai pi* (mulberry bark), *zhi shi* (bitter orange), *jie geng* (balloon flower root), *qian cao gen* (madder root), *gou teng* (gambir vine hooks), *niu huang* (ox gallstone) and *she xiang* (musk).

In the Warring States period herbal medicine practitioners began to be called *fang shi*, a term that Unschuld translates as 'prescription gentlemen'. *Shi* is an aspirational gentleman scholar, and the character *fang*, as pointed out by the US Chinese medical scholar Jeffery Yuen, also implies that these were gentlemen who were notable amongst the populace for applying a *method*, that is, they were distinguishable from simple folk herbalists by the fact that they professed to have studied a learned medical doctrine, the implication being that they were more systematic and therefore more skilled than shamans or folk medicine practitioners. Later, in the Qin and Han dynasties, it is the knowledge that circulated in these lineages that is believed to have formed the basis of Han dynasty medical texts such as the *Neijing*.

Yi Yin, legendary herbalist

Diverging away from folk herbalism, Chinese herbal medicine seems to have begun to develop as a profession for educated practitioners in the course of the Warring States period as the educated *shi* scholar classes emerging after the time of Confucius sought alternatives to superstition and folk medicine. Perhaps taking a cue from the culinary arts, medicinal herb scholars began to realise that combining substances together allowed for more skilful therapy and more complex functions than the folk medicine style of simply matching a symptom to an individual herb. This occurred in the context of the new theories of disease mechanism and therapeutics that were beginning to appear.

If the famed 'first historian of China' Si Ma-qian (writing in about −75) is correct, the move to structured herbal formulas was planted much earlier. In his *Shiji* (Historical Records), Si Ma-qian claims that the first medicinal formulas appeared at the start of the Shang dynasty (roughly −1660), and were allegedly introduced by a court chef named Yi Yin who set down his health recipes in a medicinal formulary called the *Tang Ye Jing* (Classic of Decocted Drinks, also called *Yi Yin Tang Ye*). Described as having originated from peasant slave stock, Yi Yin is portrayed as a skilled cook who had acquired his clan's medical lore early in life, a medical style Si Ma-qian described as being more sophisticated than most. Whilst it is impossible to be certain of the accuracy of this legend, many contemporary medical historians in China contend that Yi Yin was indeed a real person who explored the boundaries between food and medicine. Some credit him with the introduction of the food-based medicinal formula *gui zhi tang* (cinnamon twig decoction), a formula that also contains zizyphus dates, ginger, liquorice and peony root. This formula and its many variants were to reappear in the ground-breaking medical classic written in about +200, the *Shang Han Lun*.

夏
商
周
秦

Dawn of China's classical medical tradition

In the Shang and Western Zhou dynasties medicine in China was a mix of simple folk medicine and shamanic practices based on the appeasement of ancestor spirits. From the time of Confucius new intellectual classes appeared who, faced with the ongoing strife of the Warring States period, tended to favour rationality and scholarship, and began to create a medicine that was more in accord with their rational outlook. The medical *shi* scholars who appeared during the Warring States period took ownership of the folk knowledge and medical artisan skills gathered from the community, and combined this with the fundamental ideas taken from ancient teachings on philosophy, metaphysics and the Daoist spirit of investigation of man and nature as well as ideas and terminology borrowed from thinkers involved in statecraft and military tactics. This mix created the foundations for a more systematic and rational medicine, and the information was assembled into texts that could be brought to life when catalysed by study with an experienced medical mentor. The scene was set for the next generations of medical scholars in the Han dynasty to collate and develop these ideas by large-scale investigation that would assemble the medicine into a more coherent and complete system.

夏
商
周
秦

3

FOUNDING OF CLASSICAL MEDICINE IN THE HAN DYNASTY

The Han dynasty is divided into the Western Han (–206 to +8) and the Eastern Han (+23–221). For the most part this was a period of peace and stability that allowed civilisation to reach a high point, and such conditions also tended to be beneficial for the advancement of medicine. This period saw the founding of China's literate medical tradition, and it is also the earliest historical period from which detailed medical writings survive. Although the vast majority of Han dynasty written works have been lost, those that we have record a time when new ideas and technological innovations proliferated against the background of a new investigative spirit. Knowledge that had accumulated in previous centuries was gathered together and re-evaluated to form the background to the creation of the systematic medical tradition that has continued to evolve up to the present day. It was in these four centuries that the founding texts of this innovative medicine were compiled, the *Huangdi Neijing Suwen*, the *Lingshu*, the *Nanjing, Shennong Bencao, Shang Han Lun* and the *Jiayi Jing*, to begin a medical tradition that, stretching the word a touch, we can refer to as 'classical' Chinese medicine. This term describes a medical system that was, in the main, developed by and intended to serve the literate and ruling classes, but which drew on pre-existing medical ideas and discoveries taken from the wider community.

The Warring States period (Zhanguo, –475 to –221) had been briskly brought to a close with the founding of the brief but pivotal Qin dynasty (–221 to –206). Qin Emperor Shi Huang-di (–246 to –210) is famed for his Terracotta Army, his use of military force to unify China into one state, and for his grandiose governmental schemes. Although maligned for his tyrannical excesses, it was Shi Huang-di who was responsible for introducing a wide range of civilising and unifying measures, such as standardising the written language and regulating weights and measures across the Chinese empire, as well as for dragging the country out of its self-perpetuating strife.

Shi Huang-di was gradually poisoned and sent to an early death by consuming the toxic mercury-based immortality remedies prescribed by his Daoist court physicians, which we now know cause hair and teeth loss, mental derangement and eventually death. It is believed that his tomb, as yet unexcavated, included a landscape running with rivers of liquid mercury, a legend now supported by local soil analysis. As well as defining the country of China (named after his Qin rule), the regulation and order he imposed in his short reign contributed to the success of the following Han dynasty.

Rise of the shi scholars

The previous centuries had seen the gradual ascendancy of a class of private literati scholars called *shi* (师) whose knowledge, literacy and skills had given them increasing power and influence over rulers and the state administration. Becoming ever more arrogant and confident of their unassailable position in state affairs, eventually the *shi* saw themselves as the equals of their rulers, or even their superiors. Eventually, by the start of Shi Huang-di's Qin dynasty, it was clear that their skills had become a self-serving monopoly that fed the ongoing troubles, and their scheming and intrigues exerted a negative influence on harmonious governance. Wishing to deprive them of their power and exclusivity, Shi Huang-di's solution was to try to seize their valuable knowledge and scholarship, and so he ordered, on pain of death, that all their books be burned, with only a few texts exempt. Works that were spared included the *Yijing*, the works of Confucius and books on agriculture. However, the fact that this draconian edict did not apply to books kept in the imperial library suggests that the Qin emperor's motive was not simply a barbaric dislike of knowledge; rather, it was part of a strategy to purloin written knowledge from the literate classes and to restrict access to learning to the ruling elite. The aim seems to have been to reduce the power of those *shi* literati operating outside the Qin government circles and, probably, to stifle organised dissent. Whilst one intent of this sanction may have been to consolidate his own power by depriving potential adversaries of access to texts on military strategy, in terms of medicine this helped ensure that medical learning could also be brought under centralised control.

At first, Shi Huang-di, over the space of a few years, had seized power and unified the empire using his overwhelming military force, so as to quickly restore order to the new state of China. After this his power was built on a monumental bureaucratic state machine that functioned by regulating numerous aspects of daily life. In a draconian sanction aimed at curbing the arrogance of the *shi* literati Shi Huang-di is said to have ordered the live burial of hundreds of court scholars in the year following the book-burning episode. Some, though, claim that this atrocity was a slander invented by the subsequent Han rulers. Many of the *shi* class were professional military tacticians prized for their Machiavellian skills and for whom conflict and intrigue was a way of life; in the new unified Qin state, these specialists were now redundant and in need of something else to occupy their minds.

We saw in the previous chapter how some of the fundamental ideas of Han dynasty medicine were derived from Warring States military logic and terminology. It seems that now that the military threats had been largely extinguished by the Qin unification, court scholars quickly turned their attention to developing medicine.

In just a few years the Qin dynasty crumbled, as Shi Huang-di himself succumbed to his longevity medicines, making way for the foundation of the Han dynasty in −201 and the start of a prolonged era of peace and good government. Life became progressively more civilised and well organised as the Han dynasty progressed; glazed pottery became commonplace (typically a holly-green lead-based glaze), and water was supplied to cities and palaces using bamboo and sealed earthenware pipes. A new social order was established that was founded on the orderly rules that had been proposed by Confucius four centuries earlier, and these proved to be a very successful recipe for harmonious governance.

One aspect of this new orderly environment was an increased emphasis on rationality that helped to foster 'scientific', technological and medical investigation. Educated thinkers in the decades up to and including the Han dynasty were explicit in their desire to replace superstition with rational enquiry, and in the space of a century or two they had constructed a much more complete and coherent medical system than had existed previously. Now that the threats to life from war, famine and strife had been reduced, medicine moved up the agenda for the *shi* classes. The results of this movement to create an improved professional medicine were summarised in the *Neijing*, most of which was compiled between −150 and +100 on the basis of earlier texts and what appears to have been deliberate and systematic medical investigation. Recent textual analysis indicates that the *Suwen*, the older part of the *Neijing*, was compiled by about 30 scholars from roughly 200 older writings.

Many new medical writings began to appear in the second half of the Western Han and, in a reversal of the spirit of the book-burning episode, these were disseminated across the country and for a while were available for purchase in shops. Also at this time, various medicinal herbs became established as items of commerce that were distributed from the growing regions to other areas for use in medical practice. Those recorded include *gan cao* (liquorice), *huang qi* (astragalus) and *fang feng* (ledebouriella root). Such trade suggests a move away from folk herbalist practices, where freshly collected local herbs were more the rule, towards a more professional medicine, with standard products and commercial distribution channels serving a professional medical class of practitioners.

As we have seen, in the centuries leading up to the Han dynasty, the educated classes had already begun to develop a medicine that fitted the accepted intellectual thought of the times. Ideas were incorporated from past generations of philosopher thinkers and military strategists, and combined with the practical medical knowledge that could be gleaned from the wider community. The early Han elite redoubled this process of improving and rationalising medicine with the aim of eliminating the more irrational ideas – magic, spirit possession and so on – and replacing them with plainer explanatory models. Such models employed the *yin-yang* rationale and *wu xing* (five transitional states) and many other accepted analytical tools of the time. These were combined with experiential information drawn from the folk traditions together with knowledge based on experimentation and observation. Hoping to understand the inner workings of nature, the *shi* scholars systematised their understanding of the cosmos and brought together all available resources to create a more coherent system intended to map the relationships between all things observable in the heavens, on earth and in the affairs of mankind. To give dignity, authenticity and a little fairy dust to their endeavours, they adopted the Daoist mantle so as to imply that they were the true inheritors of ancient wisdom.

Difficulties arose from the grandiosity of the project. The Han dynasty scholars were attempting to construct a grand unified scheme that encompassed all aspects of the universe, including such imponderables as the relationship between the stars and constellations in the sky with the patterns of change on earth and on the affairs of mankind. As with most overarching theories, some useful insights emerged alongside areas that do not quite hold up to closer examination. Despite the availability of esoteric theory in the practical application of real-world medical care, I expect that most physicians would fall back on pragmatic therapies. Treating acute or life-threatening illness demands a certain pragmatism rather than fancy calculations of the cycles of the cosmos. Medical pragmatism dictates that the diagnostic methods and techniques applied must be for the most part appropriate to the clinical situation in hand in order for physicians to survive with credibility intact. It is reasonable to argue that one measure of the robustness of Han dynasty medicine is seen in its continued survival down two millennia into modern times, with numerous doctors across the world continuing to use the discoveries of these ancient physicians. We are fortunate to have acquired a glimpse of an early stage of development of the classic medical tradition with the unearthing of the Mawangdui manuscripts a few decades ago – a glorious mix of superstition, folk remedies and pragmatic therapy.

Mawangdui manuscripts

In 1973 archaeologists excavating a tomb near Changsha in Hunan province discovered a collection of medical manuscripts; some were written on silk and others on bamboo or wood. Dating to exactly −168, this find predated the compilation of the *Neijing* by roughly a century, and provided an insight into classical Chinese medicine at an earlier state of development. An overview of the silk writings unearthed is outlined in the table on the next page.

Silk Mawangdui manuscripts

Wushier Bing Fang	Prescriptions for 52 Ailments
Tai Chan Shu	Book of the Fetus and Gestation
Za Liao Fang	Formulas for the Treatment of Miscellaneous Diseases
Yang Sheng Fang	Recipes for Nourishing Life
Zubi Shiyi Mai Jiujing	Cauterisation Canon for the Eleven Vessels of the Foot and Forearm
Yin Yang Shiyi Mai Jiujing	Cauterisation Canon of the Eleven Yin and Yang Vessels
Maifa	Methods of Using Pulse
Yin Yang Mai Si Hou	Pulse Conditions Seen in Severe Cases
Daoyin Tu	Exercise chart
Que Gu Shi Qi	Key to Promoting Digestion and Strengthening the Health

One of the most interesting of these texts is the extensive *Wushier Bing Fang* which includes prescriptions for over 100 diseases; some of the suggested treatments appear to be implausible folk medicine, often based on sympathetic magic, whilst others are quite ingenious. In total the Mawangdui texts mention about 400 medicinals, from plant, animal, human and mineral sources, and record 283 medical formulas. These are crudely constructed when compared with those that would appear 400 years later, in the *Shang Han Lun*. Included too are surgical techniques, lancing, cupping and moxa treatments. Another high point of the Mawangdui find is the famous *Daoyin Tu* consisting of 44 charming illustrations of health exercises largely based on mimicking animal movements. This founded a *yang sheng* (health cultivation) tradition of callisthenics that has continued through over two millennia to the present time. Given that the Mawangdui texts seem to have been a collection of home medical texts of a noble family, the inclusion of health cultivation exercises probably reflects the great interest in keeping fit and well amongst this strata of early Western Han families of the time. Other writings focus on sexual techniques for increasing health and longevity that emphasise coordinated breathing, contracting things and counting things.

Some things are conspicuous for their absence in these writings – the focus on *yin-yang* thinking to the exclusion of *wu xing* (five phase) doctrine, for example. We know that *wu xing* theory had been in use as a political theory a few decades earlier, and that this doctrine took a prominent position only a few decades after the burial of these manuscripts. Also, the silk manuscripts advocate moxibustion on the affected channels and barely mention acupuncture needling; this may be taken to suggest that therapeutic needling was yet to develop. Alternatively, it may be that the focus of the owners of this medical library was on home remedies and health preservation, for which moxibustion was perhaps more suitable. Tempting as it is to extrapolate from relatively scant data and to take this snapshot of Han medical practice as indicative of medicine in China as a whole, we should bear in mind that this is only a handful of writings from the home library of a single early Han dynasty family. Numerous other medical writings, now lost, will certainly have existed across the country, probably including more divergent medical styles.

The other writings found in the Mawangdui burial were inscriptions on bamboo and wood, and these fall into four categories: *He Yin-yang* (Harmonising Yin-Yang), *Shi Wen* (Ten Questions), *Za Jin Fang* (Various Formulas and Contraindications) and *Tianxia Zhidao Tang* (On Statecraft Knowledge). The bamboo writings include health advice relating to sexual activity, regulated emotions, diet and advice on lifestyle behaviours that accord with the changing seasons.

In addition to the writings, the Mawangdui tombs also provided a figurine marked with 11 *mai* or circulation tracts. This shows that the characteristic Han dynasty idea of distribution of substances around the body was emerging at this time. Within a few decades the number of main circulation tracts had increased to 14, and scores of other secondary vessels had become incorporated into the system.

Mai channels

Where 16th-century Italian anatomists used knives to meticulously map the physical body, physicians in the first 150 years of the Han dynasty developed the idea of *mai* channels that served to chart and explain normal physiological function, pathological states and stimulus-response connections during treatment. This idea of *qi* and blood flow in conduits or tracts probably arose from observation of movement in the blood vessels, and from simple charting of the subjective sensations that often radiate along the limbs and body in response to the needle and heat stimulation used in acumoxa. Sensations of numbness, tingling or aching generally follow a predictable course, and so were believed to be significant. It is likely as well that early physicians had noticed the progress of lines of erythema resulting from bacterial lymphangitis, an apparently clear case of *xie qi* progressing along *jing-luo* toward the *zangfu* where, if not halted, the disease would likely take a turn for the worse. Many people must have died in this manner, especially following injuries sustained in the 200 years of the Warring States period. The *jing-luo* system could also be charted by recording patterns of referred pain following skeleto-muscular injury. All these observations were taken to indicate the existence of a communication system in the body that, when functioning properly, contributed to health and, when disrupted, led to disease or death. Accepted doctrine from long before held that things separated by distance could influence each other, and that there were mutual connections between the body surface and deeper tissues, so it made sense to meticulously map these channels of communication if medical knowledge was to advance.

The earliest known reference to *mai* channels appeared prior to the Han in the *Zuo Zhuan*, a –4th-century text where a passage describing a horse says: '[There is] wildly chaotic *qi*, *yin*-blood erupts, coursing and springing forth, ridges of engorged *mai* vessels bulge.' The original character for *mai* (脉) included the radical character component for blood (血), which, in modern Chinese, has been replaced by the flesh (月) radical. This suggests that the recognition of the movement of blood in the vascular system was a precursor to the idea of *jing-luo* vessels distributing other substances (see Daly 1999).

Almost certainly through a process of systematic observation, *jing-luo* theory continued to evolve through the first half of the Han with the addition to the system of *luo* (branch), *bie* (diverging) and *qi* (strange) *jing* channels. If the evidence that was excavated from the Mawangdui tombs can be taken to be representative, in −168 11 main *jing-luo* channels were described rather than the 12 of the subsequent classic tradition. The latecomer, the *sanjiao* (triple burner) channel, was added at some time in the following century. Early on, the *qi* in these channels was envisaged as flowing from the tips of the extremities proximally towards the body. Another view was that *qi* flowed from deep inside the body to the extremities; this was later replaced by the idea of 12 main channels flowing in a circuit up and down the limbs and body. Such divergent views may also reflect ideas prevailing in differing traditions that had yet to be reconciled, so in the first two centuries of the Han dynasty, medical theories were not fixed but were evolving in the light of further enquiry and debate.

> …the sages consider the *mai* to be precious…those who cure illness clear away excess and fill up deficiency. (Mawangdui manuscripts)

> If the *mai* are full, empty them; when they are empty, fill them. Be still in order to treat them. (*Zhengjia Shan Mai*, a *mai*-vessel text excavated in Hubei and dated to roughly −160)

Early physicians saw that disease was often associated with stasis of blood, of fluids and so on, and indeed that death was characterised by a complete cessation of bodily flows and cycles. With this in mind it was axiomatic that good health depended on the proper circulation of *qi* and blood in the *mai* vessels. Further, it was considered that these channels of blood, *qi* and fluid circulation should not only move but move in the correct direction, that they should be just sufficiently filled and not become stagnated, stuck or accumulating. In addition it was believed that the *mai* should only contain *zheng* (i.e. normal) substances and not *xie* pathogens such as the pus that might be generated following injury.

In this conception some of the prime indicators of dysfunction were seen as pain, tenderness, swelling, colour changes and alterations in temperature. The idea of close visual examination was very important, and may have originated in the face-reading techniques cultivated by court ministers with the intention of sensing intrigue and misbehaviour, both in their court circles and for use when in negotiation with officials from neighbouring states.

Various passages in the *Neijing* refer to the virtues of different styles of diagnosis used by different practitioners: '…to use vision is divine, to use palpation is skilful, to use asking is workmanlike…' This may reflect different theories developed by different lineages of pre-Han medical practice that, as we will see later, were to be incorporated into the classical medical tradition in the Han dynasty. First, though, we should consider the elite cultural environment in the few centuries prior to the compilation of the *Neijing*.

Wu xing origins

The origins of *wu xing* (five phase theory) and the details of the way it was introduced into early Chinese medical doctrine are obscure. Although in the Zhou dynasty there are some brief mentions of five-fold classifications, these are only vaguely related to later *wu xing* theories. Earlier still, Shang dynasty cosmology divided the night sky into four quadrants (*si fang*), making a five-part division by including the central pivot point – the pole star. Some see this as a precursor to the *wu xing* model. It makes more sense to take the view that the *wu xing* system was applied retrospectively onto the earlier cosmic map as this idea had been in existence for over a millennium before *wu xing* appeared. It is not until the decades before the Qin dynasty that a formal coherent model of *wu xing* correspondence and transformation begins to appear. Credit is traditionally given to the leading legalist scholar Zou Yan (−350 to −270) for developing *wu xing* theory, which he originally proposed as a system for modelling political activities. However, the first verifiable description of *wu xing* theory is found in the *Lushi Chunqiu* (Lu's Spring and Autumn Annals) written in −239.

This was a time when the literate ruling classes were interested in accessing the knowledge and trade secrets of various groups in the wider community, and so it may be that the *sheng* (generating) cycle of the five phases was originally a mnemonic device for transmitting the trade secrets used by metallurgists.

Let us speculate for a moment. Metallurgy was a crucial technology in the Shang and Zhou dynasties, especially for the production of vessels for ritual use, and in the Zhanguo period, for the manufacture of weapons and chariot bearings. These trade secrets were in the hands of castes of metallurgists, blacksmiths, craftsmen and artisans. Information about foundry work using iron, and early forms of steel (known in the China of −400), would have included proprietary secrets passed from master to apprentice in the form of secret mnemonics, an oral tradition along the lines of: take wood, build up a strong fire using bellows, add earth in the form of a metal ore which generates metal and which can then be tempered using water and wood ash. The effectiveness of such arcane alchemical protocols in creating useful items must have seemed remarkable, and it was not unreasonable to suppose that a secret of nature had been uncovered, one that was perhaps generalisable more widely to other transformations such as those seen in the body and the world at large.

Whatever its true origins, the apparent insights that *wu xing* ideas of transformation provided now gave the first generations of Han medical scholars a means of conceptualising the way that things interact and influence each other in nature and in the body. Once they had accepted the *wu xing* model as true, then the next step was to ascribe the appropriate *wu xing* attributes to all things in the body and the world, and the intricate mechanics of medical reality could be untangled. So, through the Western Han the seasons, animals, grains, foods and so on were all to be given these attributions, thereby allowing an appealing correspondence system to be built up. It allowed things to be classified with a view to modelling their interrelationships. With this new model predictions could be made about the way things would resonate together to influence each other. In terms of understanding the body, the *jing-luo*, *zangfu* and individual acumoxa *xue* points were ascribed qualities using this idea of correspondence between things having a similar nature. Throughout the Western Han the general consensus seemed to be that the *wu xing* system made sense, was insightful and provided predictive power. It appealed to the sense of coherence and correspondence that the literate elite classes saw in their newly ordered and peaceful society.

Eventually, though, some intellectuals began to have doubts about the truth of the *wu xing* model. In the subsequent Eastern Han the best-known sceptic was Wang Chong (+27–100), who ridiculed the *wu xing* system in his book *Lun Heng*, and pointed out some of the doctrine's absurd inconsistencies. The sceptics appear to have held sway because in the next few centuries *wu xing* theory, whilst not absent, seems to have been downplayed. Compared to the *Suwen*, later texts, such as the *Shennong Bencao*, give little emphasis to *wu xing* ideas, and in the *Shang Han Zhabing Lun* (+200) it is barely evident at all. It is not until the end of the Tang dynasty that *wu xing* re-appears before being further revived in the Song dynasty, when the classical Han roots were being re-investigated.

Early anatomy

It is sometimes said that Chinese medicine is characterised by its lack of interest in the detailed study of anatomy, a criticism that came to the fore in the Qing dynasty (+1640–1911). Traditionalist Qing dynasty physicians pointed out that biomedicine was equally weak in paying insufficient attention to the understanding and adjustment of function. Anatomy was the main area of medical knowledge in the 19th century that Western physicians chose to use as evidence of the superiority of their medicine over Chinese medicine. This was a time when, on the treatment side, Chinese medicine was far superior in terms of its treatment with medicinal substances. Western physicians had only a small repertoire of effective treatments compared to those in the Chinese tradition. Nonetheless, it is true that Chinese physicians had tended to neglect form in favour of function.

Chinese medicine is not devoid of anatomical study, though – even in the Han dynasty there is evidence that some efforts were made to study the physical body structure with the aim of improving medical knowledge. It is reasonable to say that for most of the past two millennia Chinese physicians' understanding of anatomy has exceeded that of the West. Doubtless too much information has simply been lost, having been held in the hands of much less literate professions, those tending soldiers injured in battle, midwives, butchers and other occupations requiring anatomical knowledge. As we will see in Chapter 6 on Jin-Yuan medicine, officials engaged in the investigation of murder and violent crimes often called on the services of those with anatomical knowledge to assist in post-mortem forensic examination.

So, even though Chinese medicine emphasised function over structure, it is incorrect to assert that anatomical knowledge is missing from the classical tradition. Even as early as –168, in the Mawangdui manuscripts, specific names appear for the individual muscle structures in the neck.

Mawangdui muscle name	Meaning	Believed to correspond to
Heng yang	Enduring *yang*	Sacrospinalis
Ce yang	Slanted *yang*	Trapezius
Ce yin	Slanted *yin*	Scalene
Qian yin	Anterior *yin*	Sternocleidomastoid

The *Neijing* makes frequent mention of the main internal organs, and there are records of human dissection in the Han dynasty. One example appears in the *Biography of Wang Mang* in the *Han Shu* (Annals of the Han Dynasty). This tells us that in –206:

> Wang Sun-jing was taken prisoner after a battle and the Emperor ordered that his body be dissected by a butcher and a court physician. The internal organs were measured and the course of the blood vessels traced with the help of a strip of bamboo. This was done with the aim of bettering the treatment of disease.

Practitioners who attended the millions wounded in battle during the Warring States period were practising a different style of healthcare to that of the literati physicians – matters requiring a detailed knowledge of anatomy were seen as largely outside the remit of most classical physicians. A similar situation prevailed in 17th-century Europe, where 'barber surgeon' existed as a profession distinct from educated physicians.

The *Neijing*, the general contents of which are sketched out later in this chapter, named the major internal organs and presented many statements about their function, such as 'the heart is responsible for blood flow' (*Suwen*, Ch 44). Reflecting on ideas such as 'the kidneys dominate water' or 'the stomach is in charge of descent', we find they generally provide accurate definitions of their functions. Out of necessity these early writings had to provide brief summaries – when writing on silk or bamboo there was little room available for expounding details. Neither was it practical to describe the methodologies by which the knowledge had been obtained; sometimes, though, we see hints of the investigative process. For example, the results of investigations into morbid anatomy that were conducted in the Han dynasty are summarised in the *Neijing*:

> The height of the sky and the extent of the earth cannot be measured by man but the eight feet of the human body can be measured on the surface and, *post mortem*, it may be dissected. Observations can be made as to the size of the organs, the capacity of the intestines, the length of the arteries, the condition of the blood and the amount of *qi*.

Much of the information presented in the *Neijing* seems to have been gained through a process of observation, inference and deliberate enquiry. The text box below provides one instance, the description from the *Suwen* of the entire length of the digestive tract derived from post-mortem investigation.

ANATOMY IN THE *NEIJING*

Qi Bo said…the tongue weighs 10 ounces, its length 7 inches and its width 2.5 inches. The oesophagus weighs 10 ounces, its width 1½ inches and its length is 1½ feet. Stretched out the stomach is 2½ feet in length, its circumference is 1 foot five inches and its capacity 3 dou and 5 sheng [about 12 litres], the small intestine has a circumference of 2.5 inches, a diameter of 0.8 inches and a length of 33 feet and a capacity of 2 dou and 5 sheng. The circumference of the large intestine is 4 inches, its diameter 1½ inches, its length 20 feet and its capacity 1 dou. The rectum has a circumference of 8 inches, a diameter of 2.5 inches, a length of 2 feet 8 inches and a capacity of 2½ ho.

The anatomy and physiology of the heart and its relation to the cardiovascular system is described in some detail in the *Neijing*, and terms for different-sized blood vessels are given.

NEIJING STATEMENTS ON THE CARDIOVASCULAR SYSTEM

'All the blood is controlled by the heart.'

'The heart regulates all the blood in the body.'

'The twelve blood vessels [in the limbs] are deeply hidden beneath muscles except those near the ankles. Those that are visible on the surface we call *luo* vessels.'

'A current of blood flows unceasingly in a circuit.'

'Blood flows continuously like a river current or the orbits of the sun and moon. It is comparable to a circle without beginning or end.'

'Blood travels a distance of three inches during inhalation and another three during exhalation, moving a total of six inches per complete breath.'

In relation to anatomy, it is unfortunate that for the best part of the next thousand years there are few, if any, records of any further efforts to advance the study of anatomy. Instead, the focus was more on functional medical study and on the attempt to abstract observations and discoveries into an overarching schema.

Acumoxa treatment in the Han

Current opinion is that in the late −3rd century the preferred *jing-luo* treatment was moxibustion. As we have seen, this is evident in the early Mawangdui texts that mostly recommended moxa to regulate the *jing-luo* and only occasionally sometimes suggest *bian* (stone needle) therapy. According to Needham and Liu, the earliest known written reference to acupuncture practised using metal needles appears in −81 in a government policy document called the *Yan Tie Lun* (Iron and Salt

Discussions), where it says that one thing people particularly dislike about doctors is their tendency to treat illness by piercing patients with needles made of stone or metal. Actual use of needles must obviously predate this reference somewhat, but the question is by how much – decades or centuries? Archaeological evidence is available in the form of gold and silver needles found in the tomb of Liu Sheng, who ruled Zhong Shang from –154 until his death in –113. The tomb also contained two arrow-shaped rock crystal lancing stones. This seems to narrow down the time window for the introduction of acupuncture using metal needles to between roughly –150 to –100, although with such sparse data it is quite possible that needles were in use before this time in other regions. The consensus seems to be that moxibustion predates the use of needles, so early acupoint stimulation was mostly with heat or massage. So, in sum, we can conclude that the finely crafted stone implements found in earlier tombs were almost certainly applied as surgical instruments for massage or pus draining, and not as part of a more systemic therapy.

Significantly, in relation to the transition from stone implements to metal needles, a passage in the Mawangdui texts is virtually identical to Chapter 7 of the *Nanjing* (Classic of Difficulties, roughly +1st century) except that the word *bian* (stone needle) has been replaced by *zhen* (metallic needle). Another change is the replacement of the word *nong* (脓, pus) in this text passage by *bing* (病, disease). This helps confirm the idea that the glorious origins of acupuncture therapy is probably amongst a group of boil-lancers rather than energy medicine physicians, and that using needles was probably introduced as an alternative to stimulating acupoints using moxa. It suggests, too, that the conception of the scope of puncture therapy had progressed from a simple and limited surgical procedure to an energetic-based treatment of a newly emerging model of body function and disease. The interest in needling may have been stimulated by observation of the mild euphoria that often follows needling, combined with its sometimes almost instantaneous pain-relieving effects.

In addition, the increased use of needles for general therapy probably contributed to the more detailed mapping of the channel system. Needle stimulation frequently causes dull aches, tingling and other sensations to radiate along specific lines, responses that are similar in different individuals. To the sceptical Westerner examining acupuncture 'meridian' charts for the first time, this system of lines along and through the body looks a touch fantastical, as if some ancient mountain-dwelling sage had taken a pen and marked them all on himself on a whim. In modern practice, though, acupoint needling frequently results in the patient experiencing these propagated sensations travelling along the course of the classic *jing-luo* system. This also happens in Westerners who are generally unaware of the classical *jing-luo* trajectories.

The reliable correspondence with the effects seen in practice today suggests that the *jing-luo* charts are the aggregated results of large-scale experimentation and clinical observation on many people. They present a map of what is experienced when you needle or otherwise stimulate specific parts of the body – in this sense, they are true even if there are no recognised distal anatomical structures that follow the *jing-luo* paths. Whilst there is still debate on the structures involved in mediating the effects observed, acupuncture tracts do not seem to exist as observable or dissectible anatomical structures. Nevertheless, when we apply procaine nerve blocks proximal to a stimulated point, then we can block the channel propagation and other effects of acupuncture. In modern terms the channels may, in my view, be best seen as an artefact of the way that the nervous system is wired in the spinal cord, thalamus, basal ganglia and perhaps the cerebellum. The acumoxa stimulus is largely mediated through the nervous system, with the caveats that there are also local therapeutic tissue injury effects and further downstream responses that are consequent on the neural effects, such as immune modification and alterations in autonomic function. It is possible, too, as some have suggested, that responses are also propagated by other tissues such as connective tissue fascia.

In addition to the primary *jing-luo* channel system, the *Neijing* mentions other channel networks in the body; these include the *jing bie* (divergent channels), the *qi jing ba mai* (eight strange channels), the *luo mai* (branch channels) and the *sun luo* (grandson vessels). This diversity reflects the fact that the *Neijing* is a compilation of medical writings derived from different Han dynasty medical lineages. Whilst the main *jing-luo* map was in all likelihood based on the investigations previously mentioned, the *qi jing ba mai* and possibly the *jing bie* maps may have arisen from the doctrines of the meditative schools of practice. Such pre-existing Daoist traditions contributed an experientially derived map where subjective currents of activity were felt during health cultivation breathing and meditation exercises.

The large *luo mai* mostly represent the Han dynasty physicians' interpretation of the network of veins near the body surface, whilst the close-to-invisible *sun luo* capillaries appear to have been used to explain observations of changes in skin tone occurring with, for example, exposure to cold, heat, pressure, bruising and erythema. Again, deliberate processes of investigation are implied by the findings presented in the *Neijing*.

Acupoints

Xue (穴) is the character that we translate as 'acupuncture point' or 'acupoint', and is one of the terms commonly used in the classical texts. As is often the case in the transmission to the West of the technical terms used in Chinese medicine, the word 'point' fails to properly convey the sense of the term. *Xue* originally meant 'cave', and so, in the context of acumoxa, it has more of the sense of a three-dimensional entity than is suggested by the word 'point'; in addition, it carries the sense of a place of access to something hidden from view, and this, too, may have been in the minds of the Han dynasty pioneer explorers of the bodily landscape. Acumoxa practitioners generally conceive *xue* as having dimensions of depth and width as well as location, and these parameters are seen as varying between different acupoints, between different people and at different times. They are revealed more by skilled palpation for location and depth than by following charts.

In Shang dynasty mythology it was believed that wind originated from caves, and this idea may have been carried forward into Warring States medical thinking – if caves are the gateways that control the semi-intangible *qi*-like winds that blow across the earth, then, at a human level, perhaps the subtle nooks and crannies to be found across human surface anatomy could be places where the body's *qi* could be manipulated. This tallies with the fact that most acupoints are found in gaps between tissues, in small anatomical depressions and in places where slight changes in the tissue structure can be felt.

The first reliable mention of the use of therapeutic acumoxa treatment, as distinct from the surgical draining of pus from wounds and sores, appears in the case records of Chunyu Yi. Two of his 28 case reports, written around –180, received moxibustion treatment, and two received acupuncture. He refers to the locations he selected for treatment not as *xue* but as *suo* (所), which means 'a place', and this has been suggested as evidence that acupoints with fixed locations had not been formally identified at this time. Obviously, though, when applying acupuncture, the place has to be quite specific, and this may have led to the identification of standard locations.

Roughly a century after Chunyu Yi, various other terms appear in the *Neijing* to indicate acupoints: *qi xue* (*qi* caves), *qi fu* (*qi* palaces) and *qi suo fa* (places where *qi* emerges). These terms help provide a sense of acupoints as places when the *qi* of the *jing-luo* system extends to the exterior of the body, and where it is perceivable and accessible to influence. The first few words of Chapter 59 of the *Suwen*, for example, read: 'There are seventy-eight *xue* that are the foot *taiyang* vessel's *qi* emission places…'; the implication was that to the Han dynasty investigators, these places were palpable, verifiable and countable.

There is an academic debate that has considered the issue of which came first, knowledge of the *jing-luo* or of the acupoints. The fact that a wooden figure recovered from the Shuangbao Shan tombs (–118) showed a scheme of 11 of the 12 main *jing-luo* channels, but with no acupoints marked, has been taken as evidence that the acupoints had not been mapped by that time. It is quite possible, though, that this figure was intended to accompany instruction on exercise or massage that entailed stretching particular bands of fascia, and for this purpose, the inclusion of acupoints may have been unnecessary. Nevertheless, even if some acupoints had been identified at this time, they were few in number and may not have been given formal names or fixed locations. Right at the other end of the spectrum of possibilities is the speculation that the tattoo marks found on Otzi (the ice-preserved body dating from –3300 found in the Italian Alps in 1991) indicated that he had received acupuncture treatment for his arthritis. The fact that no other evidence of the use of therapeutic acupuncture has been found dating to the 3000 years following Otzi's death renders this idea implausible.

The likelihood is that in the Warring States period folk knowledge accumulated in the community about points that commonly become tender in association with particular illnesses, and that it was noticed that massage, heat or needling of these points often provided relief. This is akin to the way that we are aware of tenderness and knotting in the trapezius muscles in response to stress, and that stimulation of these spots makes us feel easier. Some folk traditions explored the therapeutic uses of bleeding, or bruising therapies such as cupping and *gua sha* (scraping), and could be expected to have noted the most reliable places on the body to apply these therapies. Around –250, towards the end of the Warring States period and in the Western Han, as more medical scholars turned their hands to medicine, they added in the idea of a subtle circulation of *qi* that was like that of blood, but more subtle and followed different pathways. Over the next 200 years the deliberate investigative palpation of the *jing-luo* by numerous medical scholars seems to have then led to the identification of many acupoints. The received scholarly wisdom was that the detailed mapping of terrain had important strategic benefits in warfare, and so many of the acupoints were labelled using similar terminology: mountains, bogs, valleys, passes and so on. Many of the terms chosen highlight subtle aspects of bodily topology – acupoints on areas where the skin is naturally slightly damp, such as the cubital fossa, have names such as 'foot marsh', 'curved pond' and 'curved marsh' (Lu 5 *chi ze*, LI 11 *qu chi*, Pc 3 *qu ze*). Other point names seem to have been drawn from the esoteric traditions of Daoist adepts; for instance, the acupoint *shang xing* (upper star) near the midpoint of the frontal hairline probably reflects an interest in cosmological *qigong* practices. The diversity of the naming system that was used, along with the fact that the same acupoint often had a few different names, supports the idea that divergent sources contributed to the collation of the acupoint set in classical acupuncture.

The *Neijing* claimed that the body had 365 acupoints, but only about 160 of them are specifically mentioned here; instead, there is more frequent mention of the 12 *jing* channels as a basis of therapy than actual acupoints. The main *jing* are usually referred to using the six-channel pairs system.

CLASSICAL CHANNEL NAMING SYSTEM

Jing (channel)	Translation	Associated organ *qi*
Shou tai yang	Arm extreme *yang*	Small intestine
Shou shaoyang	Arm lesser *yang*	*Sanjiao*
Shou yang ming	Arm *yang* brightness	Large intestine
Shou tai yin	Arm extreme *yin*	Lung
Shou jue yin	Arm reversal *yin*	Pericardium
Shou shao yin	Arm lesser *yin*	Heart
Zu tai yang	Leg extreme *yang*	Bladder
Zu shaoyang	Leg lesser *yang*	Gallbladder
Zu yang ming	Leg *yang* brightness	Stomach
Zu tai yin	Leg extreme *yin*	Spleen
Zu jue yin	Leg reversal *yin*	Liver
Zu shao yin	Leg lesser *yin*	Kidney

The emphasis seen in the *Neijing* on the channel to be treated rather than on specific points supports the suggestion that channel palpation as the preparatory stage before the selection of the treatment point was still the most important acumoxa style when the *Neijing* was being compiled. The text is quite specific about the importance of palpation prior to acumoxa treatment, and this seems to be carrying on the tradition seen in Chunyu Yi's cases. It also seems to have led to the identification of more and more acupoints, so, from the end of the Western Han dynasty and through the first century of the Eastern Han, the number of points that had been identified doubled. The new points discovered after the *Neijing* were compiled into the 1st acupoint text, the *Ming Tang* (Bright Hall). This book referred to acupoints as *xian* (depressions). It is believed to have included much more by way of detailed clinical indications for the points, and added new point categories such as *xi* (accumulation points), *jiao hui* (intersection points) and *mu* (alarm points), as well as points on the heart channel that had previously been omitted. Although the original classic was lost, it is believed that most of its contents have survived due to its inclusion as an important source for Huangfu Mi in the compilation of his *Jia Yi Jing* discussed in the next chapter.

In modern times acupoints have been found to have various characteristic differences from the adjacent tissues: many points are in the fascia, they generally exhibit lowered electrical impedance, those in muscle have a higher density of muscle stretch receptors, and there are greater numbers of 'gap junction' communication points between cells. Despite these findings, skilled palpation remains as crucial for modern practice as it was in the Han dynasty.

Knowledge of medicinals

When scholar physicians proliferated in the Han dynasty, as well as adopting physical therapies such as acupuncture and moxibustion, they also borrowed knowledge of herbal medicine from the previous generations of trained *fang shi* (formula gentlemen) and perhaps from folk medicine. Three centuries before, Confucius had asserted that 'knowledge progresses through research' (*zhi zhi zai ge wu*; Confucius, *Da Xue*), and so, with Confucianism inspiring Han dynasty intellectual life, the intent was to rationalise and improve what could be gleaned from the past. Although intent on rational investigation, some folk notions would be so firmly embedded as universal cultural beliefs that they were carried forward unchallenged. Everyone knew that carrying *wu zhu yu* (fructus evodia) in your pocket was able to ward off malign influences (just as everyone today knows that Prozac cures depression), despite significant evidence casting doubt on this cultural belief. During the development of classical medicine it was necessary to retain the original folk names of the herbs, and in doing so, carry forward their old folk associations. One needed, for example, to have a means of identifying the correct substances in the absence of illustrated herbal texts, and sometimes the names themselves referenced ideas from the older medicine. So, the new rational physician classes did not abandon wholesale old ideas and the traditional folk names for the medicinals. The names could not easily be changed, and the folk knowledge deserved some respect by virtue of tradition – they were agreed truths. Instead, folk knowledge was redefined using the language of the literati, and new understandings were developed of empirical observation and experiment.

To what extent was there state involvement in the Han regulation and training of medical practitioners? It appears that the court was concerned only about medical care in the court whilst the wider population was generally left to care for itself in its own way. In –43, Emperor Yuan is known to have decreed that physicians had to sit a general scholarship exam before their appointment to court service. Notable *fang shi* physicians from the community who met suitable standards would certainly have been called into court service, employed in both teaching and medical practice. In relation to the general population there seem to have been systems for investigating injury or malpractice of physicians, and as we saw in the previous chapter, specialists and bureaucracies existed for the regulation of leprosy. In a moment, when we look at the records of the celebrated physician Chunyu Yi, we will see an example of the state officially interrogating a physician and checking his credentials.

> …[court] acupuncturists should be soft spoken, contained, skilful and attentive so they can diagnose and then regulate qi and blood circulation. Smooth talkers are appointed to teach basic theory. Those who use excessive force and break pots should practise massage! (*Lingshu* 73: 131–133)

Surgery

Written near the start of the Western Han dynasty, the Mawangdui manuscripts include a collection of numerous medical tips and tricks of varying degrees of plausibility; presumably these had been gathered from folk opinion and early professional medical sources in the wider community. Some are of very doubtful validity whilst others are quite ingenious and resourceful, such as one that suggested surgical treatment for internal haemorrhoids appearing in the *Wushier Bing Fang* (Prescriptions for 52 Ailments):

> When a 'nest' obstructs the rectum. Kill a dog, remove its bladder and insert a bamboo tube. Insert this into the rectum and inflate, then draw it out slowly so you can cut the nest off with a knife. Take powdered *huang qin* and spread it on repeatedly. If the person's anus is prolapsed and cannot be put back inside, grease the prolapsed part with lard and suspend the person upside down. Throw cold water on his heart and abdomen and it will go back inside. (Adapted from Harper 1998, p.274)

Chunyu Yi, a scholar physician at the dawn of classical practice

In the last chapter we looked at the legends of Bian Que and his clan of proto-acupuncturists from Shandong province who were transforming their minor surgical skills in abscess draining and suchlike to form the foundations of a more systematic energy medicine. This was linked to an evolving explanatory model derived from a mix of clinical experimentation and hypothesis. Unfortunately, very few medical writings survive from the period of transition that created Han dynasty classical medicine. The most important documentary insight into clinical practice at this time are 25 case histories of the literate physician Chunyu Yi that are celebrated for the very rare insights they provide into clinical practice near the start of the Han.

Chunyu Yi came from an aristocratic land-owning family claiming a 1000-year lineage in the ruling classes of what is now Shandong province, where he may have been exposed to the traditions of the Bian Que medical clan. Born in about −215, roughly a decade before the founding of the Han dynasty, Chunyu held the official local bureaucratic post of 'Director of Granaries'; this meant that he was part of a system by which the state could provide grain in time of famine. His aristocratic status allowed him time to immerse himself in the study and practice of medicine to become a *fang shi* scholar physician.

Interested in medicine from his youth, Chunyu was about 28 when he began his studies under his first formal medical tutor, Gong-sun Guang, who described Chunyu as having a scholarly and sagely demeanour. In −180, having learned Gong-sun's medical style, the 36-year-old Chunyu then apprenticed for three years with another eminent physician in his town. His new mentor, Cheng Yang-qing, was about 70 at the time, and was reaching the end of his medical career. Although he had children of his own who might have continued his practice, he had a special fondness for Chunyu Yi, and so chose him as the inheritor of his lineage.

Chunyu Yi appears to have been something of a maverick physician, with personal character traits that led him into difficulties. Drifting from one nobleman's house to another, he treated various princely families and their retinues. This allowed him to avoid becoming obligated into the service of any individual clan and to maintain his independence, an outlook that may sometimes have aroused ill feeling. Chunyu, it is said, flatly refused to treat some influential patients; perhaps he could tell that they would prove incurable and die in a manner that might compromise his future. Also, tiresome official investigations generally followed the deaths of prominent people, so for this reason, too, a prudent physician was likely to decline to treat patients who were at high risk of dying. (Later, the *Neijing* includes various tips for physicians on spotting grave cases.) In addition, Chunyu seems to have had an unfortunate tendency to criticise the work of other physicians; evidence of this is seen in some of his case histories that highlight the failures of other highly placed physicians. Other political pressures may have been at play, but the end result seems to have been that some influential people disliked him. Eventually, in the 13th year of the rule of Emperor Wendi (−167), he crossed one person too many, and was charged with a serious offence. He was arrested and then taken to Chang-an, accompanied by his daughter Ti-ying. Pronounced guilty, he was sentenced to suffer punitive mutilation, but Ti-ying presented an impassioned plea in support of her father, saying that he was a great physician and that he had carried out his official duties as Director of the Granaries very well. She offered herself as a palace slave in exchange for his release. Emperor Wendi was touched by this, and pardoned Chunyu. His evident high level of attainment in medical practice, his high status and his personal connections may also have contributed to this leniency.

Some time after his acquittal, Chunyu Yi faced officialdom again when he answered an imperial edict that appears to have been aimed at identifying able physicians in the country who were especially skilled in accurate prognosis. The renowned physicians who were summoned to court had to provide details of their training and offer a selection of case histories to provide evidence of their attainment. Some have speculated that this may have been part of an initiative to license approved healers in the community; alternatively, it may have been a means of recruiting physicians into state service, and perhaps to contribute to the development of court medicine.

The case histories Chunyu Yi presented to the hearing appear to have been chosen specifically to highlight his ability to predict fatal cases, and in seven cases he does this with accuracy, although in some cases he is proven wrong. The contributors to the *Neijing* were also often concerned with this prognosis question, so clearly it was an important issue to the early literati physicians. As a yardstick of attainment this may have been borrowed from other court scholars whose skill was attested by their ability to predict the future course of events, for example in military encounters. Also, as suggested earlier, physicians who chose to engage patients who then died shortly after the onset of therapy could find themselves in an awkward position, all the more so if they specialised in treating the upper echelons of society. Another factor of particular concern to the nobility was the need to know if you were going to die, so there was an opportunity to organise all the ceremonies and affairs expected of a noble person's burial – having accurate predictive power was an important measure of mastership and connection to the *Dao*.

Chunyu Yi explained to the authorities that he had studied at first with a local physician called Gong-sun Guang before being taken under the wing of his elderly mentor, Cheng Yang-qing, with whom he studied for three years. Cheng, he informed the tribunal, had transmitted to him various texts, including:

- *A Treatise on Medicine*

- *Huangdi Bianque Mai Shu* (a pulse diagnosis text in two parts, one part allegedly linked to Bian Que and one named after the ancient Yellow Emperor Huangdi)

- *Wu Se Zhen Bing* (Five Colours Disease Diagnosis)

- *Shang Xia Jing* (Upper and Lower Classic).

Elizabeth Hsu tells us that the *Five Colours Disease Diagnosis* text referred to probably corresponds to Chapter 49 of the *Lingshu*. Chunyu also reported receiving other texts, including:

- *Qi Kai Shu* (Points of the Extraordinary Channels)

- *Gui Tu Yin Yang* (Determining Degrees of Yin and Yang)

- *Pien Yao* (Body Changing Medicines)

- *Lunshi* (A Discussion on Minerals).

This information supports the idea that these early lineage texts were akin to individual chapters of the *Neijing, Nanjing* and *Lingshu*. Succinct and abstruse, they were intended as starting points for reflection and discussion with a mentor, and to be verified and illuminated through clinical practice. They were not intended to serve as intelligible medical textbooks – for one thing, these were trade secrets and so had to be wrapped up in coded language inaccessible to outsiders. Also, in the absence of printing and paper, it was not yet practical to write wordy explanations.

In his submission to the authorities, Chunyu Yi explained the treatment rationale for his 25 cases and justified his diagnoses. 'When treating patients,' he said, 'I always palpate their *mai* vessels first and then treat them.' We cannot be sure, but it is likely that *mai*-vessel palpation included both pulse palpation and palpation of the channels and acupoints.

Chunyu Yi appears to have been especially adept at pulse palpation, both to diagnose illness and to form a prognosis. His emphasis on pulse taking is seen in the case histories which contain technical terms describing more than 25 different pulse qualities, including most of those still in use in the modern practice of Chinese medicine.

ORIGINS OF PAPER-MAKING IN THE HAN DYNASTY

Early texts were mostly written on costly silk or on unwieldy bamboo slats bound together with string. Linen-based paper including written characters has recently been excavated from a site dating to –8, but it was the Han dynasty court eunuch Cai Lun who is credited with inventing paper in +105 using mulberry bark pulp. Cai's process was kept secret until some of China's paper-makers were captured in 751, leading to the start of an Arabic paper-making industry in Baghdad in 793. From here it reached Europe in the 12th century.

PULSES MENTIONED BY CHUNYU YI

wiry (*xian*)	big (*da*)	deep (*shen*)	even (*ping*)	intermittent (*dai*)
tight (*jin*)	small (*xiao*)	weak (*ruo*)	urgent (*ji*)	slippery (*hua*)
rapid (*shuo*)	replete (*shi*)	hard (*jian*)	scattered (*san*)	choppy (*se*)

It is remarkable that these same pulse qualities have remained the core of pulse diagnosis for almost 2200 years, with only a few alterations and additions.

Of the 25 case histories submitted by Chunyu Yi to the authorities, 14 were treated using herb formulas, two used moxa and two used acupuncture. The majority of patients were adult males, six were women and two were children. The fact that a high proportion of the cases, ten in all, proved fatal points to the likelihood that the cases had been selected to demonstrate skill in prognosis.

One patient, called Sui, himself a physician, had already applied the Daoist remedy 'five stone therapy' to treat himself. Chunyu Yi told Sui that this treatment had been inappropriate, but Sui disagreed, saying that this treatment had, in fact, been one that had been attributed to the legendary physician Bian Que. Chunyu Yi told Sui that, no matter how famous the source, it was not sufficient to simply copy treatments – a skilful physician was able to understand and apply the whole diagnostic process in specific clinical situations, to match the treatment to the case in hand and not simply to blindly apply this or that treatment. So, even at this early time in the development of classical Chinese medicine, physicians such as Chunyu Yi were wise enough to realise that the texts and explanations only came to life in response to clinical experience. Chunyu is revealed as a pragmatist who, although respecting the knowledge of his medical lineage, considered that if clinical reality conflicted with doctrine, then it was doctrine that needed to be re-considered. In the convention-based Confucian environment of the time, we can see how his maverick outlook might well have raised the hackles of officialdom.

Between −164 and −154 he continued to specialise in the care of the wealthy and powerful, but when one of his last patients, Liu Cang-lu, suffered a military defeat, Chunyu Yi may have been placed in a difficult position. After −154 nothing more is heard of him. He is said to have had five students, but virtually no trace survives of their lives, except for an indication that two of them, Gao Qi and Wang Wu, worked for Prince Ji Bei.

Having these very early case histories from an educated physician provides a unique glimpse into medical thinking of the time. Especially interesting is the insight we gain into Chunyu's methodology when he explains that a single disease might manifest differently in different individuals and therefore require different treatment. He tells us that by using the fine distinctions that can be made between patient presentations using pulse diagnosis and the other diagnostic examinations, it would be possible to discriminate a finer level of detail than simply the disease name. This is a key insight as it is the earliest recorded suggestion of a fundamental methodology that has characterised classical Chinese medicine throughout its history; namely, the distinction between *bian bing* (diagnosing the disease name, as derived mainly from a few main symptoms) and *bian zheng*. The distinctive aspect of this new classical methodology was evident in its intention to discern the patient's underlying pathological changes in energetic terms following a more penetrating clinical audit of the complete patient presentation.

The issue here is that although distinguishing a disease name might be sufficient in simple folk medicine, informed professional practice seeks to understand the deeper roots of illness. In classical Chinese medicine a high-level physician must unravel the underlying energetic pathology using individualised observation, palpation of pulses and channels, and questioning before deciding on appropriate treatment. We can thus trace the origin of the characteristic Chinese medicine concept of pattern differentiation and treatment to Chunyu and his peers who were practising near the beginning of the Han dynasty. Just as court military strategists in the Warring States period, themselves dealing with life-and-death issues, became effective by means of subtle intelligence gathering and a strategic approach, so medicine, it was believed, would be made more effective by adopting similar tactics. Just as in warfare predictable military configurations appeared for which set strategies could be applied, in the battle against disease, clinical patterns could be discerned for which skilful clinical strategies could be discovered.

This pattern differentiation idea is a key factor that distinguishes the folk medical traditions from classical medical systems. East and West folk systems seek simple remedies for individual symptoms whilst literate medicine seeks to unravel specific aetiology and pathology and to treat this. Even in Chunyu's time there was an attempt to develop an understanding of a disease process beyond the realm of individual symptoms. Patients may present with the same symptom but receive different treatment because the underlying pathology was recognised as being different. Throughout the next 2000 years we see an ongoing tension between the simple treatment of symptoms and the more demanding and intellectually rigorous process of pattern treatment. At different times in history there have been significant shifts in the proportion of professional physicians insightful enough to understand, employ and develop the classical disease differentiation model.

Further food for thought is that this idea of a need to rise above simple folk medicine, to move beyond a simple response to a presenting symptom, represents a commonality between modern biomedicine and Chinese medicine. Both seek to delve beneath symptoms to an understanding of deeper disease causality and mechanism. The difference is that where modern medicine seeks this understanding, largely by the application of technology such as microscopes and chemical testing, Chinese physicians, in the absence of such technology, looked instead to more experiential and complete clinical examination of the patient using a pattern recognition-based theory framework and a knowing sensory acuity. One medicine works at the limits of technological possibility and the other operates at the limits of human sensory perception.

The Huangdi Neijing and the principles of Han medicine

The *Huangdi Neijing* that has been transmitted to the present time is a mix of texts that have been considerably edited, amended and augmented through time, so what we have today can only partially be said to reflect Han dynasty medical thinking. It is considered to be the earliest surviving and most significant foundation textbook of Chinese medicine. This section aims to summarise some of its key themes, to discuss some of its ideas and their origins, and to highlight some of the parts that were added after the Western Han dynasty (–206 to +8).

The *Neijing* was first mentioned in the *Han Shu*, Si Ma-qian's famed *Han Dynasty History* that was completed in –91. It consists of the *Suwen* (Plain Questions) in 81 chapters of widely varying length that mainly presents the explanatory model current amongst Han dynasty medical scholars, and the *Lingshu* (Spiritual Axis), also consisting of 81 chapters, which was written in the Eastern Han (+8–221) and offered more practical information on acupuncture therapeutics. The *Suwen* and *Lingshu* were probably a single text originally, and the *Lingshu* gained its title in the 8th century, long after it was written. It has been known by different names at different times in history; the main ones are: *Jiuzhuan* (Nine Scrolls), *Zhenjing* (Needling Classic) and *Jiu Ling Jing* (Nine Spiritual Classics).

The characters chosen for the naming of these early texts have generated quite a lot of academic debate. The character *jing* (经) means 'classic text' and at the same time carries the connotations of the warp threads on a loom and, by association, the sense of the common cultural threads passed from one generation to the next.

Nei (内, inner) can be interpreted in a variety of ways. One explanation holds that this was a textbook of internal (*nei*) medicine to distinguish it from *wai* (外, external) medicine, meaning surgery, traumatology, dermatology, dentistry and so on. This idea has led some to postulate that a partner *wai* text must have existed. Indeed, we see from the medical texts listed in the aforementioned *Han Dynasty History* that there were texts entitled *Huangdi Neijing*, *Huangdi Waijing*, *Bian Que Neijing*, *Bian Que Waijing*, *Bai Shi Neijing* and *Bai Shi Waijing*. The two *Bai Shi* texts mentioned by Si Ma-qian are intriguing and suggest that a mysterious figure, 'Master White', existed who also made significant contributions to Han dynasty medicine, although next to nothing is known about him. *Nei* and *wai* may have carried other connotations – the *nei* in the title could refer to its position as court medicine as the term *nei* was used in the Han dynasty as shorthand to suggest 'inside the court circles' as opposed to the wider world. Alternatively, it may have been used to indicate 'national medicine' as *nei* and *wai* were also used to distinguish home and abroad.

> **WARP AND WEFT**
> The ancient fundamental precepts that were conceived by thinkers from the Zhou dynasty, through the Zhanguo period and the Han dynasty, such as the *yin-yang* dynamic, concepts of *qi*, movement, change and transformation and the resonant correspondences between nature and mankind, are seen as constants that pass from one generation to another, like the warp threads on a loom. This image posits each generation as a new weft thread, looping and conjoining these threads, but each adding its own embellishments to the ancient truths to weave an ever more sophisticated fabric of knowledge.

The *Neijing* is considered to present a relatively complete discussion of Han dynasty medical theory; it does, however, largely omit discussion of herbal medicine. The main focus of the *Neijing* is on acumoxa and on medical doctrine, although there are some discussions of dietary therapy and a handful of herbs and prescriptions are mentioned. We can see the creation of this book as marking the founding of classical Chinese medicine, and much of the medicine's subsequent development represents a process of reverential clarification and development of the ideas presented in this seminal text.

The fact that the existence of the *Huangdi Neijing* was mentioned in at least two Han dynasty records means that we can be certain that it is not a later forgery. It is named in honour of the legendary emperor of prehistory, Huangdi, but there is no possibility that the text could actually have been composed as early as −2680 when the legendary Yellow Emperor is said to have ruled. It was common practice to signal a hallowed text by attaching it to the name of a legendary figure from antiquity – in this case, one of the ancients most revered by the Daoist-orientated scholars who had a significant input into this classic.

The book title *Suwen* first appears in Zhang Zhong-jing's preface to his *Shang Han Zabing Lun* (+220) where he writes that his work was 'compiled with reference to *Suwen* and the *Jiujuan*' (Nine Volumes, another name for the *Lingshu*). A few decades later, Huangfu Mi, in his *Huangdi Sanbu Zhenjiu Jiayi Jing* (A–Z of Acupuncture from the Yellow Emperor's Three Books), mentioned that the *Neijing* text was made up of the *Suwen* and two sections of the *Zhen Jing* (True Classic). By the Tang dynasty the *Neijing* had become degraded. As a result of having passed for centuries from person to person in handwritten bundles, it had become incomplete and badly jumbled. In +780 its Tang dynasty editor, Wang Bing, bemoaned the fact that the *Suwen* now consisted of 'mistakes, repetitions and inconsistencies from beginning to end', and he believed that the seventh volume had been lost since before the start of the Tang. He devoted 12 years of his life to collecting and editing it, adding a commentary and re-ordering it to compile the 24 volumes that formed his edition, the *Bu Zhu Huangdi Neijing Suwen* (*Bu Zhu*, meaning 'with appended commentaries'), in 81 chapters. Wang Bing, whose work we discuss in more detail later in Chapter 4, added seven chapters that he claimed he had discovered, but which he is likely to have added himself.

Two chapters of the original *Neijing*, the 'Ci Fa Lun' ('Essay on Needle Method') and 'Ben Bing Lun' ('Essay on the Roots of Disease'), survived just as titles with no surviving text. In the Song dynasty Liu Wen-shu added another two chapters he called the 'Omitted Chapters of the *Suwen*'. Wang Bing's Tang dynasty edition was re-edited in 1057 as part of the Song dynasty efforts to rectify and clarify ancient medical knowledge. The Imperial Medical Bureau scholars Gao Bao-heng and Lin Yi published this new version under the title *Chong Guang Bu Zhu Huangdi Neijing Suwen*, and this is the earliest edition to survive to the present.

Various explanations for the title *Suwen* have been proposed, some quite abstruse. *Su* (素) means simple or plain, and *wen* (问) means question. A simple explanation of this title takes into account the fact that when training occurred in the context of a medical apprenticeship, as is believed to be usual in the Han dynasty, this involved 'receiving' texts from a mentor, after which the text to be transmitted would be copied out by the student before its meaning was explained. If we accept the view that Han medical scholars sought to promote easier access for fellow *shi* scholar officials to these hidden teachings, bypassing the secret and very selective lineage system, we can see that re-editing the source texts to include more interpretation reduced the need for the initiation rituals, exclusivity and apprenticeship that were so much a part of literati scholarship outside the court. It makes sense that the many source texts acquired from physicians in the community, together with their associated basic explanations, would be combined in a text entitled *Basic Questions*. The character *su* suggests something that is plain and unsullied and therefore a source or fount of the pure knowledge of the ancients. On a more mundane level the character *su* may simply reflect the fact that the questions discussed were those that were less profound and more amenable to short replies. Even today the text is abstruse and open to varying interpretation.

Lingshu

The second section of the *Neijing* is called the *Lingshu*: *ling* (灵) means spiritual and *shu* (枢) means pivot or axis, the still point that everything else revolves around that was seen as the position of ultimate power. The *Lingshu* is considered to have been completed in the Eastern Han dynasty, probably around +150, but with many parts being updates of much earlier material. The earliest reference to a book with this title comes from Wang Bing's Tang dynasty writings of +778. As sometimes happens with early texts, its name was altered in different eras; at the end of the Eastern Han dynasty it was referred to as the *Jiu Juan* (Nine Volumes), and a century later, in the Jin dynasty, Huangfu Mi referred to this text as the *Zhen Jing* (True Classic), and in Sui and Tang times it also appears under various other names. For a long period the text of the *Lingshu* disappeared until 1093, when a copy returned to China from Korea so the imperial library again possessed a relatively complete copy.

In 1155 Shi Song edited the nine volumes of the *Lingshu*, adding some content and commentary of his own to create a new version, now extended to 24 volumes. This newly published edition was named the *Lingshu Jing* and is the version that has passed through to modern times. In the Ming dynasty, Ma Shi wrote a further commentary on the *Lingshu*, the *Huangdi Neijing Lingshu Zhu Zheng Fa Wei* (Commentaries on the Utter Elegance of the Lingshu Patterns). The current version is based on a block-printed edition of this that was published by Zhao Fu-ju.

What does the title *Lingshu* refer to? Ma Shi wrote that *ling* indicated the most revered original celestial emperor, and that *shu* referred to the pivotal place around which the opening and closing of all events takes place. As mentioned in Chapter 2, early cosmologists were intrigued by their observation that the entire heavens appeared to revolve around a single point – the pole star – and so the idea of this implied that this point was pivotal for, and encompassed, the entire universe. The title *Lingshu* therefore carried with it the suggestion of an authoritative and all-encompassing quality to the writings. Perhaps by giving grandiose titles the authors hoped the text would be seen as especially precious and so be better placed to survive the vicissitudes of time, and this may indeed have been a factor that helped texts such as the *Huangdi Neijing* and the *Lingshu* survive into modern times.

Neijing authorship and compilation dates

Overall, setting authorship and compilation dates of the *Neijing* is problematic. The core material is believed to be an accumulation of short medical texts written by various authors during the Zhanguo (Warring States) period, the Qin dynasty and in Western Han times. Much of the content was probably completed in the Warring States period, but these writings were subsequently re-edited, updated and supplemented, first through the Han dynasty and then, as mentioned, through further edits and additions in the Sui, Tang and even the Song dynasties. These conclusions have been reached by a combination of archaeological finds and as a result of close textual analysis.

Examining the text for time clues we find signs that different parts were written in different eras. For example, in the chapters entitled 'Jingui Zhen Yan Lun' ('True Words from the Golden Cabinet') and 'Zang Qi Fa Shi Lun' ('Organ Qi Through Time'), various characters appear that indicate times of day, and these are all terms that were current prior to and during the Qin dynasty (–221 to –226). The 'Mai Jie', a section in the *Suwen* on pulse diagnosis, uses a calendar term that does not appear until after –104, and other words from the text also help fix the dates of different passages. The 'Bao Ming Quan Qing Lun' chapter of the *Suwen*, for example, refers to the people as *qian shou*, a term in use before and during the Qin. The 'Ling Lan Mi Dian Lun' chapter uses the titles of officials that were current much later, during the Three Kingdoms period in the decades after the end of the Eastern Han dynasty in +221. All this tells us that different parts of the text were written centuries apart.

The view that much earlier texts contributed to the *Neijing*'s Han dynasty compilers has fragmentary support. The *Zhouli* (Rites of the Zhou, a chronicle written in the Warring States period, –475 to –221) says: 'support the sick with the five flavours, the five grains and the five medicines'. In *Suwen*'s 'Zang Qi Fa Shi Lun' we find a related statement: 'toxic medicines attack *xie* [*qi*], the five grains support [*zheng qi*], the five fruit assist, the five types of livestock benefit and the five vegetables complement', which suggests this part has its origins in the centuries before the start of the Han dynasty.

Ancient artefacts excavated in recent years from archaeological digs also provide some evidence for the completion time of some parts of the *Neijing*. For example, the Mawangdui texts *Zu Bi Shi Yi Mai Jiu Jing* (Eleven Channels of the Foot and Arm) and *Yin Yang Shi Yi Mai Jiu Jing* closely parallel the *Jing Mai* text from the *Lingshu*. It is clear that the *Lingshu* was based on the much earlier Mawangdui writings. The text had simply been updated to incorporate 12 channels instead of the original 11, and to add in updated conceptions of the interconnections between the channels and the *zangfu*. Other records on acupuncture from the writings on bamboo discovered in *Wei Wu* (*Wei Wu Han Jian*) contained extra information beyond that in the *Lingshu*, which means that some chapters in the *Lingshu* were completed at the latest during the Western Han (–206 to +8), and possibly earlier.

The writing style of the *Neijing* is very variable. In terms of textual length, the *Suwen*'s 'Jing Luo Lun' consists of just 140 characters, but the 'Liu Yuan Zheng Ji Da Lun' and 'Zhi Zhen Yao Da Lun' chapters introduced by Wang Bing in the Tang dynasty have more than 6000 characters. In places the writing style is very simple, akin to the style of odes written during the Han dynasty, whereas in chapters such as the *Suwen*'s 'Shang Gu Tian Zhen Lun', the style appears to pre-date the Qin dynasty, suggesting that some chapters were written prior to –221.

In summary, the *Huangdi Neijing* was not completed by a single author during one period of time but compiled by different physicians working in the 400 years of the Han dynasty and in the century or so before the Han. It largely consists of the medical knowledge and theories that were current during the Warring States period and the Qin and Han times, and most of the core texts of the *Neijing* originated in the Warring States period; these were then gradually edited, augmented and amended in later times. Various additions were made by authors in the Sui, Tang and Song dynasties, and in the passage of time, the changes made have provided both loss and benefit.

Neijing style and content

A distinctive feature of the *Suwen* is its use of a question and answer dialogue in which various court medical scholars respond to questions from the mythical emperor Huangdi, thereby allowing scholars to circumvent the tiresome and demeaning process of supplicating to medical gurus in the community. The production of this book may also have been designed to take away some of the power, influence and mystique of those outside the court.

The scope for *Neijing* scholarship is almost inexhaustible, and the reader is directed to Paul Unschuld's texts appraising the *Huangdi Neijing Suwen* and the *Nanjing* for a much more scholarly analysis of these texts than is possible at my hands.

A fundamental characteristic of the *Neijing* is the dynamics of the *yin-yang* relationship, which is used to represent concepts of harmonious and disturbed states in the environment and in mankind. Axiomatic, too, are the networks of causal and resonant relationships posited between man, nature and the wider universe discussed in the previous chapter. The mechanics of change and influence that had evolved as *yin-yang* theory through the previous 1000 years included various assumptions: the idea of their mutual opposition and control, their mutually interdependent relationship, their cyclical, dynamic equilibrium, their transformation through time into their opposite and the idea that each contains some element of its opposite.

Numerous passages in the *Neijing* espouse the *yin-yang* dichotomy, and this basic doctrine is applied to many different contexts that can be seen to contain an underlying duality. Above and below, ascending and descending, outside and inside, warmth and coolness, front and back, summer and winter, hard and soft, fullness and emptiness, solidity and evanescence – these are all examples of such qualities in the body and in the world. The *Neijing* presented these as an important way of analysing the condition of man and his environment in health and disease.

In *Neijing* doctrine a disordered or imbalanced *yin-yang* relationship in the body is largely reflected in their relative excess and weakness, which manifests in illness. Basic statements on this subject appear many times in the *Neijing*. For example, Chapter 62 of the *Suwen* ('Tiao Jing Lun', 'On Adjustment of Jing-Channels') says: 'When *yang* is deficient external cold results, when *yin* is deficient internal heat results, when *yang* is in excess external heat manifests and when *yin* is in excess there is internal cold.' The chapter develops this idea and explains its relation to *xie* (pathogenic) *qi* and acupuncture treatment methods.

In another category of dysfunction, *yin* and *yang* may lose their interpenetration which, when absolute, results in death. Recovering the appropriate relative equilibrium between *yin* and *yang* is thus one of the most fundamental conceptions of the *Neijing*. At a very basic level, treating disease is to regulate *yin* and *yang*, to return the body to the healthy state of *yin ping yang mi* – *yin* level, *yang* calm. This is the condition when neither is beyond limits and both are changing in a regular and tidal fashion due to their properly ordered interrelations.

Wu xing (five phases)

Another fundamental explanatory model used in the *Neijing* to categorise transformation processes and to account for the relationships between things is the *wu xing* or five phases – wood, fire, earth, metal and water. Although nowhere near as ancient as the *yin-yang* concept, the *wu xing* idea seemed to be a self-evident truism to scholars in the Western Han dynasty. The origins of this scheme are unclear. Possibly it was received from India or, more speculatively, prior to the Han – it may even have originated as a mnemonic that summarised the trade secrets of the metallurgy masters. One of the important early technological achievements, metallurgy required a knowledge of skilfully combining and transforming various materials in the environment such as wood, fire, ores, metal and water. The holders of this expertise doubtless had a special status in the ancient world – people were dependent on metalsmiths for knives, tools, weapons, domestic utensils and ritual vessels. Possibly the *wu xing* schema was originally a mnemonic for summarising the knowledge of the metalworking trades – wood being used to generate fire that may be applied to earth (ores) to produce metal that could be cooled and hardened with water which itself nourished the growth of trees. Wood provides a source for fire and for the carbon used to temper steel.

Speculation aside, the true origins of *wu xing* theory remain obscure. In a record in the *Shang Shu Hong Fan*, a text from the Spring and Autumn period, and the earliest Chinese historical chronicle, we find what appear to be some early hints of the developing *wu xing* concept, 'Water moistens and descends, fire flames upward, wood is flexible, metal is agent of change, earth is sowing and reaping.' Actual *wu xing* theory entered late Warring States intellectual discourse when it was popularised as a political theory by Zou Yan (−350 to −270), although the first verifiable description is not found until a few decades later, in the *Lushi Chunqiu* (Lu's Spring and Autumn Annals), written in −239. Whatever its origins, the accepted usefulness of the five phase idea in politics seems to have convinced the founding scholars of Han dynasty medicine that it might also be a handy way of categorising and connecting other relationships, such as those of the body and of cyclical phenomena in the environment. It was applied to the seasonal cycles and their relationship to climate, and the apparent rotation of the heavens and their evident relation to human health and disease, such as the periodic appearance of epidemic diseases. It also allowed foods and medicinal substances to be categorised and linked to internal organs, body tissues and the *jing-luo* system, all things to be linked in a satisfying grand unified scheme.

Using analogy, *wu xing* infers properties of things, and their interrelationships using correspondences; it offered an overarching model of transformation, development and the apparently resonant causality connections between all aspects of nature. In the *Neijing* five phase qualities were attributed to the internal organs and tissues, five orifices, five complexion types, five spirits and five sounds. In the environment they corresponded with the cardinal directions and with colours, climate, plants, seasons, foods and tastes.

The *Neijing* applied this to medicine by adding the *wu xing* idea to match with their conception of the functions of the five *zang* organs: the heart, spleen, lungs, kidneys and liver. Early notions of physiological function such as 'the liver likes spread, the heart *yang* likes to be warm, the spleen is the source of generating and transforming of *qi* and *xue*, the lungs govern clearing descent, the kidney stores *jing* and governs water' vaguely reflected the *wu xing* properties and became fundamental to medical doctrine. As rather abstracted summaries of conclusions taken from lineage texts, such statements were abstruse and not easily intelligible to those outside the intended readership.

Like *yin-yang* theory, the five phase schema is dynamic and interactive – it aims to offer a holistic model of the connections, correspondences and mutual interactions both in normality and in situations where systems are disturbed. The *sheng* (engenderment) scheme describes normal cyclic transformation from one phase to the next in the order wood-fire-earth-metal-water. For example, water makes grass and wood grow, wood can burn, ash of grass and wood can transform into earth, metal and mineral hide in the earth and metal can melt into liquid. In the seasonal context the wood phase represents the growth and expansion of spring, fire the heat of summer, earth the bounty of harvest time, metal the autumn and water the cold and damp of winter.

The *ke* cycle of the five phases describes a restraining relationship in which each phase represses another. In the 'Liu Wei Zhi Da Lun' chapter (Ch 68), one of the chapters added in the Tang dynasty (about +780), the sequence of this restraining is given as 'wood restrains earth, earth restrains water, water restrains fire, fire restrains metal and metal restrains wood'. Working simultaneously, the engendering and restraining cycles are represented as functioning as a cycle to maintain a dynamic equilibrium between things. Various other *wu xing* relationships were described: 'overwhelming' and 'rebellion' refer to abnormal phenomena when one phase is overactive or underactive, causing control beyond the limits of normality such that the system's regulation breaks down. Another Tang dynasty chapter in *Suwen*, 'Tian Yuan Ji Da Lun' (Ch 66), points out: '*Wu Yun* (five movement phases of the heavens) and *Yinyang* are the way of nature, the principle of everything, the parents of change, the beginning of life and death and the abode of spirit, so they should be understood.' These Tang dynasty passages suggest a revival of interest in *wu xing* theory at that time; its popularity peaked in the Western Han only to fade over the following centuries, possibly partly as a result of its outright rejection by some influential thinkers. Many later texts, such as the *Shang Han Zhabing Lun* and *Jiayi Jing*, barely mention this aspect of theory.

Neijing and xie-zheng theory

Another important conception underlying the *Neijing* relates to the relationship between *xie* and *zheng* (normal or correct). *Xie* is a general term used to denote pathogens and is essentially any *qi* or substance present in the body that should not normally be there, any substance that is not a usual body constituent in health. *Xie* may invade from the outside, like an infection, or be generated internally as either a consequence or cause of a disease state. Phlegm is one example of a form of *xie qi* – it blocks and obstructs and is different from the normal fluids that contribute to proper function in the body. It may be generated as a consequence of an invasion of a pathogen from the environment or arise from many abnormal internal states. Set against *xie* influences are the normal body constituents that may either be substantial, palpable and obvious, such as blood, or subtle and evanescent, such as *qi*. These healthy components are all subsumed under the term *zheng qi*, and so include body tissues, organs, blood, fluids and the various categories of *qi*. So a fundamental conception of classical Chinese medicine pathophysiology is represented in the *Neijing* as a contention between *xie* and *zheng*, the aim being to seek ways of removing *xie* and (or) strengthening *zheng*.

A central part of the Chinese medicine narrative through history involved the refinement and detailing of this idea in light of clinical experience. Pathogens and their appropriate methods of elimination were increasingly clarified, and in the process their study made more complex. This was especially challenging in the case of the types of *xie qi* involved in epidemic diseases because their nature altered through history such that new methods and new theories had to be developed to meet each challenge.

When we look at some of the types of *zheng qi* described in the *Neijing*, we see evidence of the military generals' thinking, a legacy of the Warring States period's concerns. *Wei* (defensive *qi*) is conceived as guarding the body's external borders, the skin, and controlling sweating – the flushing away of invading *xie qi*. *Wei qi*, like a good fighting force, is *yang*, hot and aggressive in nature. It is well known that the ability of troops to function depends on keeping them well nourished – an army marches on its stomach – and so a *yin*-natured *ying qi* (nourishing *qi*) was also said to circulate at the exterior in a *yin-yang* mutual relationship with *wei qi*. This relationship, considered essential for proper function, was an important part of *Neijing* theory.

Zang xiang theory

Also at the core of the medicine espoused in the *Neijing* is *zang xiang* (organ manifestation) theory, an idea described in the previous chapter. The idea that health or disease of the internal organs may be inferred from the outside by knowing observation includes elements of anatomy, physiology, pathology and diagnosis. It was axiomatic in the *Neijing* that 'what is inside must show externally' (*you zhu nei bi xing zhu wai*). Originating in the *Yijing* (Book of Changes, c. –1000), the concept was used in the Warring States period when government emissaries to neighbouring states needed to develop skills in face, voice and body reading to divine possible malevolent intent. The *Neijing* authors adopted the same idea for medicine, studying the external reflections of illness they saw in their patients, linking it with correspondences such as 'the liver is manifested in the eyes', which may have come from observations such as the fact that jaundice leads to a yellow discolouration of the sclera of the eyes. Other connections emerged from the study of the *jing-luo* system, through palpation and through examination of the complexion in patients.

Generally speaking, the investigations conducted by the authors of the *Neijing* were focused more on function and dysfunction than physical structure; nevertheless, anatomy was also included as an element of *zang xiang*. The 'Jing Mai' chapter of the *Lingshu* says: 'A man of eight feet has skin and flesh [the functions of which] may be investigated from outside by measuring and palpating, [his insides] can be investigated after death and his anatomy examined.' Early conceptions of anatomy and physiology in the *Neijing* are discussed next.

Internal bodily function

The *Neijing* authors outline their understanding of the physiological function of each organ in simple terms. From a modern perspective, many of these statements are broadly accurate, others are erroneous and some appear to be nonsense on first reading but make sense on reflection or in the light of further information.

Statements such as 'the spirit consciousness travels with the blood' might be taken as a metaphysical belief until we reflect on the observation that haemorrhage quickly leads to loss of consciousness. When discussing the lungs, *qi* refers to inhaled air and its distribution through the body via the lungs. What we translate as the spleen was almost certainly also meant to encompass the pancreas and digestive function in general. 'The kidneys govern reproduction' seems off-track until we realise that in the Han dynasty the testicles were referred to as 'external kidneys'. Many of the early medical observations found in the *Neijing* are indicative of systematic 'proto-scientific' investigations that endeavoured to found a rational study of medicine.

The *Neijing* tells readers that normal *zangfu* function manifests as health whilst disturbed function results in disease. Outlining the normal signs of age-related decline, the *Suwen's* 'Shang Gu Tian Zhen Lun' chapter links them to a cycle of flourishing health in youth followed by a gradual decline of kidney *jing* with ageing. It gathers together the key signs of age-related decline, namely the condition of teeth, bone, hair and cognition, as evidence of the exuberance or debilitation of kidney *jing*. Although a proper understanding of the concept of *jing* takes some effort, these remain reasonable measures by which to gauge the growing, developing and degree of ageing of the body.

> **SOME *SUWEN* STATEMENTS ON ORGAN FUNCTION**
> The heart governs the blood vessels and spirit-consciousness. The lungs govern *qi* and control respiration together with the dissemination of *qi* and fluid. The spleen governs the post-natal movement of food and drink and its transformation into body tissues. The liver governs free movement and the storage of blood. The kidneys govern growth and reproduction as well as water metabolism. The stomach governs the intake and decomposition of water and grain. The small intestine governs receiving and transforming the bounty of nourishment.

> **JING (精)**
> The character *jing* is sometimes translated as 'essence', although it has many other connotations. It consists of 米 representing a rice grain, and 青 which means 'green' – meaning both the colour and the sense of fresh and youthful. A fresh young rice grain is soft, moist and slightly green – it contains the potential to grow. In ancient China the careful storage of grain, to protect it against rotting or other degradation, was crucial to retain its value as seed for the following year, and so to guard against famine. A function of government was to secure this. Gradually, as the year progressed, the rice grain would become harder, older and lose its vitality and potential for vigorous growth. The choice of the character *jing* suggests that in us, too, there was an essential substance that gradually declined with time and through careless neglect. Also, just as poorly nourished rice seedlings will not produce fully healthy grain, so weakened parents will have less vigorous essence to pass on to their offspring. For this reason the Han dynasty elite became obsessed with *yang sheng* – health-preservation practices aimed at carefully storing, strengthening and preserving their *jing*.

Considering the time it was written, the *Neijing* quite accurately describes the functions of the internal organs and the way these can manifest as symptoms and signs. Accustomed to observing the world in terms of complex interacting systems rather than seeing the organs as isolated entities, the medical scholars developed theories about the manner in which they integrate and coordinate to create a functioning system, akin to the way social groups or a healthy state involves coordinated harmony between its constituent parts. An aspect of this notion of organ coordination involved positing relationships between the *zang* (solid organ) and *fu* (hollow organ) into *yin-yang* pairs. Most of these make sense from the viewpoint of biomedical physiology. The pairing of the gallbladder with the liver, of the stomach function with that of the pancreas and spleen and the matching of the kidneys with the bladder all make sense, physiologically. Others are less obvious but probably reflect inferences derived from clinical observation as well as the need for theoretical symmetry and concordance with the classical medical conceptions. For example, one reason the lungs and the large intestine were probably paired was because in health they both normally send their *qi* in a downward direction, both connect to the outside and because both receive clean material and expel waste. Ultimately Chinese 'proto-science' (to borrow the great sinologist Joseph Needham's term) at this time in history was an attempt to map the intimate and resonant connections between all aspects of the world – and indeed the universe as a whole.

Many barriers exist to the interpretation of the *Neijing* and the other early medical texts. It has inevitably become corrupted by copyist errors and later additions, such as those mentioned earlier. Even if we had access to a perfect and complete original text, significant difficulties would remain – language changes with time, and cultural allusions are lost both through the passage of time and, for us in the West, as a consequence of the East–West culture gap. Detailed discussion of such issues would lead us into a mire of academic scholarship and debate that is beyond my present skills and the remit of this book. One simple observation is, nevertheless, worth setting down because it is an issue that is rarely expressed. This issue relates to the fact that any technical endeavour, such as the creation of a medical system, requires its founders to create a specialist terminology that expresses technical ideas in a shorthand form and allows effective communication with peers. When modern medicine was founded, this was achieved by adopting Latin and Greek terms to signal technical meaning. In Han dynasty China, such an adoption was not feasible – in some senses, Chinese *was* the classical language of Southeast Asia. In addition, the nature of the Chinese language meant that there were practical barriers to the creation of neologisms – if you invented a new character, how would anyone know how to pronounce it, or what it signified? Scholarly physicians therefore had to borrow their terminology from vernacular language, and give these words new meaning attributions signalled by their use in the context of professional medicine. Even today, an engineer who attempts to read a Chinese medicine text can recognise the characters but will struggle to grasp its meaning. This terminology issue means that distortions and misapprehensions inevitably arise as we ourselves attempt to interpret what the authors of ancient medical writings were actually trying to express. Western interpretations of the character *qi* (氣) as 'energy' and *wu xing* as 'five elements' illustrate this problem.

Eastern Han dynasty medicine

In total the Han dynasty lasted about 400 years, and conveniently divides into the Western Han (−207 to +8) and the Eastern Han (+3−221); between these two was the brief Xin dynasty. After famine and revolt the Western Han disintegrated into factional warfare until a southern aristocrat and committed Confucian named Guang Wu-di re-united the state and skilfully fostered a new stability. This new and civilised order included tax reform that corrected old inequities, reduced bureaucracy, measures to stabilise food prices and the establishment of over 100 state-administered educational institutes. As the dynasty progressed, state power became diluted, first, by the influence of provincial nobility and then by intrigues wrought by the emperor's wives' families, court officials, the rising power of court eunuchs and the new habit of appointing small children to the position of emperor.

Shennong Bencao

Written by unknown authors, the *Shennong Bencao Jing* (Divine Farmer's *Materia Medica* Classic) is the oldest known text in which the application of medicinal substances is systematically presented. This, the *Neijing* and the *Shang Han Zhabing Lun* are the three seminal texts of the classical medical tradition.

Shennong was one of the three legendary fathers of China's culture; reputed to have lived around −2850, he is credited with the invention of agriculture and various other aspects of Chinese civilisation. (Fu Xi, alleged inventor of the *Yijing*'s trigrams, and Huangdi, founder of state administration, are two other famous ancient legendary figures from prehistory.) It is said that Shennong selflessly researched numerous substances for their medicinal value, distinguishing poisonous substances from foods and medicines. There is no documentation to help us know whether Shennong was an actual living person, a mythical ideal ancestor or simply a respectful linguistic shorthand term for 'our long forgotten forefather healers'. The likelihood is that numerous individuals were involved in the information-gathering process needed to assemble this first *materia medica*, and that it represents a summary of the herbal lore that was circulating from the Warring States period onwards.

Because the place names referred to in the text were those current around the middle of the Eastern Han dynasty, that is, around +100, we can be sure that the *Shennong Bencao* is unlikely to have been compiled earlier than this. Study of the Daoist terminology that appears in the text also supports the idea of authorship in the Eastern Han dynasty. However, as with other early classics, much of the content is likely to have been in existence in other texts and as folk knowledge for some time before its compilation. Other *bencao* texts, now lost, were almost certainly in existence prior to the *Shennong Bencao*, and we have evidence for one of these in the Han dynasty history written by Si Ma-qian (−145 to −86), who mentions a *Yao Lun* (Essay on Medicines) but makes no reference to the *Shennong Bencao*. This offers further evidence for later authorship. Also, the *Wushier Bing Fang* (Prescription for 52 Ailments), one of the medical texts excavated from the Mawangdui tombs and therefore written prior to −168, mentions 247 medicinal substances, so herb study clearly predates the *Shennong Bencao* by centuries at least. The existence of the field of scholarly *bencao* study in the Western Han is also supported by records from the reign of Emperor Ping saying that in +5 *bencao* experts from across China gathered in the capital. There are also fragmentary mentions of medicinal herbs in texts written prior to the Western Han discussed in the previous chapter.

> *Bencao* (本草) is the name given to the strand of medical literature dealing with the properties of individual substances. *Ben* means root, both in the sense of origin and plant part, and *cao* means grass or herbaceous plant.

The fact that *bencao* study by medical specialists predates the *Shennong Bencao* by centuries can also be inferred from the very existence of literate *fang shi* experts in early Western Han, Qin and Warring States times, as well as by mentions of the use of herbal prescriptions by the physician Chunyu Yi in roughly −180.

The *Shennong Bencao* details a total of 365 medicinal substances including their indications, taste, toxicity, dosage, identification and sources. Of the total, 252 are plant-derived, 67 from animal sources and 46 are minerals.

The text classifies substances in various ways, for example by its main taste. The authors will have assumed that the reader had prior knowledge of the properties associated with each flavour, as outlined in the *Neijing*.

Flavour	Classical therapeutic effect
Pungent	Dispersing and moving *qi*. Untying exterior blockage. Often affecting the lung domain
Sour	Contracting and holding in. Affinity for the liver domain
Sweet	Harmonising and supplementing. Mainly affecting the spleen and digestion
Bitter	Drying and often cooling. Affecting the heart domain
Salty	Softening and descending. Moving to the kidneys

The tastes that were assigned in this way allowed readers to form a broad idea of the effects of substances on the body. Given that the tastes ascribed broadly match the actual taste, these properties were doubtless identified following experimental observation. It is also a relatively straightforward task to investigate basic bodily responses to the substances being studied – a pungent substance, for example, was one that, taken in sufficient quantities, would induce sweating. This meant that it reached the skin via the lung domain. According to the *Suwen* it was axiomatic that pungency affected the lungs, and the lungs were considered to be linked directly to the exterior of the body, so many of the substances that affect the lungs or the sweat pores on the body surface are said to 'enter the lungs'. Pungent substances were also considered to be expansive, influencing *qi* to move outward to the surface of the body and envigorating *qi* that had become stagnant in the digestion or elsewhere. Substances that were bitter were said to be often cold in nature and downward moving – they were able to treat what we would today consider to be bacterial infections. Interestingly, many modern antibiotic drugs have a very bitter taste.

Also, in line with *Suwen* doctrine that hot diseases be treated with cooling substances and vice versa, the *Shennong Bencao* gave the substances it described a temperature attribute. A fifth quality was 'balanced' or 'neutral', suggesting that the substance was neither hot nor cold.

It is believed that in the original Han dynasty version there was no discussion of the affinity of medicinals for particular *jing-luo* channels (*gui jing*), although *zangfu* and other body parts affected by them are mentioned frequently. Many of the refinements of *bencao*, such as the *gui jing* (channel affinity) concept, appeared in the Jin-Yuan dynasties roughly a millennium later, particularly, as we see later, through the work of Zhang Yuan-su. The *Shennong Bencao* makes few direct links between the qualities of taste and temperature described for each herb and its stated clinical indications, suggesting that these were largely pragmatically derived rather than the result of theoretical speculation. As well as symptom indications there is mention of effects on the patient's *qi*, blood, *yin* and *yang*, but it remained for later authors to refine and systematise the information in light both of clinical experience and theoretical speculation. A sense of the *Shennong Bencao* style can be drawn from the quotations given below.

> *Du huo* (Angelica pubescentis root) is pungent and balanced. It mainly treats pain in the lower back and knees, strengthens the centre, increases *jing qi*, strengthens tendons and bones, fortifies the *zhi* (will), dispels damp itching in the genitals and urinary dribbling. Taking it long term makes the body light and slows ageing. It is also known as *xi xian* (missing the immortal). It grows in mountains and valleys.

> *Da huang* (rheum palmatum root) is bitter, cold and toxic. It is chiefly used to descend blood stasis and blockage due to cold or heat. It breaks up *zheng-jia* accumulations and gatherings [abdominal lumps and swellings], lodged phlegm and retained food. It flushes out the stomach and intestines and liberates the movement of water and grain, regulates the centre and transforms food. It calms and harmonises the five *zang* organs. It grows in mountains and valleys.

Readers of the *Shennong Bencao* are warned against certain combinations of medicinals that were deemed incompatible, risking adverse clinical responses. Also included was some basic practical and theoretical guidance on the way the substances could be matched together for strategic pharmacotherapy. A scheme for understanding beneficial relationships between the medicinals was outlined as on the next page.

Xiang xu	Mutual reinforcement	Mutual strengthening of similar medicinals
Xiang shi	Mutual benefit	Strategically matched pairs
Xiang wei	Mutual awe	The taming of one substance by another
Xiang e	Mutual disempowerment	Mollifying effect of one substance by another
Xiang shi	Mutual killing	Negation of effect by one substance by another
Xiang fa	Mutually incompatible	Unsuitable or harmful combinations
Dan xin	Simples	Substances used singly

This idea of mutual relations between pairs of medicinals, although containing some logical flaws and inconsistencies, became a key part of the discourse in the historical tradition and one that lives through to modern times.

Another basic organisational thread running through the text categorised the substances using a three-fold system: upper, middle and lower grades.

- *Shang pin*: Upper-grade medicinals correspond to heaven and were those considered to 'nourish life'. Safe, nourishing and relatively non-toxic, they could be consumed to treat mild disease patterns and be taken long term as part of a regime to aid longevity. Examples of the 120 herbs falling into this category included *huang qi*, *ling zhi* and *chai hu*. Prolonged ingestion of many of the herbs from this class were often said to 'make the body light', probably a reference to the Daoist quest for fostering a weightless and therefore more spiritual body form with the intention of achieving an immortal spirit. Some substances in this category, such as mercury, lead and arsenic compounds, turned out later to be more toxic than life-enhancing.

- *Zhong pin*: 120 middle-grade herbs corresponding to 'man' were considered safe and to possess useful therapeutic properties in the treatment of disease, although the implication was that these were unsuitable for use in the absence of specific clinical indications. They were to be viewed more as tools for illness treatment more than aids to general health. Examples include *wu zhu yu*, *shan zhi zi* and *dan zhu ye*. With modern eyes the boundaries appear somewhat arbitrary, with many substances now considered to be safe tonic herbs included in this category.

- *Xia pin*: Linked to 'earth', the lower-grade herbs were considered harsh or even drastic in their action, but they could be useful short-term therapy for the treatment of acute or life-threatening illness. Perhaps emblematic of this category is *ba dou* (croton seeds), considered a 'drastic purgative' in Chinese herbal medicine – consumption of just a few of these leads to significant fluid escape via the rectum, and few situations warrant such drastic action – one being ascites due to late-stage liver disease where the kidneys are unable to excrete water rapidly enough.

Later authors, in the Tang dynasty and especially those from the Song dynasty onwards, found this three-part division into *shang pin*, *zhong pin* and *xia pin* insufficient, and so devised more refined classification systems.

It was the *Shennong Bencao* that provided instruction on the way that individual herbs can contribute strategic functions within a prescription, designating these components as sovereign, minister, assistant and emissary (*jun*, *chen*, *zuo* and *shi*). This was valuable in providing a systematic framework for formula construction, guiding physicians into a habit of structured and logical prescription writing, and helping to lift medical practice above the application of single substances to treat individual symptoms. This sense of structure is evident in the formulas appearing in Zhang Zhong-jing's *Shang Han Zhabing Lin* of +220.

Function in formula	With the aim of
Sovereign	Treating main pattern
Minister	Supporting or moderating the sovereign
Assistant	Control side effects and treat symptoms
Emissary	Harmonise and direct the formula to a specific area

The original edition of the *Shennong Bencao* was lost, so the version we have today comes courtesy of the 5th-century Daoist alchemist Tao Hong-jing (discussed in the following chapter) who copied the text verbatim into two of his works. These, too, were lost, but thanks to extensive quotations of Tao Hong-jing's work in other texts, such as those by Sun Si-miao, scholars in the Song dynasty were able to reconstruct the ancient classic.

Han dynasty strip writings

Among the bamboo slips (*jian*) excavated in 1983 from a Han dynasty grave at Zhang Jia Shan two medical texts were found: the *Mai Shu* (Pulse Book) and *Yin Shu* (Book on Guiding [*Qi*]). This *Mai Shu* included similar content to some of the texts written on silk that were excavated from the Mawangdui tomb, namely the *Yinyang Shiyi Mai Jiu Jing* (*Yin-Yang* Eleven Channels Moxa Classic), the *Mai Fa* (Pulse Method) and the *Yinyang Mai Si Hou* (*Yin-Yang* Death Pulse Signs). These Zhang Jia Shan finds helped fill in some words in the text that had become deleted or changed from the Mawangdui version. The find also corrected the previous misapprehension that the first of these three might be a version of *Zu Bi Shi Yi Mai Jiu Jing* (Foot and Arm Eleven Channels Moxa Classic). The section discussing the 11 channels and their death signs later reappeared as the 'Jing Mai' chapter of the *Lingshu*; this added weight to the assertion that much of the material presented in the *Lingshu* was recycled material from the writings of previous centuries.

The *Yin Shu* (Guiding Book) is closely related to the silk picture known as the *Dao Yin Tu* (Guiding Teaching Diagram) recovered from the Mawangdui tombs. The

漢

Dao Yin Tu diagram presented the various aspects of the *qi*-guiding exercises in a picture format whilst the *Yin Shu* explained the same activities in words and described their applications in treating specific diseases – together, they clarify each other.

These health exercises, the forerunners of *taijiquan* and *qigong*, were popular amongst the ruling classes in the Han dynasty for whom it seems to have been fashionable to emulate the health practices of the *shi* scholar adepts in the community. Also popular amongst educated people were other longevity and health practices, such as special sexual practices borrowed from the Daoist adepts and diet balancing using Han dynasty ideas of matching diet and activity according to season and individual body condition. The secrets of the adepts were now more widely available to the educated classes.

> **YIN SHU AND DAO YIN TU CLARIFY EACH OTHER**
> For example, when we look at the action of *yin tui* (leading and declining) in the *Dao Yin Tu* illustrations, the arms are dropped, the knees slightly bent, the right leg to the front and the left to the back. In the *Yin Shu* text the action is explained: 'the left hand leans against left thigh, the left leg bends forward, the right leg extends backwards, bend the right arm, look to the left three times; then put right leg to the front, left leg at the back, look to the right three times'.

The *Yin Shu* text also offered a succinct view on an aspect of disease causality: 'The reason people become ill is because summer heat, dampness, wind, cold, rain or dew [disturb] the opening and closing of the pores and the interstitial tissues (*cou li*). Alternatively, illness develops when the diet is not harmonious or [a person's] lifestyle does not properly correspond to warm and cold [climatic] conditions.'

Descriptions of illness and treatment in the Eastern Han

In 1972 various early Eastern Han medical writings, pre-dating the *Shennong Bencao*, were excavated in Wu Wei in Gansu province, including one consisting of 78 wooden slips and 14 wooden tablets. This text has been now been named as *Zhi Bai Bing Fang* (Prescriptions for Treating a Hundred Diseases). It records about 100 herbs and 30 medicinal formulas that are matched to symptoms and disease names. Dosages, together with preparation methods, are described, and guidance on use of the prescriptions recorded in detail. Acupuncture points and some contraindications of acupuncture and moxibustion were also described. The names of diseases recorded included internal medicine, external medicine, gynaecology and ear, nose and throat (ENT) medicine.

ILLNESSES IN *PRESCRIPTIONS FOR TREATING A HUNDRED DISEASES*

Internal medicine	Chronic diarrhoea, abdominal distension, abdominal masses
External medicine	Incised wounds, carbuncle, dog bite
Gynaecology	Various gynaecologic conditions, breast growths (*ru yu*)
ENT	Throat obstruction (*hou bi*), sore throat (*yi tong*), toothache, deafness

The Wu Wei writings name illnesses in descriptive or energetic terms such as 'uprising *qi* due to chronic cough', 'sound in throat like a hundred noisy worms', 'chills in the shins' and 'hoarse voice'. Many other physical symptoms were more plainly described, such as: headache, nasal obstruction, pain in the flanks, abdominal distension, swelling, haematuria, urinary difficulty and pus and bleeding following an incised wound.

TECHNICAL MEDICAL TERMS IN THE WU WEI WRITINGS

Shang han	Acute cold
Qi xiang	Seven types of injury
Da feng	Stroke
Bi zheng	Arthritis
Fu liang	Mass between the heart and the navel
Chang pi	Dysentery
Wu long	Five types of dysuria
Ru yi	Breast growth
Hou bi	Throat obstruction
Yi tong	Sore throat
Men	Stuck emotional feeling in the chest

Most of these terms are still current in the technical terminology of modern Chinese medicine.

The concept of differential pattern diagnosis is evident in these writings as different formulas were prescribed according to the pattern diagnosis. For example, for an externally contracted *shang han* (cold attack) pattern, the formula recommended was *zhi shang han zhu feng tang* (treat cold attack and expel wind decoction) which employs the herbs *fu zi* and *shu jiao* (aconite tuber and Sichuan pepper), both of which are pungent hot herbs to dispel cold.

Readers are advised to give warm kidney supplementation for cases of body wasting due to *yin* (cold internal injury), for the 'seven injuries' and also for *yang wei* (impotence), *yin shuai* (consumption) and *jing zi chu* (spermatorrhoea). Other medicinals suggested are *rou cong rong, du zhong, xu duan* and *niu xi*.

The Wu Wei text discusses 61 plant herbs, including *chai hu* and *dang gui*, animal substances such as *long gu* (fossilised vertebrate bones) and *zhe chong* (an insect), minerals such as *ci shi* (haematite) and *fan shi* (alum), as well as other substances such as *chun jiu* (distilled alcohol). Various preparation methods for medicinals and forms of administration are also detailed including decoction (*tang*), pills (*wan*), syrups (*gao*), powders (*san*), tinctures (*li*), drops (*di*) and suppositories (*shuan*). Instructions for making pills from powdered herbs describe the use of honey as a binder, a method that has remained in continuous use until today. Various pill sizes are detailed such as those akin to red beans, sheep excrement, cherry, walnut and coins. Directions were given for use such as 'take after food' and 'avoid eating at night or drinking water at dawn', and advice also often gave the time of day to take the medicine. Numerous other methods of medicine administration were recommended such as swallowing with alcohol, vinegar, rice milk or soya milk to guide the herbs to a particular area or to augment the effect of the prescription. Various methods of external application were advocated including eye washes, plugging the ears with herb mixtures, rubbing substances into the skin with a finger, irrigating the nose or preparation of medicines with other substances such as alcohol. Various contraindications when taking medicine were mentioned such as avoiding fish, meat, rich dishes, alcohol and spicy food. All this suggests a rather sophisticated approach to professional medical practice in the first few decades of the first millennium.

Acupuncture in the Eastern Han

Details of individual medical practitioners from this era are sketchy. One of the most renowned Eastern Han dynasty physicians is Guo Yu, who was born in Sichuan province and who is believed to have learned medicine from a retired government official called Cheng Gao. Cheng, in turn, had gained his medical instruction from Fu Weng (Old Man Fu), a recluse who fished on the River Pei and who was known for his habit of providing treatment to local peasants in exchange for food, treatments that were reputed to be often instantaneously effective. Although a penniless recluse, Fu Weng was said to have written two widely read textbooks, one on pulse diagnosis and one on acupuncture called *Zhen Jing* (Acupuncture Classic); this, along with over 90 per cent of the medical texts mentioned in ancient library inventories, is now lost.

From Cheng Gao, Guo Yu is said to have learned channel palpation, diagnosis, acumoxa and herb formula construction, and in around +89 had risen to prominence sufficiently to become personal physician to Emperor Hedi when the emperor was aged about ten.

Wishing to put his physician's skills to the test, the playful child Emperor Hedi arranged a trial in which Guo Yu had to feel the pulse of one of his concubines from behind a curtain. Unknown to Guo, one of the arms actually belonged to a soft-skinned court eunuch. Physician Guo was confused by this trickery, and declared that one of the pulses seemed to be that of a man, but that he could not see how that could make sense. The emperor was impressed. Later it was noticed that Guo's success rates were higher when he treated commoners than when he treated people at court, and the emperor arranged another trick for his physician. An aristocrat was disguised as a poor commoner and placed in a hovel to be attended by Guo Yu – the treatment worked extremely well, and later he was called to explain the discrepancies in effectiveness to the emperor.

'Why are your treatments less effective on the rich?'

'It's simple,' said Guo Yu. 'The effect of treatment depends on the physician's mental state at the time. This aspect is quite subtle; one skill in acumoxa is to adapt treatment to match the individual's *qi* and blood circulation – small changes can have large effects. The understandings that are needed for good acupuncture are hard to put into words. Poor patients usually have more respect for, and belief in, doctors; in this case the physician is more comfortable and finds it easier to bring all his knowledge and skill to the treatment. Wealthy aristocrats are often arrogant and ignore guidance and so doctors feel stressed and distracted from their practice. Deep needling has a different effect from shallow needling and good timing gives better outcomes than bad timing. Diagnosis, too, requires the physician's careful attention, so when a patient's attitude distracts us it is harder to treat effectively. This is why my treatments for the wealthy and high-born tend to be less effective.'

Zhang Zhong-jing (+150–221)

Now we come to the author of one of the most revered and seminal texts of Chinese medicine, the *Shang Han Zhabing Lun* (Essays on Attack by Cold Pathogens and Miscellaneous Diseases). After the *Neijing*, most see this as the second most important work in the early history of Chinese medicine. One measure of its influence is reflected in the fact that it has been the subject of hundreds of commentaries since the Song dynasty, and it continues to be the subject of scholarship today.

Zhang Zhong-jing (aka Zhangji) was a native of Nanyang in present-day Henan province where some sources say he held the inherited post of 'Chamberlain of Revenues'. Little reliable historical detail is known about his life, but in the foreword to his *Shang Han Zhabing Lun* he tells us that as a child he saw two-thirds of his village and extended family die in the space of a decade from epidemic febrile diseases. It was this, he said, that drove him to study medicine and to devote much of his life to improving the diagnosis and treatment of acute febrile disease. Zhang Zhong-jing is said to have learned medicine from Zhang Bo-zu, but soon excelled him.

One traditional measure of mastery in a *shi* scholar was the ability to interpret subtle changes in a manner that allowed accurate predictions to be made. One story, probably untrue, says that Zhang Zhong-jing met the young Wang Zong-xuan, the emperor's minister, then aged about 20. Making a visual diagnosis he told him that, if he did not take 'five stone decoction' now, in 20 years his eyebrows would fall out and six months later he would die. Wang did not take this advice and, sure enough, aged 40, Zhang's prediction came true. There are many reasons for us to see this story as mythological but, nevertheless, it illustrates the qualities expected of an adept. Given that five stone decoction was quite toxic, Wang may well have died much earlier had he followed the advice.

Zhang studied the classical medical literature available at the time, mostly now lost, and gathered the experience of contemporary physicians to develop novel methods of examination and differentiation of disease. The 'Shang Han' section of his book detailed his understanding of the examination, treatment and consequences of attack by external pathogens, especially wind and cold. The other part, which was later re-titled the 'Jingui Yaolue', deals with general illness. Some authors also credit him with writing three other texts: *Liao Furen Fang* (Fine Formulas for Women), *Kou Chi Lun* (On Mouth and Teeth) and *Huang Su Fang* (Huang Su's Formulas).

For his cold attack theories Zhang adopted a differentiation system based on the six *jing* channel pairs as a framework with which to codify the depth of penetration of the pathogen and to delineate its clinical manifestations. His point of origin was a passage from Chapter 31 of the *Suwen*, namely:

> The Yellow Emperor said: 'I wish to hear about the symptoms [of acute febrile disease].'
>
> Qi Bo replied: 'When cold *xie* attacks the body the *taiyang* is injured on day one leading to symptoms such as headache, dorsal neck pain and stiffness of the lumbar spine. The *yangming* will be affected on the second day with symptoms of hot body, eye pain, dry nose and an inability to lie down. This is because the *yangming* is in charge of the flesh, its channel meets the nose and is linked with the eyes. On the third day the *shaoyang* will be affected which controls the gallbladder whose channel travels along the ribs to connect with the ears so the symptoms include chest and rib pain with deafness. The three yang channels are diseased but the illness has not yet entered into the *zang* so it can be cured by inducing perspiration.
>
> The *taiyin* is affected on the fourth day leading to symptoms such as abdominal fullness and dry throat because the channel of *taiyin* spreads over the stomach and joins with the throat. The *shaoyin* will be affected on the fifth day. Its channel passes the kidneys before joining with the lungs and meeting the root of tongue, hence the symptoms include dry mouth and tongue and thirst. On day six the *Jueyin* will be affected whose channel passes the sex organs to meet with the liver and hence the symptoms include feeling miserable and congested with contraction of scrotum.'

Zhang appears to have taken this rough scheme from the *Suwen* and refined it in light of the clinical pictures evident in his febrile patients, carefully noting the distinctions that could be made in signs such as sweating and either co-opting existing prescriptions or designing new formulas to match.

Energetic layer	Channels	Typical pattern
Tai yang	Bl and SI	Fevers or chills, sweating disturbance, aches and pains
Yang ming	St and LI	High fever, thirst, constipation, heavy sweats, agitation
Shao yang	GB and SJ	Phased alternate chills-fevers, nausea, bitter taste in mouth, irritable
Tai yin	Sp and Lu	Poor appetite, chilliness, loose stools
Shao yin	Kid and He	Various patterns of debility
Jue yin	Liv and Pc	Collapse, mixed heat and cold, pre-fatal signs

Many of the prescriptions set down by Zhang are technically brilliant in a way that is probably unimaginable to those not well versed in Chinese medicine thinking and strategy. So consistently brilliant are these prescriptions, and the implicit explanatory model that underlies them, that it is evident that most were probably handed down in a scholarly tradition that is now lost. As we saw in the last chapter, some formulas used by Zhang, such as *gui zhi tang*, may have existed centuries before his time; this idea is supported by his foreword where he mentions having received instruction on ancient formulas. Writing less than a century later, Huangfu Mi (c. +281) said that the *Shang Han Lun* was based on an earlier text, now lost, called *Yiyin Tangye* (Yiyin's Decocted Drinks), something that was alluded to in the previous chapter. So it is likely that Zhang was able to draw on a range of written and oral teachings that no longer survive – the terseness of the text left Zhang's sources unacknowledged.

The *Shang Han Zhabing Lun* is sometimes identified as the earliest surviving example of the application of *bagang* (eight-principle) differential diagnosis and the origin of the idea of *bian zheng lun zhi* (treatment based on pattern differentiation). Zhang's writings assume that the mechanisms underlying any main complaint can be different in different cases, and so the same symptoms may require different treatment. Also, later analysis in the Song dynasty demonstrated that the thinking that informed Zhang's approach to medicine was based primarily on distinguishing heat and cold, excess and weakness, and interior and exterior. However, the realisation that pattern differentiation was the key to medical sophistication is also evident in earlier writings such as the *Neijing* which itself was concerned with *bian zheng* pattern differentiation, and the idea could be seen even centuries earlier in the work of Chunyu Yi. Some insist that pattern differentiation was not introduced until the +12th century, and, whilst it is true that the idea was more formally described at this time, my reading suggests that *bian zheng lun zhi* existed as a key concept at the beginnings of the classical tradition. It has continued to develop and become gradually more explicit and more formalised through most of the past 2500 years.

Zhang Zhong-jing's prescriptions

Roughly 25 per cent of the key formulas in the modern *fangji* (prescription) literature come from Zhang Zhong-jing's writings, many more than from any other single author or text. They form the foundation of classical prescription writing. These ancient formulas are characterised by a succinct and distinctive style that employs few but well-chosen herbs with a sophisticated sense of strategy. Zhang often combines herbs that have contrasting qualities – combining warm with coolness, *qi* ascent with descent, expansion with contraction and supplementation of *zheng* with draining of *xie*. Relative doses and the preparation methods used are carefully considered with the aim of maximising effect. *Shan Han Zhabing Lun* study therefore forms the bedrock of Chinese herb education.

Some of the more famous formulas from the text are shown in the table on the next page:

漢

Bai hu tang	Treats *yang ming* channel fever – thirst, high fever, sweating, constipation
Bai-tou-weng tang	For dysentery with pus and blood
Ban-xia hou-po tang	For feeling of stuckness in the throat, due to *qi* stagnation and phlegm accumulation
Ban-xia xie xin tang	For chronic digestive imbalances, with tight bloating and rumbling diarrhoea, greasy tongue coating with mixed heat and cold
Chai-hu jia long-gu mu-li tang	A *shen* calming formula for *yin-yang* disharmony at the *shaoyin* level
Da chai-hu tang	A formula for a digesting pattern with nausea and vomiting
Da cheng qi tang	For fever with severe constipation due to intestinal heat
Da-huang fu-zi tang	For severe cold-accumulation constipation
Da-huang mu-dan tang	For what we now recognise as early appendicitis
Da jian zhong tang	For severe stomach pain due to cold in the digestive system
Da xian xiong tang	Chest tightness due to wrong treatment of *shang han* disorder
Dang-gui shao-yao san	Chronic, mild abdominal pain and cramps due to liver-spleen dysharmony
Dang-gui si ni tang	For chronic cold hands and feet due to blood deficiency
Fang-ji huang-qi tang	For *qi xu* leg oedema, especially in women
Gan mai da-zao tang	For anxiety and restlessness
Gegen huang-lian huang-qin tang	Dysentery with pus and blood
Ge-gen tang	For fever and chills without sweating, and stiff neck
Gua-di san	For phlegm obstruction where emesis is the only way to eliminate
Gua-lou xie-bai bai-jiu tang	For angina due to cold and phlegm in the chest
Gui-zhi tang	Fever and chills with sweating and no resolution due to *ying-wei* dysharmony
Gui-zhi fu-ling wan	Abdominal pain and mild uterine bleeding due to blood stasis in pregnancy
Gui-zhi jia long-gu mu-li tang	*Yin-yang* disharmony with dreams and sperm loss
Gui-zhi shao-yao zhi-mu tang	Painful obstruction syndrome, arthritic pains
Huang-lian e-jiao tang	Insomnia and vexation due to *yin xu* heat
Jiao ai tang	Uterine bleeding with blood *xu*
Jin gui shen qi wan	Kidney *yang* weakness with polyuria, oedema, chilliness, apathy

Ju-pi zhu-ru tang	Chronic *xu* rebellious stomach *qi* – nausea, hiccoughs, etc.
Ling gan wu-wei jiang xin tang	Cold phlegm-damp cough
Ling gui zhu gan tang	*Lu tanyin* (phlegm-fluid accumulation), breathlessness
Li zhong wan	Spleen *yang xu* and cold, *taiyin* disorder
Ma-huang tang	Acute *shi* exterior wind cold
Ma-huang xi-xin fu-zi tang	Wind cold with pre-existing *yang xu*
Ma xing shi gan tang	Lung heat asthma
Ma zi ren wan	Dry intestine constipation
Mai-men-dong tang	Lu and St *yin xu* dryness
Shao-yao gan-cao tang	Abdominal cramps
Si ni san	For cold extremities due to liver constraint
Si ni tang	For collapse and coma due to severe *yang xu*
Suan-zao-ren tang	Liver blood *xu* insomnia with heat
Tao-he cheng qi tang	For acute abdominal pain due to heat causing blood stagnation, appendicitis
Tao-hua tang	Chronic dysentery due to *yang* deficiency cold
Wu ling san	Cold oedema
Wen jing tang	Blood *xu* and cold menstrual pain and irregularity
Wu-mei wan	Digestive roundworms
Wu-zhu-yu tang	Cold stasis in liver channel; headaches, genital pain
Xiao chai-hu tang	For *shaoyang* disorder, liver-spleen dysharmony
Xiao jian zhong tang	Cold and *xu* abdominal pain
Xiao qing long tang	*Lung yang xu* wheezing with *tanyin*
Xiao xian xiong tang	Phlegm-heat clumping in chest with discomfort
Xie xin tang	For strong internal heat and damp heat
Xuan-fu dai-zhe tang	For rebellious stomach *qi*
Yin-chen-hao tang	Jaundice due to damp heat
Zhen wu tang	Oedema due to kidney *yang zu*
Zhi-zi dou-chi san	Post-fever irritability due to retained heat in chest
Zhi gan-cao tang	For heart arrhythmia due to *yin* and *yang* deficiency
Zhu-ling tang	Oedema with heat or *yin* deficiency
Zhu ye shi gao tang	Residual *qi* level heat

Zhang Ji's original work, the *Shang Han Zhabing Lun*, is today published as two texts. This is because, a century after the original work was written, the pulse expert Wang Shu-he split the text into two sections, the *Shang Han Lun* on cold attack and the *Jingui Yaolue* (Prescriptions from the Golden Casket) that discusses general internal disease. After this edit Zhang Ji's works fell into relative obscurity for over

700 years before they were re-discovered by medical scholars looking for promising guidelines on the treatment of the epidemics ravaging the country at that time. Up until the new intensive medical scholarship drive in the Song dynasty, the few who came across the text found it difficult to make sense of – it was written in a very abbreviated style with little by way of explanation. Its existence was occasionally mentioned in the Tang dynasty, for example, by the great Tang dynasty medical scholar Sun Si-miao, but even he gave it little attention. We detail the progress of this important text a little more in the two chapters that follow.

Hua Tuo

Hua Tuo (style name Yuan Hua) was a native of what is now Hao county in Anhui province. He lived roughly between +108 and +203 and became one of the Eastern Han dynasty's most renowned doctors. As a youth he studied in today's Jiangsu province, and at an early age is said to have completed the standard classical scholars education and to have been a skilled naturalist. Not motivated by fame or riches, Hua Tuo is said to have declined invitations for official government posts on many occasions. Despite his high level of scholarly attainment, Hua Tuo generally practised in the unassuming manner of a folk doctor, and was content to provide medical services to ordinary people across Anhui, Shandong, Jiangsu and Henan, where he became deeply respected. No reliable writings of his survive, so legend has to fill the gaps.

One surviving text, *Zhong Zang Jing* (Divinely Responding Classic), has been attributed to Hua Tuo on the basis of a preface attributed to someone calling himself Hua Tuo's nephew and who claimed that this book had been found in the master's bedroom after he had been executed. Although interesting, especially for its emphasis on *zangfu* differentiation using *yin-yang*, *shi-xu* and hot-cold, this book is almost certainly not Hua Tuo's work. Its language is odd, and it is now felt to have been written centuries later, and sanctified by the use of Hua Tuo's name. Its style and content place it probably somewhere between the end of the Tang and the start of the Ming dynasties – between the 9th and 14th centuries, long after Hua Tuo's death.

Famous for his proficiency in both internal and external medicine as well as gynaecology, paediatrics and acupuncture, Hua Tuo was legendary for his reputed pioneering surgical skills. In particular he is said to have developed a narcotic formula called *ma fei san* (numbness powder) as a general anaesthetic for abdominal surgery. Modern authors speculate that this probably included substances such as opium, hashish and aconite tubers. According to the *Hou Han Shu* (History of the Later Han): 'For the internal diseases that needles and medicine are unable to reach, administer *ma fei san* together with alcohol. When the patient loses consciousness make incisions in the abdomen or back to excise the accumulations and masses, [and the patient] will recover within a month.'

Hua Tuo is said to have used mulberry bark fibres as sutures for the wounds after surgery. Surgery under anaesthesia was essentially unknown in China and the world as a whole, so Chinese medicine celebrates him as the original heroic pioneer surgeon, despite little documentary evidence of his exploits.

Later in life Hua Tuo was summoned to treat Emperor Cao Cao's headaches but he was reluctant to accept the case – he is said to have made his excuses and returned home, saying that his wife had been taken ill. Repeatedly refusing to go back to attend to the emperor he was eventually arrested and condemned to be executed on the orders of Cao Cao. Before the sentence was carried out, the story is that Hua Tuo handed his medical case notes and writings to his jailer so that his wife might make them available for posterity. Afraid for his own safety, the jailer refused to accept them and, instead, all Hua Tuo's writings and case notes were burned.

Most modern commentators generally dismiss the story of Hua Tou's surgery and anaesthesia exploits as improbable myth and legend. There is certainly little likelihood of supporting textual verification coming to light, but it is worth bearing in mind that it was during Hua Tuo's time that surgical techniques were being introduced from India by Buddhist mendicant missionaries. Hua Tuo may have apprenticed with some of these specialists, and this would have created a new imperative to develop better anaesthesia. It is not inconceivable that he did achieve effective anaesthesia by employing existing herbs in the *bencao* and using traditional investigative methodologies. The story of Seishu Hanoaka (born in 1760) in relatively recent history attests to this possibility.

Seishu Hanoaka was a Japanese doctor who is likely to have been aware of the Hua Tuo story, and who carried out some remarkable research into surgical anaesthesia using Chinese herbs. He had trained in Chinese medicine and had also studied Western anatomical sciences and surgery with Dutch surgeons in Japan. Impressed with their anatomical knowledge and surgical skills, Seishu Hanoaka was disturbed that the Dutch surgeons conducted surgery without anaesthetic, thereby inflicting terrible pain and suffering on their patients. Aware that some of the medicinals used in Chinese medicine had a numbing and narcotic effect, he undertook a series of experiments to create his own version of Hua Tuo's *ma fei san*. He undertook 20 years of trials using different herbs, doses and formulas, testing them first on cats and dogs, and then on himself and his family. Getting the right herb ingredients and the right dosage was a difficult problem as the most effective substances were also quite toxic, with a narrow therapeutic range. Nevertheless, he finally succeeded in creating an effective formula that was safe to use on patients. His formula, which he called *tsusensan* (*chu shen san*, leave consciousness powder), included *wu tou* (aconite), *man tuo luo* (stramonium – formerly datura), *chuan xiong, bai zhi, dang gui* and *tian nan xing*. In 1804 he successfully performed surgery to remove a breast malignancy using his *tsusensan* formula, and over the following years surgeons flocked to his surgery to see him administer his anaesthetic in the course of more than 150 operations. Because of Japan's isolation, very few from the outside world came to hear of his innovation, which was then overshadowed in 1853 with the discovery in the West of ether and chloroform as an inhaled general anaesthetic. What is interesting is the fact that he was able to arrive at an effective Chinese herbal anaesthetic by simple low-technology experimentation. This allows at least the possibility that Hua Tuo could have followed a similar path and made a similar discovery in the early days of Chinese medicine.

Hou Han Shu (History of the Later Han) and *San Guo Zhi – Hua Tuo Zhuan* (Records of Three Countries) claims to document some of Hua Tuo's cases illustrating his advanced level of diagnostic skill and treatment methods. One of these patients who suffered from an inability to swallow was diagnosed as having an intestinal worm disease; for this he was prescribed finely chopped garlic in vinegar. The patient immediately vomited a snake-like worm and then recovered. In another case the imperial officials Ni Xun and Li Yan both suffered from what appeared to be identical headaches and fever. After conducting his pattern differentiation, Hua Tuo concluded that Ni Xun had an external excess pattern whilst Li Yan had an internal excess pattern. On the basis of his diagnosis he applied exterior release by diaphoresis in the first case and interior precipitation by purging for Li Yan, and both cases were resolved. This case may have been recorded as a public relations device aimed at illustrating the assertion by scholars that scholarly medicine was more sophisticated than, and distinct from, simple folk practices.

In another case the wife of a certain General Li was suffering a post-partum illness. Hua Tuo took her pulse and concluded that she had been carrying twins and that one had been delivered but the other foetus was unable to come out and had been retained and died, causing the illness. This is claimed as the earliest record of this situation in Chinese medicine.

Hua Tuo also used emotional therapies. One patient, for example, had been ill for a long time such that his *qi* and blood had become very stagnated. Hua Tuo considered that only a bout of rage would have the power to rid him of his disease, so he deliberately induced a state of fury in his patient sufficient to induce vomiting. The patient is reported to have vomited stagnated black blood before making a full recovery.

The historical records also characterise Hua Tuo as a highly skilled acupuncturist. Emperor Cao Cao's head wind disease, mentioned earlier, had been treated by court physicians for a long time without success, but the pain was eventually relieved after Hua Tuo administered acupuncture. According to *San Guo Zhi* (Three Kingdoms History, +221–280), written 20 years after his death, Hua Tuo obtained good results using very few points for acumoxa treatment. He advised that 'if moxibustion is indicated use no more than one or two points, and on each point use no more than seven or eight cones and the disease will be cured. Acupuncture should also be applied at no more than one or two points.' The biographies also tell us that Hua Tuo was especially skilled at propagating the acupuncture *qi* sensation along the channels.

On the basis of its first appearance in the controversial *Zhong Cang Jing* (Central Treasury Classic), Hua Tuo is credited with inventing the formula *wu pi san* (five peel powder), a diuretic for heavy dampness conditions where weak digestive function has allowed damp to infiltrate into the tissues. *Shi xiao san* and *an tai tang* are attributed to him.

The *hua tou jiaji* (Hua Tuo's along-the-spine) points, a group of 24 acupuncture points adjacent to the spinous processes on the back, were introduced later in history but named in honour of Hua Tuo.

Hua Tuo believed in preventative medicine for which he often advocated physical exercise, and for this purpose he is credited with inventing the calisthenic 'five bird play' (*wu qin xi*). He is said to have trained three students. One of these, Wu Pu, who wrote the *Wu Pu Bencao*, stayed healthy into his nineties with the help of Hua Tuo's animal exercises and by taking his master's longevity formula *qi ye qing shu zhen* which includes the herbs *qi ye* and *huang jing*. Another of his students was Li Dangzhi, who is credited with writing a text called *Li Shi Yao Lu* (Master Li's Medical Records). His third student, Fan E, is said to have focused on acumoxa treatment. All were famed as great physicians and for their own contributions to Chinese medicine.

The Han dynasty was a remarkable era for the development of medicine as it was the time when classical Chinese medicine was founded. Much knowledge on medicine and health that had previously circulated in the community amongst the *shi* scholar community as well as the folk healers, shamans, trauma and sores specialists, midwives and the like was collected by scholars inside and outside the imperial court. This information was sifted, re-ordered and re-crafted to make it congruent with the currently accepted framework of ideas on natural philosophy, together with the time-worn strategies and terminology of politics and warfare. The generally peaceful conditions of the Western Han dynasty fostered this move away from conflict and towards healthcare. The Daoist outlook that continued to flourish alongside Confucianism encouraged a spirit of investigation, and some effort was diverted away from esoteric and introspective studies to more pragmatic and vaguely scientific study and classification of substances and phenomena in the world. This included concerted efforts to understand the body in health and disease. This new medicine was codified into a new technical language schema that was borrowed from court military scholars and other sources, and in this way, Western Han medical thinkers provided the basic paradigm set for classical Chinese medicine. Then, in the course of the Eastern Han, the knowledge was consolidated with the compilation of the *Nanjing*, the *Lingshu*, the *Shennong Bencao* and the *Shang Han Zhabing Lun*. Much of subsequent Chinese medical history rested on the sanctity and assumed veracity of the Han medical classics, and much of the medical scholarship of the next two millennia simply involved closer and closer examination and elucidation of individual statements from the early classics.

As history progressed, Chinese physicians tried to fit new observations into the existing theory base from the classics and by reconciling differences; when this proved impractical, they developed new doctrines in the spirit of the old. If differences were irreconcilable, the failing doctrine was quietly dropped from the new version to maintain harmony of the texts. This dynamic tension between stolid reiteration and re-interpretation of revered ancient doctrine and the occasional revolutionary innovation is, in part, the story of Chinese medicine.

4

POST-HAN AND TANG DYNASTIES

Three Kingdoms, Northern and Southern, Sui and Tang dynasties

With the repeated appointment of child emperors placed at the centre of power but subjected to competing pressures from relatives, court eunuchs, ministers and warlords, the Eastern Han court slid into ever-increasing intrigue. State revenue declined as corruption reigned, leading to unrest and rebellion, and eventually central authority broke down, leaving three separate kingdoms. This led to over three centuries of strife

> **POST-HAN PERIOD**
> Three Kingdoms, 221–280
> Jin dynasty, 265–479
> Northern dynasty, 478–502
> Southern dynasty, 502–581
> Sui dynasty, 581–618
> Tang dynasty, 618–907

interspersed with periods of stability. Ironically, by the Jin dynasty (+265–479), this factionalisation had fostered a cultural diversity that allowed Daoism, Buddhism, philosophy and the arts to flourish, and even the emperors themselves fell under the charm of the Buddhist spell. Further dynastic changes, invasions, mismanagement, insurrection and geographic splits were then eventually resolved with the founding of the Sui dynasty (+581–618), during which the adept Buddhist Emperor Wendi re-unified China to restore peace and stability. It only took a few decades for this dynasty to disintegrate under the mismanagement of his successor son before the founding in 618 of the Tang dynasty – which is seen as a sustained highpoint of peace and high culture lasting three centuries. Skipping over the complexity of the background history of this time and its many dynastic changes, perhaps clumsily I refer to it as 'post-Han'.

Early post-Han medicine

After the demise of the Han dynasty in 221, few physicians practised using the classical styles that had been laid down in texts such as the *Neijing* and *Shang Han Lun*. One reason was that the *Neijing* did not function especially well as a guide to clinical practice; its layout was unsystematic, its language obscure, the acumoxa points were only vaguely described and, although replete with theories, it provided few clear pointers for the practical business of diagnosis and treatment. This is akin to the problems facing European acupuncture pioneers in the 1970s who had access to a partial translation of the *Suwen* but few clues on how to make sense of the information or how to translate it into practice. Speculation, interpolation and guesswork filled the void.

The first post-Han historical figure to address this difficulty was Huangfu Mi who completed his *Zhenjiu Jiayi Jing* (Systematic Classic of Acumoxa) in +280, a work that is discussed in more detail later in this chapter. As we have seen in the previous chapter, the *Shang Han Lun* was rarely transmitted or copied at this time, and so had little influence on medical practice prior to the start of the Song dynasty in +960. Access to written information by those interested in medical study was restricted by the fact that medical texts were still rare, handwritten and so costly or not freely circulated. State sponsorship of medicine was also weak in the centuries after the Han – times of warfare, lack of government revenue and political strife are times when organised medicine tends to be less of a priority. Most of those who wished to formally learn professional medicine were taught in exclusive master–disciple relationships, a factor that tended to reduce the scope for larger-scale collaborative ventures and the wider peer-to-peer debate that can serve to refine and critique knowledge.

The master–disciple system had various other drawbacks – for example, it allowed medical knowledge transmission to be subject to the vagaries of individual interpretation and in this way maverick theories could easily be introduced and be promulgated. Apprentice physicians would be selected on the basis of family ties or their ability to pay tuition fees and not necessarily on intelligence or aptitude, and medicine was a much more lowly calling than government service. However, the oft-held romantic image of the one-to-one master–student apprenticeship may not be quite accurate – the more successful physician mentors were effectively running small private colleges as businesses, with student numbers running into the dozens.

The mentor system, regulated only by 'survival of the fittest' rules, also meant that low-level provincial medical practitioners, perhaps mixing useful basic remedies with a significant element of superstition or nonsense, could represent their ideas as revered ancient and secret doctrine. A free-for-all risks sullying the scholarly medical tradition with folk medicine speculation and superstition, which explains some of the nonsense component to be found in the ancient literature. Somewhere in the mix of sense and nonsense are grey areas such as the Daoist adepts' delight in the use of elixirs containing toxic minerals such as arsenic and mercuric sulphide (cinnabar), many of which possessed significant biological effects but not always to the therapeutic benefit of the end user.

In one ironic and tragic example of this, the toxic effects of poisoning by mercury compounds turn out to be a close match to the symptoms of *jing* essence weakness. These cause the very symptoms that the heavy metal Daoist elixirs were intended

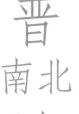

to cure: falling out of hair and teeth, mental decline and insanity. Spermatorrhoea, the inappropriate and uncontrolled loss of semen, can also result from mercury poisoning or appear as a symptom of schistosomiasis, and these two factors offer possible explanations for the prevalence of this symptom historically. The wealthy patrons of Daoist healers, claiming profound connections to the Dao, would thus be prescribed increasing doses of poisonous minerals to counter the ever-worsening signs of their *jing* deficiency. One example of this occurred with the Qin dynasty Emperor Qin Shi Huang, famed for unifying China in −221, who died prematurely as a result of consuming mercury-based longevity drugs.

With the importation of Buddhism from the Indian subcontinent and the continued fascination with Daoism, the influence of Confucian thinking declined. However, Daoists, with their magical ideas and their longevity practices and elixirs, came under some critical attack, and advocates of Buddhist spiritual ideas were not without their critics. The respected scholar Fan Zhen (+450–515), in his 'Shen Mie Lun' essay ('Disintegration of Spirit with Body'), refuted the Buddhist idea of reincarnation, saying:

> The *shen* is the body, the body is the *shen*… When the body disintegrates so does the *shen*…and so having *shen* is a consequence of having a body. The *shen* to matter is like sharpness to a blade… There is no blade without its sharpness and no sharpness without its blade… It is impossible for a *shen* to exist without its body. (Translated by Nathan Sivin)

Court scholars debated this problem at length, but failed to defeat Fan Zhen's rationale, so to resolve matters and bring things to a satisfactory conclusion, he was denounced as a heretic and exiled. Other sceptics of the Buddhist beliefs popular at the time included Lin Zong-yuan who wrote *On Vitality* and Liu Yu-xi who developed a theory that was tagged 'Heaven and Man Prevail Alternately'. Still, despite the reservations of some, the strong humanitarian outlook of Buddhism provided something that was weak in Confucianism, namely hope in the face of suffering, and so it continued to grow in popularity throughout the post-Han period.

The dominant political and sociological outlook in the preceding Han dynasty had been rooted in the ideas of Confucius, who emphasised ritual and proscribed correct behaviour by citizens. This ethic was effective in maintaining social harmony by promoting good order and relations between people; the stability and peace it fostered probably contributed to the longevity not only of the Han dynasty but also of subsequent Chinese culture as a whole. In their proto-scientific observation of nature and medicine, many of the Han dynasty elite had striven to rise above irrationality; philosophers and thinkers often denounced superstition and popular shamanic notions of ghosts and spirits in favour of more tangible realities. This outlook had already been developing amongst the *shi* scholar classes in the Warring States (Zhanguo) and Qin dynasties in the centuries leading up to the Qin and Han dynasties, when the great legalist philosopher and political thinker, Han Feizi (−280 to −234), famously declared, 'It is stupid to claim certainty without corroborating

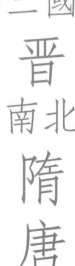

evidence.' This, taken together with our previous discussion of official Han medical jurisprudence, helps to highlight a rational tendency in thought around the time of the inception of the classical medical tradition. Superstition, though, always lurks on the medical fringes, perhaps to provide inspiration and intellectual light and shade. Most of the great physicians of Chinese medicine history specifically intended their work to be rational and pragmatic, but few were able to escape the pressure to accept cultural shibboleths such as belief in spirit realms.

Now, after the fall of the Han dynasty, Buddhism steadily gained a place in popular and elite culture following its introduction from the Indian subcontinent in the 1st century. As Daoist magic and Buddhism flourished, its tendency towards mysticism had an inhibitory effect on the Confucian outlook, and they continued to influence medical thinking and the way that medicine was practised through the subsequent seven centuries. One manifestation of this is in the popularity of incantation medicine and the use of charms and talismans in which special characters are carried on one's person, or are ritually burned or swallowed to protect against spirits or treat illness. The good thing about medicine of this nature is that it requires little investment by way of gruelling and expensive education.

The beneficial aspect was the creative and inquisitive mindset that formed part of the Daoist outlook, and this led to an expansion of alchemical investigation in the Tang dynasty. It was Daoist alchemists who introduced many of the techniques that were much later to become standard in the science of chemistry, such as distillation, filtration, evaporation, precipitation and sublimation. They were especially interested in studying change and transformation, including those seen in chemical reactions, where one substance can be transmuted into another. This held an obvious fascination. Especially beguiling was the observation made by metallurgists centuries before that heating mercuric sulphide, itself blood red in colour, released liquid metal in the form of *jing* essence-like elemental mercury. The observation that during a blood haemorrhage our spirit and consciousness went with it was taken to suggest that the human spirit and consciousness was contained in the blood. It seemed as if mercury was the spirit contained in the blood-red cinnabar, and that it could be magically released by heat generated by the alchemist's bellows.

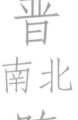

Chemical transformations such as these were allied to their interest in spiritual development and longevity, and so increasingly influenced medical studies. The air bellows of the lungs could be directed down to focus on the *dantian* (the 'cinnabar field' below the navel) to release *jing* and cultivate more *shen* and perhaps generate superhuman states such as immortality. The influence of Daoist bodily alchemy had both positive and negative aspects. They encouraged experimental investigations into mankind and the study of phenomena in nature, but at the same time, from a modern perspective, their investigations were muddied by the inclusion of layers of speculative mysticism that was not especially well grounded in pragmatic reality. Without this befuddlement the ancient thinkers would have got closer to true science, but perhaps at the cost of the strategic systems thinking that gives Chinese medicine some of its appeal today.

As well as the Buddhist and Daoist influences in the centuries after the Han dynasty, trade and cultural links with surrounding countries increasingly flourished. Diverse new ideas were imported that provided a stimulus to China's intellectual life, bringing poetry and a heightened aesthetic sense, seen, for example, in the remarkable ceramics of this era. Towards the end of the Tang dynasty ideas flowed outwards too, notably as a result of the translation into Arabic of China's medical and scientific writings, an endeavour that brought chemistry, mathematics, medicine and science to the Middle East and from there to Europe. Also, at the end of the Tang dynasty, the Confucian outlook began to re-emerge, although the full impact of this was not seen until the introduction of a revised form of Confucianism in the subsequent Song dynasty.

So it was that many of the medical authors in the Sui and Tang dynasties exhibited both Daoist and Buddhist tendencies; their alchemy and mysticism coloured their medical writing and practice. It can be argued that the greatness of some of the medical scholars of this era, such as Sun Si-miao, rested on an ability to root their thinking in pragmatic real-world rationalism tinged with a creative mysticism, a thinking style that also characterised some of the founders of Western science such as Sir Isaac Newton and Niels Bohr, as well as some of the architects of Chinese medicine.

Renowned post-Han medical thinkers
Ge Hong (+281–341)

Ge Hong was born in Ju Rong near the city of Nanjing in today's Jiangsu province, the son of an official of the Wu state. Unfortunately, his father died when he was 13 and the family library was destroyed by military action during the chaos of the first few years of the Jin dynasty (+265–479). With the family now experiencing hard times, Ge writes that he was forced to labour through his teens as a woodcutter in order to fund his education and to buy scholars' tools such as textbooks, ink stone, brush and paper. After a hard day's physical toil, he relates how he was forced by his circumstances to borrow from neighbours to make his own copies of textbooks. His self-penned tales of hardship may have served to demonstrate that he paid his academic dues by dedicated study in the face of adversity. At this time in history the typical classical education was still founded on study of the five Confucian classics, but from the Jin dynasty onwards, these texts were increasingly overshadowed by the more beguiling esoteric Daoist arts and sciences.

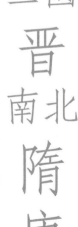

> **THE FIVE CONFUCIAN CLASSICS**
> *Yijing* (Classic of Changes)
> *Shujing* (Classic of History)
> *Shijing* (Classic of Poetry)
> *Liji* (Book of Rites)
> *Chunqiu* (Spring and Autumn Annals)

So, as well as his studies of the ancient classic literature, Ge Hong was exposed to Daoist theories, longevity techniques, alchemy and meditative breathing exercises. In his mid-teens he studied under a close friend of his family, the very elderly and accomplished classical scholar Zheng Yin, who headed his own academy catering to the educational needs of more than 50 students. Zheng Yin introduced Ge to numerous rare Daoist texts, almost all of which are now lost. As well as studying and copying texts as part of the tuition and transmission process, daily life at this private academy included mundane chores such as chopping wood and sweeping. It may have been that undertaking these chores provided a discount on tuition fees, which may be what Ge Hong was referring to when he said that he had to undertake menial work in order to continue his studies.

Through his late teenage years Ge Hong continued his enthusiasm for alchemy with his circle of Daoist knowledge-seekers consisting of relatives and colleagues. One of the quests of scholars such as Ge Hong, his mentor Zheng Yin and his uncle Ge Huan involved attempts to formulate the *jin dan* (golden elixir), a chemical aid to personal transcendent transformation and immortality. This is perhaps the source (via the 9th- and 10th-century Arabic translation of Chinese classics) a millennium later of the mediaeval European alchemists' search for a process able to transform base metals into gold, thereby confusing transmutation of the soul with transmutation of the wallet.

In +302 Ge Hong was appointed to a military post that placed him in charge of quelling one of the many violent rebellions that were rife at the start of the Jin dynasty. Later, when ruler Sima Rui founded the Eastern Jin dynasty, Ge Hong was given a senior military post in Guangzhou in the south. This allowed him to escape the turmoil in the north of the country, and gave him an opportunity to study the herbs and medical knowledge of south China, including that of Yunnan province and Vietnam. Later in his life Ge Hong declined all honours and offers of high office from the imperial court, and from +306 to +314 he retired to become a recluse on Mount Luofu in Guandong province. Here he befriended a fellow Daoist scholar called Bao Jing from whom he acquired further esoteric knowledge and medical skills. Now able to devote his time to writing, Ge Hong's scholarly endeavours were prolific and wide-ranging, including books on politics and statecraft, poetry, literature, medicine and warfare. Most of these writings are now lost, and those that do survive are so riddled with copyists' errors and later additions that it is almost impossible to discern the contents of the original.

Ge Hong is viewed as a talented and eclectic scholar with a very broad view of the world and its possibilities. Alongside his military career he continued his early interest as an alchemist in search of longevity drugs and investigating the chemistry and medical effects of mineral drugs using alchemical techniques such as distillation and sublimation. Daoists were intrigued by minerals, both geological and those derived from animal shells. They saw these as a secret sixth element of the *wu xing* (five phase) scheme, lying between metal and water, at the polar opposite of the fire element. Daoist adepts thus saw minerals as the ultimate *yin* substances. They were fascinated, too, by the manner in which water could seemingly be transformed into solid mineral material, something exemplified by the formation of the calciferous shells of shellfish. Ge Hong's experiments with substances such as cinnabar, sulphur, potassium nitrate, realgar, magnetite, mica, iron and tin are recorded in his *Baopuzi Nei Pian* (Inner Writings of Baopuzi, his Daoist name, meaning 'one who embraces simplicity') and his *Baopuzi Wai Pian* (Outer Writings of Baopuzi). In these writings he also explored the properties of herbal medicines such as *sheng di huang*, *huang lian*, *da huang*, *shan zhi zi*, *fu ling* and *yu zhu*. Together, his *Nei Pian* and *Wai Pian* texts discussed approaches to preventative medicine based on adhering to a moderate lifestyle – avoiding excessive eating and drinking, getting chilled and over-exertion. Ge Hong also advocated Daoist breathing exercises and the consumption of tonic foods and herbs for health maintenance when appropriate.

Ge Hong's more clinically orientated writings include his first-aid manual, *Zhouhou Beiji Fang* (Emergency Prescriptions to Keep Up Your Sleeve), a practical handbook of medicine that focused on cheap and practical therapy using acumoxa, cupping, massage and fumigation. Here Ge also included the herb formulas that in his experience had proved to be the most useful and effective. The *Zhouhou Beiji Fang* is notable for providing quite accurate descriptions of various diseases such as cholera, typhoid, malaria, dysentery, erysipelas, dysentery and leprosy. Ge Hong is also credited with the first clinical description of smallpox.

Disease	Description in *Zhouhou Beiji Fang*
Smallpox	'Recently people have suffered from epidemic sores attacking the head, face and trunk which then quickly spread to affect the whole body. They look like burns covered with a white starchy material; this dries up whilst a fresh crop appears. If not treated immediately patients usually die and those who do recover are afflicted with purplish scars that can take a year to fade. This is due to a toxic *qi*. It is believed to have been introduced by prisoners when Emperor Qian Wu was fighting the Huns at Nanyang so it has been named *Hun Pox*.'
Pulmonary tuberculosis	'…gives rise to high fever with sweating, weakness, diffuse pains making all positions uncomfortable; it gradually causes wasting and death. The disease transmits to relatives until the whole family is wiped out.'
Beriberi	'…[this] is not contagious, the patient experiences frequent indeterminate pains, has leg swelling, a sudden weakness on rising, tingling and numbness of the lower abdomen and sometimes feels excessively hot or cold. Unless treated early the disease affects the abdomen and the patient dies.'
Prisoner jaundice (hepatitis)	'…the illness begins with lassitude of the limbs, then the eyes become yellow and the discolouration progresses to cover the whole body. The patient's urine gives white paper the colour of the sap of the shoots of young plants.'

An interesting observation arising from these writings is the fact that Ge Hong implicitly recognised the transmissibility of contagious diseases by recommending

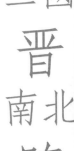

the quarantining of those affected, although as we have seen, this sanction was also evident centuries before in the official instructions relating to leprosy. Notable, too, is Ge Hong's emphasis on the importance of preventative strategies in maintaining resistance to epidemic diseases; at the same time he had powerful strategies up his sleeve for fulminant acute disease. For example, he was the first to describe the strong antibiotic prescription *huang lian jie du tang*, although the modern name of this formula did not appear until the publication of Wang Tao's formula compilation text, *Waitai Miyao Fang*, in +752.

Ge Hong also compiled a formula text called *Jin Gui Yao Fang* (Golden Casket Formulas Synopsis). In addition to his medical works, as a committed Daoist Ge Hong also wrote a number of philosophical works, including *Shenxian Zhuan* (Biographies of the Immortals).

> ## GE HONG'S SURVIVING TEXTS
> *Baopuzi Nei Pian* (Baopuzi Inner Writings)
>
> *Baopuzi Wai Pian* (Baopuzi Outer Writings)
>
> *Shanxian Zhuan* (Biographies of the Immortals)
>
> *Zhouhou Beiji Fang* (Emergency Prescriptions to Keep Up Your Sleeve)
>
> Some of Ge Hong's Daoist writings appear in the *Zheng Tong Dao Zang* (A Compendium of Daoist Orthodoxy)

Huangfu Mi (+215–282)

Born in the Jin dynasty, Huangfu Mi came from a humble background in a remote part of what is now Gansu province in northwest China. It is said that as a child Huangfu was ridiculed for being dim-witted and lazy, but when aged about 20, he suddenly started to blossom intellectually, and began to study the classics assiduously. Unable to afford private tutors or books, he borrowed them from neighbours, and read them in between farming work; thus by dedication and self-study he rose to fame as a scholar with a deep insight into classical learning.

Having become an established historian, poet and writer, Huangfu then developed a disabling illness (either a stroke or severe arthritic illness) when he was 42, and this prompted him to investigate the acumoxa tradition. These studies eventually culminated in the compilation of his masterwork, *Zhenjiu Jiayi Jing* (A–Z of Acupuncture and Moxibustion, often shortened to *Jiayi Jing*). At 54 he consumed a popular Daoist mineral remedy that brought him very close to death, and the additional ill health that this brought almost led Huangfu to take his own life. Instead, it inspired him to write a monograph (now lost) on the perils of Daoist formulas containing toxic minerals and to redouble his studies of medicine.

Collecting and systematising the classical literature on acumoxa, Huangfu compiled his encyclopaedic *Zhenjiu Jiayi Jing* (originally titled *Huangdi San Bu Zhenjiu Jiayi Jing* – Three Parts Huangdi's Acumoxa – An A to Z). Huangfu wrote the 12 volumes and 128 chapters of the *Jiayi Jing* between +256 and +282, the final 26 years of his life. The first known practical and comprehensive manual on acumoxa, the *Jiayi Jing* clarified the many confusing and contradictory conceptions

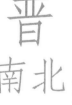

of anatomy, physiology and therapeutics found in the *Suwen*, the *Lingshu* and the *Mingtang Zhenjiu Zhi Yao* (Principles of Acumoxa Treatment from the Bright Hall). This last text was referred to by earlier authors but has been lost, apart from those parts that were copied by Huangfu into his *Jiayi Jing*.

Elucidating channel theory, Huangfu updated the descriptions of the *jing-luo* system including the *qijing ba mai* (eight extraordinary channels) and the *luo mai* (minute channels). He provided much more exact descriptions of the locations of the acupoints together with their basic indications, and appropriate acumoxa stimulation methods. Many practical aspects of treatment were also made plain such as the number of moxa cones to apply to different points and in different illnesses. Where the *Neijing* had only hinted at the way acupoints could be paired together, for greater effect Huangfu provided much more detail on this aspect of clinical practice. The clarity and pragmatic style of his work suggests that much of the knowledge he set down was the fruit of his own experience and scholarship rather than just theoretical speculation. In terms of disease pathology, Huangfu explained many disease patterns seen in various branches of medical practice, including gynaecology, paediatrics and external and internal medicine. The *Jiayi Jing* was the earliest known work of its kind, and is considered to be the single most significant book on the practice of acupuncture written before the Song dynasty.

Huangfu's contribution to the study of acupoints was especially important. The *Suwen* claimed the existence of 365 acupoints but, in fact, it mentioned only 160, and then provided few pointers on their locations and uses in clinical practice. The *Jiayi Jing* discusses a total of 349 points and offers much more clinically relevant detail on their application. Of particular value was Huangfu's work in standardising the location of the acupoints and refining the application of *jing-luo* theories as a method to explain illness and its treatment. Without this foundation in place, the development of acumoxa, and perhaps even the whole of Chinese medicine, would have been much less coherent. As Yang and Chace (1994) say in the preface to their monumental translation of the *Jiayi Jing*, 'It is not unreasonable to say that Huang Fu-mi's work defined acupuncture as we know it today.' The *Jiayi Jing* became the definitive acumoxa text not just for future Chinese acupuncturists through the Tang and beyond, but also for China's satellite cultures in Japan, Korea and Vietnam.

JIAYI JING

The *Jiayi Jing* was based on previous texts such as the *Suwen*, *Zhen Jing* (Acupuncture Classic) and *Mingtang Zhenjiu Zhi Yao* (Principles of Acumoxa Treatment from the Bright Hall). Much content also came from the *Nanjing*, augmented by some further refinements of acupuncture practise that had appeared after the Han dynasty. To the mix of classic source texts Huangfu Mi added his own clinical experience, and the doctrine that is presented in the *Jiayi Jing* is taken to be a comprehensive account of the dominant style of acumoxa practised by the elite physicians of the time. Its very practical approach to therapy meant that it soon became the prime manual for acumoxa practice in the subsequent centuries.

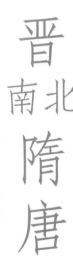

In his preface, Huangfu Mi told readers that, even in his time, much of the content of the *Neijing* had been lost, disordered or corrupted. The ideas presented in the *Neijing* were, he wrote, ancient and profound, but although it was strong on theory, it was weak as a guide to practical clinical medicine. The content of the three versions of the *Neijing* he had obtained included many repetitions and was riddled with errors – Chapter 9, 'The Profound Meaning of the Original Channels', he found to be almost unreadable. Seeing that its usefulness as a clinical manual could be made much more transparent, he devoted himself to reorganising and clarifying the text. Huangfu succeeded in balancing proper respect for the text with a degree of criticality for some of the opinions in his source material: 'The original text makes sense but what is said is not always in accord with more recent opinion. It is best, though, not to delete these older views.' Ideally, Huangfu believed, the essential core teachings should also be distilled out to create a new textbook, but this task, he said, would have to be left to a later date. Unfortunately, Huangfu was unable to complete this objective but he was successful in the task of clarifying and systematising acupuncture methodology. Before the *Jiayi Jing* was written, acumoxa practice had deviated from its connection with classical theory, but from now on most educated acupuncturists based their practice on *Jiayi Jing* opinion. By the Tang dynasty it had become the standard textbook.

JIAYI JING CONTENT AND STYLE

Huangfu Mi gives detailed practical information on locating acupoints, insertion depth, types of needles, the use of moxibustion and advice on suitable needle retention times. Volumes 7–12 are practical guides to the points and methods for treating various diseases and the appropriate acupuncture manipulation methods.

Huangfu's editing process aggregated previously scattered sources to reach a clearer consensus of opinion. His *Jingshen Wuzang Lun* (Essay on the Spirit and the Five Zang) drew on at least six chapters from the *Neijing* and *Lingshu*. His presentation of needling methods summarised the content of a range of writings from the *Suwen* and *Lingshu* and so allowed practitioners to gain a better understanding of needling methods, needling sensation, contraindications and the use of strengthening and draining manipulations.

Besides offering a systematic re-editing of the classic text, the *Jiayi Jing* also gave practical details and expressed the classical acumoxa concepts in more precise terms. The contemporary medical historian Fu Wei-kang provides examples of the numerous discrepancies that were rectified by Huangfu such as confusion as to whether the abdominal pathway of the *chong mai* extra channel follows the stomach channel or the kidney channel.

The hand *shaoyin* (heart) channel points that had been omitted from the *Neijing* were now fully described in the *Jiayi Jing*. Further innovations introduced by Huangfu Mi included the idea of *jiao hui* (intersection) points that joined the *jing-luo* together such as *sanyinjiao* (Sp 6). The inclusion of these new ideas support the idea that acupuncture theory was continuing to develop after the end of the Han dynasty,

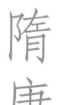

suggesting that this remained an actively evolving medicine rather than one frozen into simple reiteration of ancient doctrine. Some points were even relocated from one channel to another in the light of experience: *tian rong* (SI 17) was on the GB channel in the *Neijing* but in the *Jiayi Jing* it was re-assigned to the *sanjiao* channel. Later generations moved it again to its current location on the small intestine channel. Further developments through the Wei and Jin periods (+220–420) provided new indications for the points such as the new use of *renzhong* (GV 26) to treat epilepsy and *lie que* (Lu 7) to treat exterior patterns. By recording these new advances as well as systematising classical knowledge, Huangfu created a new benchmark reference text for subsequent generations of acumoxa practitioners.

As the great sinologist Nathan Sivin has pointed out, the history of Chinese medical scholarship is a history of attempts to make sense of the classics. Working at the end of the great founding era of classical Chinese medicine, Huangfu Mi was one of the earliest exponents of this endeavour.

Wang Shu-ho (+265–317)

Little is known about the life of Wang Shu-ho (Wang Xi) except that in his later years he is said to have held a senior post as physician in the imperial medical service. He is best known for composing the ten-volume *Mai Jing* (Pulse Classic) in which he summarised the knowledge on pulse diagnosis that had accumulated over the previous five centuries. Included are 24 pulse qualities that are essentially the same as those mentioned by Chunyu Yi in about −180 and used by subsequent practitioners. In the *Mai Jing* Wang Shu-ho described the different positions and depths in radial artery pulse diagnosis, their *zangfu* resonances and their diagnostic significance. His systematisation of pulse diagnosis set the foundation for pulse study in subsequent Chinese medical practice and became the standard text on the subject.

In Wang's scheme, the left *cun* (distal) pulse reflected the *qi* of the heart and small intestine whilst that on the right corresponded to the lungs and large intestine. The left *guan* (middle position) indicated the state of the liver and gallbladder, and on the right was the spleen and stomach. Both *chi* (proximal) pulses reflected the kidneys and bladder. This arrangement was the subject of much debate and variation through the subsequent history of the classical medical tradition, the dominant version today being based on the Ming dynasty physician Li Shi-zhen's interpretation.

As well as his work on pulse diagnosis, Wang is also notable for undertaking the earliest known attempt to rescue and re-construct Zhang Zhong-jing's *Shang Han Zhabing Lun* (Treatise on Cold Attack and Miscellaneous Illnesses). Taking what was originally a single text, he was the scholar who divided it into two sections: the *Shang Han Lun*, which schematised externally contracted illness, and the *Jingui Yaolue* (Prescriptions from the Gold Casket) that focused on the differentiation and treatment of many internal conditions. With the original version of the text now lost, it was Wang's preservation of this crucial early classic that ensured its survival for posterity.

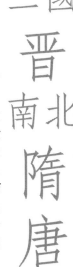

A later pulse text, *Mai Jue* (Pulses in Rhyme), appeared in the Five Dynasties period (+907–960) just prior to the Song dynasty, and this has sometimes been confused with Wang Shu-ho's pulse classic. It was *Mai Jue* that was translated into French in 1735 by the missionary Julien Hervieu and then re-translated into English by Richard Brookes in 1736. The availability of these translations led to a fad for diagnostic pulse taking amongst European physicians. Divorced, though, from any true scholarly understanding of Chinese medicine theory and practice, it can have made little sense to them. Many Western intellectuals of the time had a vague sense of the high medical attainment of Chinese physicians but, due to the language and other barriers, they were unable to access the knowledge base required to benefit from China's medical tradition. Despite the significant lack of insight, new fashions appeared in medical circles both for acupuncture and moxibustion, the latter being especially known in London society around this time for its success in treating gout.

Tao Hongjing (+456–536)

Born in Jiangsu, Tao Hongjing was inspired to become a scholar when, at the age of ten, he read Ge Hong's *Shenxian Zhuan* (Biographies of the Immortals). Emulating Ge Hong, he soon became a polymath Renaissance man with interests not only in medicine but also in calligraphy, music, chess, astronomy and geography. His remarkable genius was recognised when aged only 20 Tao was appointed to a high official post, a position he resigned in his middle years to become a mountain recluse. Even though he lived as a hermit in the remote countryside, he nonetheless wielded significant power and influence, and was often consulted for his opinion on official government affairs, earning himself the epithet 'the Prime Minister in the Mountains'.

Writing on numerous subjects including history and Confucian philosophy, Tao Hongjing is best known for his revision and updating of the *Shennong Bencao Jing*, the original Han dynasty *bencao* classic. Especially helpful was his innovation of highlighting the original textual quotes by writing these in red ink and appending his own commentary in black. This habit proved valuable to later scholars because it sidesteps a problem that often arises when exploring old medical classics, namely the difficulty of distinguishing original source material from later additions and copyist errors.

Tao expanded the *bencao* contents to over 700 substances, and enlarged the entries to include more detailed information on their properties, identification and harvesting. He also introduced a new method of categorising the *bencao* materials that used a seven-part distinction based on their origin: stones, plants, creatures, fruits and vegetables, grains and substances. Newly introduced substances he considered should be placed in a special probationary category pending further observation; these he designated as 'recognised but not [yet commonly] used'.

Tao also revised and enlarged Ge Hong's *Zhouhou Beiji Fang*, calling his version the *Zhouhou Beiji Fang* (100 Emergency Prescriptions to Keep Up Your Sleeve). This

三國晉北南隋唐

collection of prescriptions became so renowned by the end of the 6th century that the text was engraved for posterity on stone tablets in the Dragon Gate (Longmen) caves near Luoyang in Henan province. This benevolent enterprise sponsored by the imperial court aimed to preserve knowledge on medicine and many other subjects for the benefit of future generations. In an era before China's invention of printing, the only way to spread medical texts was to hand copy them; this enabled scholars to take rubbings for easier dissemination of medical knowledge. The Dragon Gate texts were innovative because physicians now had access to what in effect were basic medical library copying facilities.

Tao also wrote the *Ming Yi Bie Lu* (Transactions of Famous Physicians' Prescriptions) and various other medical texts that are now lost. Tao Hingjing was another physician whose outstanding characteristic was his pragmatic approach; his main interest was the actual effect of medicinals in clinical practice rather than predictions based on theoretical speculation. In summarising and systematising previous texts, Tao helped to set a precedent for future medical scholars, showing the value of developing and refining the tradition in a straightforward and practical way, even if the focus was on a simple matching of formula to main complaint.

Other early post-Han writings

We know from library records and mentions in surviving texts that many writings on acumoxa appeared in the period between the end of the Han and the start of the Tang dynasty, but only a small proportion have survived into modern times, survivors being *Zhen Jing* (Acupuncture Classic) which was later to be known as *Lingshu* (Spiritual Pivot) and *Nanjing* (Classic of Difficult Issues). There are records of the transmission of various other works into post-Han times, such as *Pei Weng Zheng Jing* (Peng Wei's Normality Classic, Han dynasty), Lu Guang's *Yu Gui Zhen Jing* (Jade Box Acupuncture Classic, Wu dynasty) and *Mingtang Zhenjiu Zhi Yao* (Principles of Acumoxa Treatment from the Bright Hall). All of these, including Hua Tuo's *Zhen Zhong Jiu Ci Jing*, are lost, although some parts of the *Ming Tang* have been preserved in Huangfu Mi's *Zhenjiu Jiayi Jing*.

Surgery before the Tang

Jinshu (History of the Jin Dynasty) mentions a surgical operation carried out in the 5th century to repair a cleft lip. At the end of the 5th century Gong Qing-xuan also recorded his own surgical exploits in a text called *Liu Juanzi Guiyi Fang* (Lui Juan-zi's Ghost Legacy Formulas), which is China's oldest surviving text on surgery. Included in this book are discussions on the treatment of wounds as well as abscesses and other skin lesions. Here we find discussions of the use of an ointment based on mercuric chloride that was used for the external treatment of skin conditions. Much later, following reports of its efficacy, calomel was introduced into Western medical practice for the external treatment of sores and syphilitic chancres. So successful was

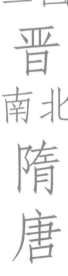

this therapy that some Western physicians felt that it must also be beneficial when administered internally – leading to many deaths. It has been claimed that during the US civil war more people died of physician-inspired mercury poisoning than were killed as a result of the fighting.

Sui and Tang dynasties

In +581 the founding of the Sui dynasty overturned the previous Southern dynasties, and improvements in infrastructure, government and military organisation soon followed. These included the founding of the cities of Luoyang and Changan and the construction of new waterways. The Sui regime initially ushered in a brief period of good governance and social order, but progress was cut short in only a few decades. Although Wendi, the founding ruler, was benevolent, his son was despotic, and so the peasantry revolted, and this, together with conflicts with the Koreans, soon led to its downfall. Order was then restored with the founding of the Tang dynasty in +618. The outlook of this new regime included a greater court interest in medicine that led to the founding of a state medical school, albeit for the benefit of the elite, and some state-sponsored initiatives to revive neglected classical texts.

The Tang emperors were able to enact many of the civic reforms and civilising projects that had been planned by the Sui government. Both in court circles and in the population at large Buddhism flourished, and this blended with the existing Daoist traditions to contribute to a new flowering of Chinese culture. The distinctive Chan (Zen in Japanese) Buddhism was created, and the imperial outlook became more outward-looking and more receptive to foreign interaction. This cultural flowering manifested in a proliferation of poets and painters, and the creation of stunning ceramics epitomised by three-colour (*san cai*) glazed pottery figures of horses, camels and people.

The important acumoxa text *Huangdi Ming Tang Jing* (Yellow Emperor's Enlightened Hall Classic) had appeared early in the Tang dynasty, and this was augmented by the physician Yang Sheng-shang who added new chapters on each *jing* channel and on the *qijing ba mai* (eight extraordinary channels) to create a new edition. Unfortunately most of this material is now lost apart from the preface and first chapter, which has surfaced in Japan. In about +600 Yang Sheng-shang wrote *Huangdi Neijing Taisu* (The Grand Basis), which was a revision of the *Neijing*.

Interactions with neighbouring states

During the Tang dynasty the Chinese interacted with neighbouring cultures, both on intellectual and commercial levels, trading goods, medicines and thoughts with Japan, Persia, Tibet, India and other countries in the region. In relation to medicine, one example of this spirit of receptiveness to new ideas and outside influences was the publication of *Hu Bencao* (Tartar *Materia Medica*) containing descriptions of medicinals from the 'barbarian' regions to the north and west. Exchanges also took place with what are now Vietnam and Korea, leading to the introduction of new herbs to the Chinese *bencao* such as *chen xiang* (Eaglewood, Lignum aquilaria) and *su he xiang* (liquidambar Taiwanense sap).

The transmission of Chinese medicine to Japan had begun prior to the Tang when, in +552, the emperor presented the Japanese emperor with a copy of *Zhen Jing* (Acupuncture Classic). A decade later, Zhi Cong, from Jiangsu province, travelled to Japan, taking with him a selection of medical works, and later, in +608, two Japanese monks travelled to China to study medicine; in +632 various texts were taken to Japan including Wang Shu-hu's *Mai Jing* (Pulse Classic). At the start of the 8th century the Japanese introduced laws intended to regulate medical education and practice – these rules emulated China's Tang dynasty regulations. In +702 the Japanese founded a medical college modelled on China's state medical academy, Tai Yi Shu, with Chinese classic texts such as *Mai Jing* listed as required reading.

In the time of the Tang dynasty (Emperor Gao Zong, +649–683), China's trade and other interactions with other countries increased significantly, allowing its medical, technological and proto-scientific knowledge to spread to other neighbouring countries, notably India, Persia and other Arabian countries. The spread to the Arabian and Byzantine cultures then went on to exert a significant influence on learning in Mediterranean and European cultures. Later we will see specific instances of the way China's medical knowledge went on to inspire Arabic medical writings that were themselves to influence mediaeval European medicine. From these interactions Chinese culture and Chinese medicine itself benefited from the acquisition of some of the medical substances important in Arabic medicine, such as *mo yao* and *ru xiang* (myrrh and frankincense) and *xiao hui xiang* (fennel seeds), as well as *sha ren* (cardamom) from India, *mu xiang* (costus root) from the Himalayas and *xi honghua* (saffron) from Tibet. From Korea came *yan hu suo* (Corydalis tuber) and *bai fu zi* (Typhonium tuber). These became treasured items of trade and a new focus for investigation by Chinese physicians wishing to understand their effects so as to slot them into their own medical tradition. Around this time the poet Li Xun compiled a *bencao* of the newly introduced medicines called *Hai Yao Bencao* (Overseas Medicines *Bencao*). This book was lost at the end of the Song dynasty and was later reconstructed from quotes in other texts.

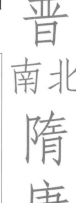

IMPERIAL COURT INTRIGUE

We can get a snapshot of the typical plotting and intrigue that went on in imperial court life by diverting for a moment to Tang Emperor Gao Zong's court. On accession to the throne, Gao Zong took one of his father's ambitious concubines, Wu Zetian, as his own. She then murdered her own new-born baby and succeeded in having Gao Zong's wife Wang blamed for the crime. Just to be sure, she then murdered Wang and took the position of empress for herself. Usurping her husband, Wu appointed her own supporters to high office and brutally disposed of her opponents. Wu Zetian's expansionist tendencies were the driving force that led to Korea being conquered by the Chinese as well as the wider contacts with Arabia and India.

Tibet, too, was a beneficiary of the Tang spirit of interaction. In +641 the Chinese princess Wen Cheng was dispatched to marry a Tibetan king, taking with her a statue of the Buddha and various medical texts that had been translated into Tibetan, including *Mai Jing*. The next hundred years saw further exportation both of Chinese brides and medical knowledge, and in return Chinese medicine benefited from the introduction of some indigenous Tibetan herbs, such as *xi honghua* and *dong chong xia cao* (Cordyceps caterpillar fungus).

The spirit of cultural exchange is also well exemplified by Jian Chen (born in 688, family name Chunyu), a man who was highly educated in a range of subjects including Buddhism, the arts and medicine. Jian spent the final decade of his life in Japan introducing the prevailing Chinese medical knowledge as well as Buddhism and many other aspects of Chinese culture.

The continuing rise of Buddhism in the Tang dynasty created a fashion for pilgrimages to India, and this, too, allowed cross-fertilisation of medical ideas to take place as a by-product of this interchange. Some Indian medical texts were translated into Chinese, and a wave of Indian physicians came to China to practise. Wishing to embody the Buddhist spirit of compassion and beneficence, they brought with them new medical skills, notably cataract surgical techniques, that, according to Wang Tao's *Waitai Bi Yao* (Essential Secrets from the Imperial Library, 752), were taught to Chinese physicians. However, the fact that six centuries later a comprehensive Ming dynasty text on ophthalmology fails to make any mention of this cataract surgery suggests that the technique had by that time probably fallen into obscurity. It may have dwindled away as a result of becoming a secret speciality or, more likely, Chinese patients were less tolerant of the risks of infection and permanent injury than patients in India. Even today signs of this two-way medical exchange in the Tang dynasty are evident in the fact that the current *Unani* medical tradition of North India retains some of the characteristic hallmarks of Chinese medicine, such as its use of Chinese-style pulse and tongue diagnosis.

In the early Tang dynasty, as a result of Buddhist ideas of benevolence, other charitable medical endeavours were established: monasteries began to offer treatment to lay people and pharmacies for the poor were set up – although the imperial state itself still took very little responsibility for public health. The Buddhist benevolent spirit was kept alive and was expanded by the subsequent Song dynasty to become a continuing aspect of court policy after the fall of the Tang dynasty.

Chinese medical practices were also affected by the introduction of Buddhist beliefs, such as the notion that health problems might result from adverse Karma inherited from a previous life. Other new ideas appeared, such as treatment by Buddhist spiritual healing, prayer and chanting, and Tang monasteries began to deliver their own brand of healthcare using these techniques and the prescription of proprietary temple herb formulas. The temples even systematised the provision of herbal medicine using a kind of divine lottery where the sick would randomly select bamboo slats indicating the formula to be taken, thereby relying on luck and faith for treatment. This was not especially helpful for the pragmatic development of the classical medical tradition. Classical physicians and scholars expressed dismay at this style of practice, but so pervasive was the Buddhist philosophy in imperial circles that critics faced repression and punishment.

Wealthy patients could afford to spread their healthcare bets by consulting trained doctors and temple healers at the same time. Indeed, it is common throughout history for well-heeled patients to consult a few doctors simultaneously, choosing to follow the treatment of the one who seemed the most convincing. Sometimes patients were more convinced by the physician who offered more expensive care or prescribed anodyne remedies than those who offered more gruelling treatments. Refined people might prefer to be prescribed rare and expensive tonics than more gruelling emesis, purgation or acupuncture. Later, the renowned Jin-Yuan dynasty physician Zhang Cong-zheng was to point out the folly of this for patients whose condition, he believed, warranted more aggressive treatment.

Tai Yi Shu (imperial medical service)

As we have seen, medical skills were often acquired through family lineages, by master–apprentice relationships and by the study of texts, and, as a rule, the more wealth or influence you had, the better the education you could acquire. Under some imperial regimes from the Eastern Han dynasty onwards, medical education for an elite handful of individuals could be sponsored by the court, but more commonly, prominent physicians were simply appointed from the community to serve the thousands of people in the court. Some would be appointed not so much to serve as practitioners but to supervise other court physicians.

For much of history imperial interest in medicine has tended to concern itself primarily with provision for the court; it is difficult to get an overview of the degree to which the state took responsibility for medical practice, although this does happen from time to time. Generally the peasantry had to look after their own healthcare. When we look back to the descriptions of Chunyu Yi's medical apprenticeships in about −180 we see suggestions, even at this early time, that the state took an interest in regulating medical practice – at least of those physicians serving the nobility. In +5 court physicians were specifically required to demonstrate their proficiency in herbs and formulas, but at this time there was no known officially sanctioned medical educational training. Across history the requirements for physicians both inside and outside the imperial court seem to have altered decade-by-decade and dynasty-by-dynasty, according to the outlook of the particular regime, with periods when state sponsorship of medical training flourished and others when it withered away.

Outside of imperial influence, in the centuries after the Han and leading up to the Tang dynasty, many medical families existed which persisted for generations, with each generation inheriting the fame, texts and lineage style of the last.

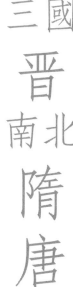

Eventually, for one reason or another, the lineage would wither away. We know of one prominent and long-lasting medical family that specialised in acupuncture of the post-Han period, a lineage that was founded by Xu Xi in the 4th century and continued through to Xu Min-qi in the 7th century. Thousands more unrecorded and now unknown will have existed alongside the Xu family.

Wealthy gentlemen scholars often kept private libraries that included medical works, but most were limited in scope and variable in quality. State-sponsored and institutionalised medical learning had obvious advantages, with its potential for access to the best literature, availability of scholars able to explain the texts and clinicians to demonstrate how medicine worked in practice. The problem was persuading emperors of the value of investing in such endeavours. This is exactly what happened in +443 when the Jin dynasty Emperor Wendi's physician Qin Cheng-zu successfully lobbied for the founding of a state medical school. Called Tai Yi Shu, this pioneering initiative unfortunately petered out after Wendi's death in +453, and in the face of more pressing political problems caused by revolts.

A little over a century later the resolution of military conflicts allowed the Sui dynasty (+581–618) to give attention again to the need for state regulation of medical education and so, in +581, the Tai Yi Shu idea was revived and styled as the highest state medical education authority. One graduate of the Tai Yi Shu was Chao Yuan-fang, lead author of the most important early work on aetiology and pathology, *Zhubing Yuanhou Lun*, a crucially important text discussed later in this chapter.

The Tai Yi Shu continued to mature in the decades after its founding, and it survived into the subsequent Tang dynasty when it included many departments with numerous high-level teaching staff and clinical facilities. In +624 it was formally established in the capital Chang An (today's Xian). There were four main medical departments: internal medicine (*yi*), acupuncture (*zhen*), massage-traumatology (*anmo*) and incantation (*zhujing*). The internal medicine training lasted seven years; five years were required for surgery and paediatrics training; and ENT physicians trained for four years. Ophthalmology and various other sub-specialities were also taught. Admission to the Tai Yi Shu medical faculty was through entrance examinations that were officially considered equal in standard to the *Guo Zi Jian*, the highest-level state officials' exams. The true status of medical graduates, though, remained well below most other court scholars and officials – medicine was not a calling for ambitious young men.

Scholar physicians of various official grades were involved in supervising the four medical departments, each of which was headed by a professor aided by a team of lecturers, practical teachers and teaching assistants. The inclusion of a department for incantation reflects the strong Buddhist and Daoist influences of the time. The use of charms and prayers to the deities was especially popular in the general population, but should probably be seen as a fringe activity in relation to the main classical medical tradition.

三國
晉南北
隋唐

STAFF AT THE TANG DYNASTY TAI YI SHU

Job title / Department	Professor	Senior Lecturer	Lecturer	Worker	Students	Pharmacists
Medicine	1	1	20	100	40	2
Acupuncture	1	1	10	20	20	
Massage	1		4	16	15	
Incantation	1		2	8	10	

In total Tai Yi Shu employed about 360 staff, making this a fairly large institution requiring significant investment in terms of finance and administration. Students were subjected to rigorous assessment in monthly written exams that were marked by the departmental professors. Quarterly exams were marked by the imperial physicians, and the annual exams marked by the highest-ranking imperial medical consultant. Clinical skills were also formally assessed, and those who graduated with the highest marks were assigned to senior medical postings in the imperial medical service. There was a clearly proscribed schedule of rewards and punishments stipulated depending on exam performance. Any student whose knowledge and skills exceeded those of his tutors could be invited to replace his tutor, whilst those who failed to meet the standard required for graduation within nine years were expelled. In this way students' knowledge and progress was strictly assessed; the most talented were recognised and promoted and the less gifted were excluded from further study. Those who were expelled would still have been well placed to follow medical careers in the community, akin to the owners of the medical brass plates seen a few decades ago in some cities in India that make proud declarations such as 'Dr Sunil Bharti MBChB, London University (Failed)'.

TEACHING AT TAI YI SHU

All four departments in Tai Yi Shu based their teaching on a structured curriculum designed to integrate theory with practice, so a significant part of the training involved clinical placement. In the internal medicine department tuition was given by senior physicians holding the rank of 'chief 8th grade scholar' or higher. Their work was supported by assistant lecturers who were required to hold a rank above 'sub-9th grade scholar'.

General medical theory was studied from the main classical texts of the time, such as the *Suwen*, *Shennong Bencao Jing* and Wang Shu-he's *Mai Jing*. Having mastered the basics of medicine students then progressed to more specialist study in departments such as internal medicine, surgery (mainly traumatology and the care of sores and swellings), paediatric medicine, and 'ear, eye, mouth and teeth'. Those studying internal medicine were required to be skilled in identifying the *bencao* substances as well as knowing their properties, and so students were made familiar with the dried pharmacy materials and with herb cultivation in the pharmacy gardens.

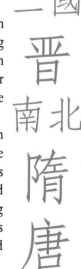

三國晉北南隋唐

The chief acupuncture physician professor was supported by acupuncture lecturers and teaching assistants. Subjects studied included the *jing-luo* channels and acupoints, the illnesses associated with the individual pulse pictures and the various acupuncture needling methods used for supplementation and draining. In their studies of pulse and channel palpation the students learned the classical literature on the subject in addition to taking each other's pulses to experience and learn the various qualities. They were taught to identify *shi* excess and *xu* vacuity of the five *zang* organs in order to determine the appropriate methods to apply. Set texts for acupuncture students included the *Lingshu* (Spiritual Pivot), Huangfu Mi's *Jiayi Jing* and *Ming Tang Mai Jue* (Vessels from the Bright Hall). The curriculum also stipulated that students should learn the *Liu Zhu Yan Ce* medical cosmology diagram, *Chi Ma Lun* (Red Horse Canon) and the *Shenzhen* (Spiritual Needle) text. To learn point location acupuncturists studied *Ming Tang* charts and were also required to demonstrate their ability to locate acupoints on live subjects.

The *anmo* (massage and traumatology) training lasted a total of seven years and was taught by specialist physicians with a specific rank – 'below sub-9th grade'. The physical therapies taught in this course of study were applied mainly in rheumatology and to relieve the 'eight illnesses': namely, those caused by wind, cold, heat, dampness, hunger, overeating and 'disharmony of work and rest'. A key aspect of the theoretical doctrine used in *anmo* study was that physical illness resulted from blockage of the *jing-luo* channels of the limbs or, sometimes more deeply, of the *zangfu* of the body. Massage and physical therapies functioned to disperse and guide *qi* and blood so that internal illness could not become established and so that exterior attack and injury could be resisted. One style of treatment was the 'instructing–inducing' method that originated in Chao Yuan-fang's *Zhubing Yuanhou Lun*. This was an extension of massage for physical injury and consisted of various physical therapeutic manipulations that are akin to osteopathic or chiropractic manipulation methods used today.

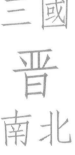

Incantation medicine, based on Buddhist and Daoist beliefs, was taught by specialists whose instruction was founded on the notion that these methods were able to treat some illnesses by expelling malign spirits or by making appeals to the medicine Buddha. It is likely that a high proportion of the cases deemed appropriate for this approach would involve neurological and psychiatric conditions such as epilepsy and psychosis as well as clinical situations that were refractory to other methods. Doubtless this alternative psychotherapeutic approach delivered useful results in suitable cases or gave succour to the terminally ill.

Pharmacy section

Tai Yi Shu employed two officials in overall charge of pharmacy management; four librarian clerks managed documentation and books, and eight chief pharmacists and 24 youth pharmacists were assigned to menial tasks such as slicing and grinding herbs. A 50-acre herb garden was established so that pharmacists could be trained in the cultivation, identification and optimal harvesting and storage of medicinal substances. Students at Tai Yi Shu also went on field excursions to collect special wild substances that needed to be collected from the mountains and remote regions. On graduation they had the chance of being selected for official positions as Tai Yi Shu masters.

A product of the economic stability, political will and good organisation of the time, Tai Yi Shu was the world's first state-sponsored medical school; it operated on a scale and organisational level that remained unmatched anywhere in the world for centuries. It arose partly as a development of the ongoing success of the imperial examinations system as a way of creating a well-governed and ordered society administered by gentlemen scholars, an approach that may have gradually filtered westward to influence mediaeval European political organisation. Two centuries later, in 9th-century Italy, Salaro Medical School was founded, but this small-scale endeavour took a further two centuries to reach maturity. The idea of state-regulated medicine, along with other Sui and Tang ideas for the creation of a harmonious society, were carried forward into the subsequent Song dynasty where they continued to expand and develop under imperial auspices. (These later developments are discussed in the next chapter.)

In addition to the creation of the imperial Tai Yi Shu, in the first century of Tang rule attempts were also made to improve the quality of healthcare for the wider population by setting up provincial medical schools to train local doctors. These altruistic efforts were intended to provide further training to existing physicians and to treat local people, but they proved difficult to maintain, largely because it was difficult to recruit and motivate provincial professors and tutors who were designated as office managers, the lowest possible status that the imperial medical service offered.

In another public-spirited initiative Emperor Xuan Song (ruled +713–755), presiding at the peak of Tang imperial grandeur, personally arranged for the distribution of a *bencao* text and a formula collection (*Guang Zhi Fang*, Formulas for Widespread Benefaction) to the provinces. Despite the fact that the state was now facing escalating challenges to its governance, benevolent attempts to improve public health continued, and in +796 Emperor De Song personally compiled a formula text, *Chen Yuan Guang Li Fang* (Satisfying Prescriptions for Widespread Benefit), for dispatch to every prefecture. The belief was that the availability of better medical literature would improve the health of the population and demonstrate that the ruling classes cared about people in the provinces, thereby contributing to the stability of the regime. Ironically this desire to disseminate China's classical medical heritage turned out to be more successful in spreading knowledge to surrounding countries than to its own people.

The Japanese had previously been exposed to acupuncture in +562 when the physician Zhi Cong went to Japan, taking with him various textbooks on the subject. A year or two later Liang dynasty Emperor Wendi presented the Japanese court with a copy of Huangfu Mi's *Jiayi Jing* (A to Z of Acumoxa). Then, in +608, a delegation of Japanese scholars came to China to study medicine for 15 years before

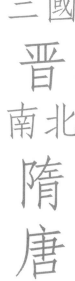

returning home with many texts, including Chao Yuan-fang's pathology text and Sun Si-miao's *Qianjin Yao Fang*. These interactions helped establish traditions of Han and Tang dynasty medicine in Japan, an influence that has survived to the present day. As a result of such interactions, some medical writings that have been lost in China have been preserved in Japan. As well as its transportation eastwards to Japan, Chao Yuan-fang's pathology text was also amongst those selected for translation by Arabic scholars in the 9th century. Next we examine the lives and work of some medical scholars of this era, starting with Chao Yuan-fang.

Key figures in Sui and Tang medicine
Chao Yuan-fang (+550–630)

Chao Yuan-fang authored one of the most outstanding contributions to medical literature in the Sui dynasty and became Emperor Yang Di's chief physician. In +610 Chao was appointed as chief of an editorial board at Tai Yi Shu, and was ordered to compile a comprehensive textbook on the aetiology and pathology of disease. The resulting 50-volume work was entitled *Zhubing Yuanhou Lun* (Treatise on the Origin and Symptoms of Diseases). It is also known as *Chao Shi Bing Yuan* (Master Chao's Origins of Illness), and is Chinese medicine's earliest surviving medical encyclopaedia detailing general disease aetiology.

Zhubing Yuanhou Lun

Using the language and ideas of Han dynasty classical medical doctrine, Chao and his team collated and systematised what was known about the pathogenesis of 1739 symptoms and diseases up until the Sui dynasty. They classified illness under 67 categories such as internal medicine, surgery, gynaecology, paediatrics, ophthalmology, dermatology and ear-nose-throat-teeth medicine. These writings provided detailed and generally quite accurate descriptions of many illnesses including a range of epidemic, parasitic and infectious diseases. The wide-ranging discussions of aetiology combine classical theory with the innovative thinking arising from the clinical experience of Chao and many other contributors to the work. Just as Tao Hong-jing had done before him, Chao condemned the use of the toxic mineral longevity elixirs that continued to be advocated by Daoist practitioners.

Building on Ge Hong's descriptions of epidemic diseases, Chao recognised that, in addition to the traditional climatic attack category of diseases, some acute epidemic illnesses (then called *yi li* and *shi qi*) were transmitted from person to person. These illnesses were characterised by their tendency to indiscriminately affect both young and old, and by having a pattern of more or less identical symptoms and signs.

In his section on parasitic diseases, Chao wrote that 'roundworms may be six to twelve inches in length; they gravitate to weakened organs causing abdominal pain and swelling and excessive salivation'. 'Pinworms,' he wrote, 'are smaller in length and also proliferate when the *zangfu* become weakened.' Chao described many other types of parasitic infection. Discussing schistosomiasis (*shui du hou*, water toxicity disease), he said the disease was prevalent 'east of San Wu [in today's Jiangsu province] and in the streams and valleys of the southern mountain areas'. He said that it was contracted by 'bathing in contaminated waters in the summer, the pathogen hibernates in the soil in winter', and by 'paddling or bathing in water in summer, or when rain water floods into people's houses…'

On the clinical picture of acute schistosomiasis Chao says:

> …at onset the person feels chilly and has a mild headache with pain around orbit and an anxious feeling internally… They suffer in the morning and by the evening symptoms become severe…including bloody diarrhoea… Some have a high temperature, abdominal discomfort, they stop eating and begin talking madly, the stools become like rotten liver.

Chao detailed the sources and routes of spread of many types of wound infection. One example, he observed, occurred when toxins entered the skin through a wound, '[for example] the patient may develop an open sore from horse riding. The mixed toxins from sweat, dirt, urine and stool on the horse's fur enters the sore; initially this causes pain and fever and this eventually causes death.' Tetanus was identified as a specific illness that, Chao said, was associated with incised wounds, or due to peri-natal infection, especially in infants who developed umbilical infections. *Zhubing Yuanhou Lun* also outlined the points of differentiation that allow the distinctions to be drawn between tetanus, stroke and epilepsy.

Chao recognised that allergic diseases were sometimes related to individual constitution. For example, on lacquer dermatitis he wrote, 'Whether male or female, young or old, there are some who are intolerant to lacquer becoming poisoned immediately on exposure to paint or newly painted furniture. Others though are tolerant to lacquer paints and are able to boil them everyday without any adverse reactions.'

In urology Chao said that the kidneys were the origin of *shi lin* (stone dysuria), and that this in turn was the result of disorders of body metabolism. He wrote, '*Lin* disease with the passing of stones is called *shi lin*. The kidneys are in charge of water. Fluids can precipitate stone and grit which then reside as guests in the kidneys.' Discussing causes of infertility, Chao maintained that the fault was not, as was often assumed, with the wife; in some cases, the dysfunction was on the male side. The section on scabies says, 'The itchy scabies sores (*jie chuang*) always contain a tiny worm. We can extract it with a needle and see its worm-like shape when it is dropped into water… More often than not *jie chuang* first appears between the fingers and toes. Babies often acquire it from the mother if she herself is infected.'

Apart from the above, numerous other diseases were described in detail, including: stroke, rheumatoid arthritis, tuberculosis, acute febrile diseases, scarlet fever, cholera, smallpox, leprosy, malaria, oedema, ascites, jaundice, diabetes, beriberi, mental problems, haemorrhoid, irregular menses, vaginal discharge, uterine

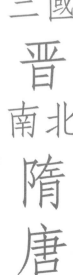

三國晉北南隋唐

prolapse, mastitis, morning sickness, retained lochia, cystitis, anal fistula, carbuncle and many more. Many of those described were conditions that previous medical writers had either failed to identify or had described poorly, so this work represented a considerable advance for the classical medical tradition.

Chao delineated the symptoms of acute stroke: '*Zhong feng*: loss of consciousness, noises in the throat, stiff tongue, inability to speak, absence of sweating, stiff body.' Outlined, too, were the sequelae of stroke: 'Hemiplegia, muscle atrophy, speech often unchanged, this is not a psychiatric disorder.' He said that '*pian feng hou* [wind hemiplegia sequelae] means that the wind pathogen is confined to one half of the body... It is like numbness, unable to feel itching or pain, along with slowness.'

Describing leprosy, Chao said, 'It passes unnoticed when it first enters the skin, it then circulates around the limbs and incubates in the *jing-luo* system, on the face, chest or neck. The skin then begins to feel numb or is itchy as if a worm is wriggling beneath. Objects in front of eyes start to appear smoky.' When leprosy becomes fully established, 'there is widespread itching, sores appear on the face, the body swells and deep pains develop in the bone and marrow... Progressing further the eyebrows and eyelashes fall off, the nasal bridge collapses and the joints begin to come apart... When it erupts from the body there are boils on the face and head the size of walnuts or dates.' Chao said that if symptoms primarily involved 'stiffness with difficulty bending, inability to move hands and feet, pallid complexion, and the patient seems in a trance this is called *zhu dian hou*'. In modern medicine this type is called neuro-leprosy.

In his discussion of diabetes, he wrote that 'the disease called *xiao ke* involves unremitting thirst with polyuria... Those suffering this disease tend to develop carbuncles and gangrene... This is a disease with sweet urine that often begins to develop in those who become obese having overindulged in sweet and rich food.' Written 1400 years ago this description, like so many others in this work, could safely be copied into a modern biomedical textbook.

Discussing beriberi, Chao said:

> ...this is caused by contracting an acute toxicity (*feng du*); normally it is not felt initially...[but as it progresses] symptoms of numbness start in the lower legs with symptoms similar to *bi* (arthritis). There may be a sensation like worms moving, the toes and shin may tingle, the feet may feel too weak to walk or be slightly swollen, bitterly cold, painful, slow and paralysed or stiff and spastic... It may feel as if a finger was moving up from the calf towards the heart or it may involve fever and headaches, or cause palpitations... If treatment is delayed it spreads up to the abdomen, which may or may not be swollen, and there may be distension in chest and hypochondria. When the *qi* sensation travels upward the patient may soon die. In acute cases this will be within the day; if it is chronic then death may be in one, two or three months.

Chao recognised the characteristic hallmark of this disease as:

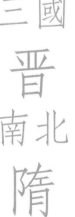

usually progressing from the bottom and moving upwards, so the feet become weak first. The poison follows the course of the *jing-luo* channels before slowly entering the organs; the organs then show signs of *qi ni* (rebellion and counterflow) when attacked by pathogenic *qi*. Because this disease starts in the feet it is called *jiao qi* (foot *qi*).

On scarlet fever:

Fire toxicity attacks the body when it is weak and emerges from the skin. The skin eruptions and rashes (*ban zhen*) have the appearance of brocade; in severe cases the throat and mouth become affected by sores.

Discussing threatened miscarriage in pregnancy, Chao said:

…if a pregnant woman is weak and thin, or has another illness that puts her body in a state that is unable to properly support the foetus so that the pregnancy threatens to harm the woman, the body takes action to get rid of it.

In a quite remarkable section entitled 'Incised wounds that have severed the intestines', *Zhubing Yuanhou Lun* includes a reference to abdominal surgery. Here Chao advised:

For those who have suffered a severed intestine caused by an incised wound we need to investigate to discover if the wound is shallow or deep… When we find the two cut ends of the intestine this must be dealt with very swiftly. First use a needle and thread to connect the severed intestine, then use chicken blood to rub the suture so as to prevent the *qi* [in the intestines] from escaping, then push the intestines back into place.

Another section headed '[Blood] vessel injury following tooth extraction' said:

…if the extraction of a tooth damages the blood vessels then non-stop bleeding occurs. The result is that the *zang* organs become weakened and [the person] will feel dizzy.

Further examples of Chao's innovations are seen in the chapter on 'Pudendal polyps', where the growths are described as 'looking like the nipples of mice'. This describes either vulval warts or perhaps the polyps of the uterine cervix. Another example of Chao's broader systematic approach is seen in his classification of gynaecological diseases. These he put under five headings: general problems, pregnancy disorders, problems at the onset of labour, difficult labour and post-natal complications. This created a structure for disease classification that was used by later generations.

Actual clinical case histories from the Tang dynasty are scarce, but Chao's work is useful because it shows us that medical treatment at that time encompassed dental extractions, emergency surgical procedures and gynaecological examination. And because meticulous care was being applied in describing and differentiating disease

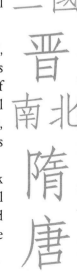

states, medical conditions were not simply characterised in the classical terms of *yin-yang*, *qi*, hot-cold, *jing-luo* and so on.

Another innovation of *Zhubing Yuanhou Lun* was that it provided schemas that allowed symptoms and diseases to be clearly ordered and categorised; this was valuable because it helped clinicians to more easily find information relevant to a case on hand. As medical knowledge expanded and textbooks became more densely content-rich reference texts, there was a need to find ways of indexing the information. One sign that this issue was uppermost in Chao's mind was his placement of discussions on acute and emergency illnesses at the front so that it could be more easily found in emergency situations. He put the discussions of diseases into clear and well-ordered categories, and separated these from the chapters on *zangfu* pattern differentiation. For example, he discussed *xiao-ke* (diabetes), *jiaoqi* (beriberi) and jaundice as individual diseases in separate chapters; elsewhere spleen-stomach disorders such as vomiting and indigestion were collected together.

The remarkable achievement we see in *Zhubing Yuanhou Lun* demonstrates that Chao and his team of medical scholars had very clear and well-developed ideas about the ways that illnesses could be systematically classified using both disease differentiation (*bian bing*) and pattern discrimination (*bian zheng*). The fact that he was able to make these distinctions is important because it clearly demonstrates that Chinese medicine is primarily a practical and rational medicine and not primarily a medicine of speculative metaphysical doctrine. It shows that both *bian bing* disease differentiation and *bian zheng* pattern differentiation were recognised as parallel models serving medical practice, and that both were appropriate dimensions of diagnosis and treatment. And also, that skilled practice involved an understanding of the relationship between these two – an understanding that is often missing in modern Western practice of Chinese medicine. This important insight counters the suggestion by modern commentators that classical Chinese medicine was concerned purely with speculative and metaphysical abstractions and did not understand real illness and its treatment. Chao focused heavily on accurately describing and differentiating real diseases and guiding physicians toward pragmatic medical practice.

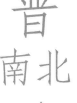

Zhubing Yuanhou Lun covers a vast array of material – its content is complex and varied. It focuses less on therapeutics and more on detailed descriptions of symptoms that were gathered both from historical texts and from the experience of his peers. Applying an encyclopaedic yet discerning approach to his subject matter, Chao exerted a significant influence on later generations by adding a new level of clarity and criticality to medical study. Many important medical writings that appeared subsequently, such as Sun Si-miao's *Qian Jin Yao Fang*, Wang Tao's *Waitai Miyao* and the early Song dynasty *Taiping Shenghui Fang* (Taiping Era Formulas from Benevolent Sages, Wang Huai-yin, 992), quoted Chao's discussions and opinions either directly or indirectly.

As one of the most important medical texts of the Sui and Tang dynasties, the value of *Zhubing Yuanhou Lun* was soon recognised, and it became one of the main textbooks used to teach medical skills in the Tang and Song dynasties, and so it strongly influenced the subsequent course of Chinese medical history. Indeed, as touched on earlier, the influence of *Zhubing Yuanhou Lun* was not limited to medical scholarship in China; the medical knowledge it contained was exported to Japan, and its contents travelled westward, where it made a significant contribution to the medicine espoused by the Arabic scholar Ibn-Sina (+981–1037). Avicenna, as he is also known, used Chao's pathology text as a major source in writing his *Al-Qann fi al-Tibb* (Canon of Medicine) that was completed in about +1025. Subsequently then translated into various European languages, the *Canon of Medicine* came to influence the understanding of pathology in Europe in early mediaeval times when it was a required text for many European universities, until the 18th century. Another text accessed by Avicenna's text also presented information on pulse diagnosis that was taken from Wang Shu-he's *Mai Jing*, and 24 of the pulse types described in his *Canon* are the same as those used in Chinese medicine. The Arabic route also brought writings on medical jurisprudence from China to Northern Europe; this is discussed in Chapter 6 on Jin-Yuan dynasty medicine.

Sun Si-miao (+581–682)

Sun Si-miao, also known as Sun Zhen-ren (True Man Sun), was an eminent Daoist and Buddhist who was later to be immortalised in Chinese culture as a god of medicine. Born in what is now Shaanxi province, Sun began formal education aged seven and studied medicine from the age of 18. Legend has it that within two years he was practising on his neighbours. Later in life, partly as a result of his deep understanding of Daoism, Buddhism and Confucianism, Sun was offered a post as medical adviser by the Tang Emperors Taizong and Gaozong, but he soon resigned, saying he preferred to continue with his medical studies and writing. Many case histories appear in his writings, although it is now thought that Sun devoted more of his attention to studying medicine and collecting information than to practical clinical practice. In the course of his work he made numerous important contributions to the medical tradition – indeed, his intellectual power and scope verges on the superhuman, so we should devote some space here to detail his contributions.

Sun Si-miao is revered for compiling the major medical classic of the Tang dynasty, *Qian Jin Yao Fang* (Prescriptions Worth 1000 Gold Pieces), a title shortened from *Bei Ji Qian Jin Yao Fang* (Formulas for Every Emergency Worth a Thousand in Gold). The 'thousand in gold' title concept refers to Sun's view that human life was as precious as gold. Completed in +652, this 30-volume encyclopaedia of existing medical knowledge contained descriptions of the medical practices of the time including herbal treatment, acumoxa, massage, dietetics, physical therapies and *yang sheng* (health-preservation practices). Drawing on numerous sources, Sun listed herb formulas and techniques also gleaned from his study of folk practitioners' methods. Many of the herbal formulas he cites are still in use today, one example being *wei jing tang*, which remains a key prescription used to treat early-stage lung abscess.

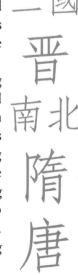

三國晋南北隋唐

Later, towards the end of his life, Sun produced another 30-volume sister text, *Qian Jin Yi Fang* (Wings to the Thousand in Gold Prescriptions), that corrected omissions from his first book and added two chapters that present Zhang Zhong-jing's *Shang Han Lun*. Both works include material on incantation and therapeutic magic, reflecting the fact that Sun could stand comfortably with one foot in plain rationality and the other planted in the arcane world of Daoist and Buddhist mysticism. Sun is credited with writing various other texts, but these are thought likely to have been retrospectively attributed to him. The character *yi* in the title of the second book means 'wing', and the two books together Sun envisaged as the two wings needed for medicine to take flight.

As we will see, when discussing general pathology and medicine, Sun described and classified a wide range of disease entities, thereby advancing the understanding of disease differentiation (*bian bing*). Basic pattern differentiation (*bian zheng*) approaches using *zangfu shi* and *xu* and heat-cold concepts are mentioned, and Sun advocated the use of the four diagnostic methods (*si zhen*, namely looking, asking, listening and palpation). He wrote that physicians should initially listen to the patient's voice, then observe their complexion, and then take their pulse.

> ### QIAN JIN YAO FANG: MAIN CONTENTS
> Gynaecology
>
> Paediatrics
>
> Diseases of the seven orifices
>
> Wind toxin *jiao qi* (foot *qi*)
>
> Various wind and *shang han* formulas
>
> Formulas for *zangfu* diseases
>
> *Xiao-ke* (diabetes)
>
> *Lin* and other urinary tract diseases
>
> Edema, boils, swellings, carbuncles
>
> Haemorrhoids
>
> Toxin resolving
>
> Emergency medicine
>
> Dietary treatment
>
> Temperament cultivation
>
> Pulse diagnosis
>
> *Ming Tang* (Bright Hall)
>
> 5300 herb formulas are included
>
> 232 acupoints described

SUN SI-MIAO AND INFECTIOUS DISEASES

Sun is one of the very few pre-Song physicians to make any mention of the *Shang Han Lun*. He divided externally contracted febrile illnesses into 12 types based on their clinical appearance, and recommended specific *Shang Han Lun* formulas for their treatment. For cold attack, he said that *ma hang tang*, *gui zhi tang* and *qing long tang* were the main formulas. Apart from acute exterior conditions, Sun advocated other *Shang Han Lun* formulas such as the harmonising formula *xiao chaihu tang* for use when the three methods of attack (emesis, purgation and diaphoresis) had proved ineffective. Also in the style of the *Shang Han Lun*, he wrote that *taiyang* stage disease could be subdivided into syndromes such as *gui zhi tang* pattern, *ma huang tang* pattern, *xiao qing long tang* pattern, *xiao chai hu tang* pattern and others. Included, too, were the more internal *shang han* patterns – *yangming*, *shaoyang*, *taiyin*, *shaoyin* and *jueyin* – and he gave his opinion on the applicability and contraindications of the various treatment methods described in the *Shang Han Lun*. Sun discussed the appropriate use of the three methods of pathogen removal (exterior release, emesis

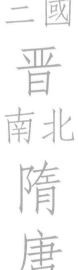

and draining downwards), when it was appropriate to use warmth or to clear fire and so on; he also mentioned the applicability of acupuncture and moxibustion in *shang han* illness. Given that for much of Chinese medicine history the *shang han* methodologies were generally considered part of herb practice, Sun's discussions demonstrate that acupuncture was also applied in the Tang dynasty for these illnesses. Keen to promote practical medicine, Sun included analyses of patients' symptom changes to be expected in response to diaphoretic, emetic and purgative treatments.

Sun Si-miao's writings show remarkable insights into some of the ways that infectious illnesses were propagated. He said that diseases such as cholera and dysentery were caused not, as some believed, by malevolent spirits, but by contaminated food and drink. For this reason he advocated preventative measures such as the disinfection of well water, eating properly washed and cooked food, fumigation of the air in sickrooms, and urging people not to spit. From today's health and safety perspective his choice of sterilising agents such as arsenic and mercury compounds, although probably effective, was perhaps a little suspect.

He considered pulmonary tuberculosis to be an infectious condition of the lungs. In other types of infection he employed herbs now understood to have antibiotic and anti-inflammatory properties, such as *huang lian* (Rhizoma coptidis) and *bai tou weng* (Pulsatilla root) to treat dysentery, and *chang shan* (Dichroa febrifuga root) to treat malaria. These are all herbs that have been found to be pharmacologically effective today. In the footsteps of Chao Yuan-fang, Sun concurred, saying that diabetic patients were especially prone to skin infections, and for this reason Sun said that these patients should avoid being given acupuncture. He also advised that patients with oedema should avoid salt, and advocated the activation of blood circulation for those with late-stage oedema. Again, in the light of modern medicine, we can appreciate this generally sensible advice today. Also sensible, and in line with his 'be prepared' philosophy, Sun advocated having ready-made medicines ready for emergency use to avoid delays in starting treatment.

NUTRITION AND DIET

Sun Si-miao was also interested in nutritional factors in disease development. He realised that some illnesses were due to dietary deficiencies and, once again, many of his conclusions are remarkably accurate.

Sun treated goitre (*ying* disease) with seaweed and shellfish, and advocated that these be transported to inland and highland areas where iodine deficiency goitre was endemic. For other thyroid deficiencies he prescribed preparations made from animal thyroid glands, and for poor night vision he recommended increased dietary intake of liver. To treat beriberi he used substances now known to contain high levels of vitamin B such as grain husks and herbs such as *du huo, han fang ji, fang feng, ma huang* and *wu zhu yu*. Sun believed that diet was the foundation of good health – diet, he said, should be the medicine of first resort, and drug treatment should begin when dietary regulation had failed. One chapter in Sun's *Qian Jin Yao Fang* describes the medicinal properties of foods; here he says that learning the positive

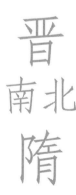

and negative effects on the body of the five tastes was key to a balanced diet. In Sun's view, a really excellent physician was able to bring together skills in dietary treatment, drug therapy and acumoxa. One of Sun's followers, Meng Shen, further developed his master's ideas in a text devoted to dietary therapy.

SUN SI-MIAO ON DIET

'…food can dispel pathogens and harmonise the *zangfu*, delight the spirit, relax mood and support blood and *qi*. Those who have the ability to remove illness and relax mood with diet can be called good doctors.'

'The foundations of health must come from diet.'

'…doctors should first know the course of the illness, treat it first with diet, then give medicine.'

'Do not eat excessively, too much food causes accumulation, drinking too much causes phlegm…chronic alcohol drinking rots the intestines and stomach, soaks the marrow and steams the tendons, harms the spirit and reduces life span.'

'…after a light breakfast use warm hands to rub your stomach, take a fifty-yard walk and then rest. After lunch, again use warm hands and walk one or two hundred yards, going slowly and taking time; do not let the *qi* rush. After walking return to bed to lie down, spread hands and feet, don't sleep; in a minute the qi becomes sufficient, then sit up… When the stomach feels empty attend to this instantly, don't be starved… During autumn and winter we should keep a warm stomach. If stomach feels upset take *hou po sheng jiang* decoction. Keep to a lifestyle like this and we avoid premature death.'

Medical teachings such as those collected by Sun Si-miao are unlikely to have been reached by random guesswork or superstition; some form of rational and investigative process is implied. It is unfortunate for modern perceptions of the medicine and proto-sciences in ancient China that the actual methods of discovery and investigation used to make these discoveries were generally omitted in these texts. With textual space at a premium, the important thing to convey was the knowledge itself, the utility of which could be re-checked in clinical practice. As the later Zhou dynasty founder of Daoism Zhuang-zi said, 'When the rabbit is caught you can forget the snare.'

Sun Si-miao and gynaecology

Sun Si-miao believed that the care of women and babies was of prime importance, so he placed these discussions prominently at the beginning of his books. The first book included discussions on fertility, pregnancy, obstetrics, post-partum deficiency diseases, menstruation, discharge, growths and tumours and miscellaneous diseases in gynaecology. He also introduced a 'women's facial formula' for beauty therapy.

Sun Si-miao pioneered the study of gynaecology and obstetrics, and wrote extensively on these subjects, offering rational advice and treatment in relation to menstruation, pregnancy and delivery. The chapter on fertility said that low male fertility resulted from a decline in *jing qi*, which could be treated with *qi zi san* (seven seed powder) or *qing zi san* (child celebration powder). Poor fertility in women, Sun said, was due to various *xu* and *shi* diseases, such as the 36 *xia jiao* (lower burner) ailments, treatable with formulas such as *che zeng wan, da huang wan, bai wei wan* and *qin jiao wan.*

He advised that pregnant women should 'bide their time in a simple and peaceful place…with a regulated heart *shen*, maintaining a harmonious mood, avoiding overindulgence and cravings so that everything is peaceful'. During labour itself, Sun said, 'it is important to discourage observers from attending; a couple of people to hand is quite sufficient'. He also discussed Xu Zhi-cai's *Zhu Yue Yang Tai Fang* that advocated supportive care that altered month-by-month based on the idea that each month a different *jing* channel provides

SUN SI-MIAO'S FOETAL NOURISHMENT THEORY	
Month	*Jing* channel active
1	Liver
2	Gallbladder
3	Heart
4	*Sanjiao*
5	Spleen
6	Stomach
7	Lungs
8	Large intestine
9	Kidney

nourishment for the foetus. Much later this theory was to be derided as nonsensical by Wang Qing-ren in his *Yi Lin Gai Cuo* (On the Correction of Medical Errors) of 1810.

Sun lists many formulas for obstetric disorders including eclampsia, dead foetus, retention of the placenta, miscarriage, abortion, lactation promotion, retention of lochia, and profuse uterine bleeding in pregnancy and delivery. The treatments he assembled helped inform future developments in obstetrics and gynaecology for Chinese medicine.

PAEDIATRICS

Sun was also a pioneer in paediatric medicine and gave practical and sensible pointers on the care of the newborn child and infant. The discussions on paediatrics in *Qian Jin Yao Fang* cover breastfeeding problems, neonatal disorders, children's fright epilepsy (*jing xian*), 'guest unruliness' (*ke wu*), neonatal *shang han* attack, cough, elusive mass and accumulation (*pi jie*), carbuncle and *zu* (*yong zu*) and lymphadenitis (*luo li*), as well as various miscellaneous paediatric ailments such as enuresis.

Written much later in his life, his *Qian Jin Yi Fang* aimed to cover the omissions in *Qian Jin Yao Fang*; it added more information on children's physiology and diseases of the eyes, nose, ears, mouth and throat. Sun's unceasing innovative spirit, evident in both texts, introduced numerous new ideas to the classical medical tradition. As soon as a baby was born, he advised, 'Wrap your finger with cotton and wipe away any old blood from the baby's mouth and tongue… Failure to do this immediately means that as soon as the baby cries the material will be swallowed and may cause various diseases.' Advising on neonatal care, Sun wrote that 'the flesh and skin of neonates is not yet mature; the baby should not be wrapped in very warm clothes which will make the sinews and bones weak. Instead, it is best to expose the baby

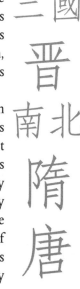

三國晉南北隋唐

to the wind and sun now and then. If this is not done the flesh and skin may become brittle and soft and vulnerable to attack. It is better to use clothes made of old material that has been worn soft rather than new cotton.' Also: 'If the weather is warm and not too windy, mother should take her baby to play in the sunshine allowing it to be exposed to gentle sun and breeze.' In relation to breastfeeding he advised, 'Don't overfeed babies; an overfed baby will vomit. If the baby vomits due to overfeeding use an empty breast to feed the baby and the vomiting will stop.' It is very likely that much of this wisdom had been gleaned from midwives, and suggests that one of Sun's skills was the ability to charm tips and trade secrets from experts in the wider medical community.

Regarding children's fevers he wrote, 'Infants do not venture into the frost so they are less prone to *shang han* (cold attack), but if the weather is abnormal they may contract such illnesses. Sometimes though, when a baby is delivered during epidemic years, he may develop a rash straightaway. Treatment is same as treating adults except that the dosage must be small.' Sun's descriptions of asphyxia and children's skin problems are very practical and sensible, and his writings on paediatrics inspired later Chinese childcare specialists including the great Song dynasty paediatrician Qian Yi in the writing of his famed *Xiaoer Yaozheng Zhi Jue*.

TRAUMATOLOGY

Qian Jin Yao Fang includes discussions on traumatology including a resuscitation method for 'sudden death' taken from Zhang Zhong-jing. He describes the use of compresses to relieve pain and cautery (*shao luo*, burning and ironing) to stop bleeding due to trauma. He describes improvements to Ge Hong's treatment of simple fractures using splints, and added new methods of setting and reducing dislocated fractures and the reduction of dislocation of the mandible. *Qian Jin Yao Fang* also introduced some massage techniques (*lao zi*, massage) that are still applied in orthopaedic departments in Chinese hospitals today.

GENERAL MEDICINE

In Sun's writings on general internal medicine practice, we find an early form of *zangfu* pattern differentiation that categorises illnesses into 11 groups, according to which five *zang* and six *fu* needed regulating to correct the patient's illness. For example, illnesses that manifest the presence of hard masses and accumulations pointed to a need for treatment of the liver; chest *bi* (obstruction) suggested a need to treat the heart; dysentery belonged to the liver; vomiting blood belonged to the gallbladder; *jing dian* (fright and withdrawal) belonged to the small intestine; and cough, phlegm and thin mucus illnesses belonged to the large intestine. The merits or otherwise of this system were a subject for debate amongst later generations of physicians.

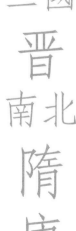

Sun Si-miao and acumoxa

Whilst the bulk of his writings present herb prescriptions, Sun Si-miao advocated both acupuncture and moxibustion therapy, saying: 'It is mistaken to employ just acupuncture and neglect moxibustion and vice versa; it is also wrong to use these and neglect medicinals and vice versa.' 'A good physician,' he continued, 'knows both acupuncture and herbs.' He is credited with making some important contributions to acumoxa practice, and some credit him with devising the proportional measurement system that enabled acupoints to be accurately located regardless of body size and physique. Chapters 29 and 30 of his *Qian Jin Yao Fang* focus on clinical acumoxa. Assuming access to Huangfu Mi's *Jiayi Jing* and existing basic knowledge of acupuncture in his readership, the text omits explanations on how to locate acupoints; instead Sun focuses on practical applications, such as the clinical use of the five *shu* points and specific guidance to the selection of the most appropriate acupoints. Incorporating many extra points outside the *jing-luo* system he also stressed the importance of identifying *ahshi* (spontaneously tender) acupoints in practice. Advocating moxibustion as a mainstay of preventative medicine, he said that it could be used on points such as *zu san li* for maintaining health and preventing disease. Again, these are important aspects of modern practice.

Sun Si-miao's contributions to herb and formula study

A natural investigator and polymath, Sun personally researched many aspects of herbal medicine and its prescriptions. Not content with fluency in the medicine of his time, he was driven to seek improvement. His *Qian Jin Yao Fang* includes a *bencao* section consisting of over 700 substances arranged according to the *Shennong Bencao* classification of upper, middle and lower class herbs (a scheme discussed earlier in Chapter 3). He embarked on mountain herb-collecting field expeditions to research and improve the identification, cultivation, harvesting, quality control and processing of hundreds of herbs. Sun realised that without accurate identification of the correct substances, the value of the herbal medicine tradition would be lost; this realisation meant that his understanding of pharmacognosy was by far the most detailed, systematic and penetrating of his time. As a result of this obsession, Sun acquired in his lifetime the informal epithet 'King of Herbs'.

In Sun's opinion, the efficacy of herbal medicine is directly related to the correct timing of herb collection and to the use of appropriate methods of processing: 'Herbs collected without proper knowledge of timing are no better than dead wood, they are a waste of labour and have no effect.' Physicians, he said, had a responsibility to know the source of the medicinals they prescribed. Accordingly, *Qian Jin Yi Fang* mentions the provinces from which most substances originated, and categorised roughly 800 of them according to function, together with data on the collection, processing and applications for 238 of these.

Sun also contributed to systematising the understanding of the dynamic relationships between herbs in formulas. These were discussed in the terms used in the *Shennong Bencao* such as mutual engenderment (*xiang sheng*) and mutual killing

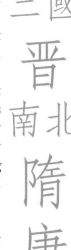

(*xiang sha*), as well as the prescription organisation schemes based on the roles played by chief herbs, assistants and envoys.

SUN SI-MIAO ON THE HARMONIOUS PAIRING OF MEDICINALS

Sovereign and minister manage each other; assistant and envoy support each other. Some doctors, in ignorance of the classics, make modifications as they see fit, such that herb and mineral suppress each other. Rather than treating diseases, when ingested, they add to the fight. Herb and mineral can oppose each other, making the patient confused with a force even stronger than knife and needle. When [formulas are] mixed and harmonised properly, even if the disease is not cured, still the five organs are calmed [and at least] the disease is not made worse.

Sun wrote that established formulas should be modified flexibly according to the patient's *zheng* pattern as opposed to the habit of some physicians to prescribe fixed formulas for main complaints. In other words, he advised formulas matched to the individual rather than simply aimed at the disease condition. For instance, when discussing Zhang Zhong-jing's *xiao jian zhong tang*, used to warm and harmonise the stomach, he created new variants based on subtypes he had seen of the main patterns, thereby applying the principle of treating the same basic *bing* disease with different formulas. He also gave many examples of the inverse principle of treating different conditions using the same basic formula. In total, Sun's two main clinical manuals describe roughly 6500 formulas.

Sun set down numerous ancient formulas that he had gleaned from both the classical and folk traditions, and so

---

SUN'S VARIATIONS ON XIAO JIAN ZHONG TANG

Qian hu jian zhong tang

Huang qi tang

Nei bu dang gui jian zhong tang

Nei bu xiong qiong tang

Da bu zhong dang gui tang

---

helped save them for posterity. Examples include *xijiao di huang tang* and *zi xue dan*. Some of Sun's formulas were later to form the basis of new formulas; his *nei bu san* (internal tonic powder), for example, was the source of Liu Wan-su's *di huang yin zi* in the Song dynasty, and Sun's *di huang wan* was to inspire the various sweet-cold fluid-nourishing formulas developed by the Qing dynasty *wen bing* febrile disease school roughly a thousand years later.

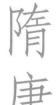

Notable Sun Si-miao formulas	Used for
Ding zhi wan	Settling disturbed emotional states
Du-huo ji sheng tang	Wind-cold-damp arthritis with *xu*
Wei jing tang	Early stages of lung abscess
Wei-rui tang	Exterior wind fevers
Xiao xu ming tang	Stroke due to wind-cold invasion with *xu*
Xi-jiao di-huang tang	High fevers

ETHICS

Sun Si-miao is also remembered for his humanitarian and ethical stance in relation to medical practice. 'Life,' he said, 'is more precious than a thousand gold coins and to save a life is to do good that is worth more than a thousand gold coins' – hence the titles of his books. He is reputed never to have refused to treat a patient and to have treated rich and poor with equal respect. Sun provided Chinese medicine its own version of the Hippocratic oath when he wrote:

> Physicians should respond to requests for help by making no distinction between rich and poor, young and old, refined or lowly, friend or foe, foreigner or native, wise or simple. Treat people in the same way you would treat your own family – without discrimination… Treat enthusiastically, regardless of your own fatigue, hunger and thirst, whether by day or night, summer or winter. Show genuine sympathy for the sick and provide care as if you yourself were stricken. Do not be hindered even by high mountain and rugged paths.

Sun's strong Buddhist and ethical outlook served to inspire a higher level of responsibility in medical practice. He demanded that physicians be exemplary in character by avoiding overindulgence and excess of all kinds and by resisting sexual temptation in clinical practice.

Sun believed that physicians should study the Confucian classics including *Yijing* (Classic of Changes) as well as the writings of the founders of Daoism such as Laozi and Zhuangzi. Physicians, he said, should understand the importance of the Confucian virtues of *ren* (benevolence) and *yi* (insightful thought). He summed up his understanding of the essence of medicine in a Chinese pun, saying 'medicine is *yi*' (*yi shi yi*); by this he meant that at the core of good medical practice was a special type of insightful, reflective, holistic and strategic thought process. This is reflected in Volker Scheid's translation of Sun's quote as 'medicine is a way of thinking'.

Born into a time where intellectual proto-scientific endeavour included alchemical experimentation, the investigation of transformation processes, Sun also dabbled in this. In his pursuits as an alchemist he mixed saltpetre, sulphur and charcoal together in what has since been acknowledged as the earliest known recipe for gunpowder. He is also believed to be the first to use arsenic as a treatment for malaria, but recognising its potential for toxicity, he preferred to use arsenous trioxide compounded with Chinese date paste, which functioned both as an antidote and a slow-release method. This he prescribed in gradually increasing doses until the effect was sufficient, but with the minimum adverse effect.

Such was Sun's influence that his innovations and his investigative spirit

SUN SI-MIAO (TRANSLATED BY SABINE WILMS)

Whenever people don't live out their lives or the life is cut short, it is always caused by not loving or cherishing themselves, they exhaust their emotions, push their sense of purpose to the extreme, pursue fame and profit, collect poisons and attack their spirit, internally damaging the bone and marrow and externally spoiling the sinews and flesh. The *qi* and blood perish, the channels and the network vessels become congested…

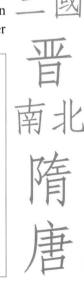

inspired many physicians in China and abroad in countries such as Japan and Korea. Sun's achievements and his contribution to Chinese medicine were so great he comes close to superhuman, and provided inspiration for many generations of physicians and medical thinkers to come.

Wang Tao (+702–772)

Wang Tao was born in 702 and lived to the age of 70. Coming from a distinguished Shaanxi family, Wang Tao's father was a very high-ranking government official, which allowed him to obtain a good education and high official position. As chief curator of the imperial library for 20 years, he could indulge his personal interest in medicine, an interest that is believed to have stemmed from his frequent illnesses as a child and his obligation later in life to care for his ailing mother. His access to the well-stocked Hong Wen library in the imperial palace allowed him to draw on an unequalled range of rare source texts to advance his own scholarship.

As a government official and not a practising professional physician, Wang Tao's contribution was founded more on textual study than clinical practice, so his work is weak on original clinical insights. His strength lay in an ability to collate information from a wide range of sources in a cogent manner. With the outlook of a gentleman scholar he avidly collected prescriptions not only from the Hong Wen library but also from the libraries of local physicians and friends. The eventual outcome of Wang Tao's researches was the completion in 752 of an imposing formula collection, *Waitai Miyao* (Medical Secrets of an Official), an encyclopaedic 40-volume text running to 1140 chapters and containing almost 10,000 formulas. The text covers virtually all branches of medicine and includes most of the treatment methods used in classical medicine up to that time.

Wang Tao opens each chapter with a discussion on the pathology of the disease in question, information that he derived mainly from Chao Yuan-fang's pathology text. This is followed by a listing of the numerous prescriptions he had collected that aimed to treat each condition. Many of the prescriptions he included came from Sun Si-miao's *Qian Jin Yao Fang*, but many others were copied from texts now lost, and this provides the main value of the compendium.

One important scholarly innovation introduced by Wang Tao was the referencing of sources; indeed, not only does he name the source text for each piece of information, he also cites the volume or chapter title where it is to be found. This referencing of his 20 or so main source texts, only five of which survive today, has allowed subsequent generations to access writings from many texts that would otherwise have been completely lost. One interesting example involves a technique that originally came from a text called the *Bi Xiao Fang* (Prescriptions of Certain Effect). This was a way of monitoring progress during the treatment of acute jaundice by soaking white cotton thread in the patient's urine every day. Reduction in colour intensity of the dried threads enabled objective monitoring of improvement or worsening of the condition, thereby facilitating optimal adjustment

三國
晉北
南隋
唐

to treatment. In Volume 11 Wang Tao discusses the diagnosis of diabetes based on testing the sweetness of the patient's urine, a method that had been derived from two lost texts, *Jin Xiao Fang* (Close-by Effective Formulas) and *Gu Jin Lu Yan* (Old and New Effective Records). Volume 29 of Wang's text describes the fixing of fractures using bamboo splints, a method Wang noted had come from *Zhouhou Beiji Fang* (Emergency Prescriptions to Keep Up Your Sleeve) and the *Qian Jin Yao Fang*, but this section has been lost and is no longer found in the surviving editions of these texts.

Wang Tao's section on acumoxa therapy (Volume 39) is noteworthy for presenting an overarching summary of the indications for each point and channel. As well as the 12 main channels, the points on the Ren and Du channel points are discussed and appear here as an appendix to the discussions on the kidney and bladder *jing-luo*, suggesting that, at this time, they were seen as extensions of these channels.

An especially significant aspect of Wang Tao's *Waitai Miyao* (Gatherings of a Frontier Official) is the observation that little or no classical doctrinal information is provided to justify, support or explain the selection of points. This supports the suggestion that the Tang medicine style tended to focus on symptomatic relief by matching disease condition to treatment rather than matching treatment to pattern diagnosis. Significant, too, is the fact that Wang Tao, when discussing acumoxa, advocated moxibustion treatment rather than needles, which suggests that society physicians and their patients, at that time, seem to have become wary of the use of needles.

The *Waitai Miyao* includes medically accurate descriptions of various contagious diseases such as pulmonary tuberculosis, malaria, smallpox and cholera. Patients suffering from tuberculosis, it says, would experience tidal fever, night sweats, afternoon flushes and gradual emaciation; if the condition worsened, then the ominous signs might include dark reddish stools and fluid accumulation in the abdomen. Wang Tao also reported the treatment of oesophageal foreign body obstruction in paediatrics, as well as mentioning some of the ophthalmology treatments that had arrived from India, such as cataract surgery.

The *Waitai Miyao* also gives some good descriptions of the ability of some individual herbs to treat particular diseases, such as the ability of *chang shan* and *shu qi* (the roots and leaves, respectively, of Dichroa febrifuga) to relieve malaria. Many of the formulas suggested for malaria used this herb. In modern times the alkaloids in Dichroa have been found to be about 25 times more potent than quinine as an anti-malarial. This herb had been previously recorded in *Shennong Bencao Jing*, in *Jingui Yao Lue* in the 2nd century and later in Sun Si-miao's *Beiji Qian Jin Yao Fang*. The star anti-malarial herb uncovered from the Chinese tradition by modern Chinese pharmacology researchers turned out to be *qing hao* (Artemesia annua), which has recently become an important part of today's battle against malaria because of its strong effect in killing the malaria plasmodium combined with its very low toxicity. According to the medical journal *The Lancet*, *qing hao* extracts are currently saving the lives of roughly 195,000 African people every year.

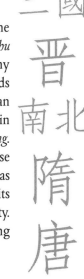

三國晉南北隋唐

As mentioned, in compiling his book Wang Tao was fortunate to be in charge of the Hong Wen library and so could draw on a vast library resource. Working against him, however, was the fact that he was not a trained physician, and because of this his work includes many misconceptions. 'Needles,' he wrote, 'can kill people and are unable to save them from death', which is why his acumoxa discussions were strongly biased in favour of moxibustion. No doubt there had been some notorious adverse events that led to this view.

Waitai Miyao was another of the texts that became widely known and that helped disseminate Chinese medicine, especially to Japan and Korea, and it was this book that contributed most to the establishment of moxibustion as a key therapy in these countries.

Although an enthusiastic and monumental work, Wang's *Waitai Miyao* suffered from a lack of the kind of pragmatic editing and clinical focus that comes from the hand of a trained and experienced physician. Large quantities of information are pasted together to create a vast and unwieldy encyclopaedia, but there is little discussion of theoretical underpinnings. There is no guidance, either, for the practising physician as to what treatments actually work best in practice and why. Other texts from the Tang era suffered from the same flaw – a voluminous tradition was respectfully preserved but with little innovation, editing, critical appraisal or practical focus. The assumption was that medicine could move directly from simple disease identification to treatment without going to the trouble of differentiation of the individual condition or applying the deeper understandings inherent in the classical tradition. It seems likely that Wang Tao did not understand the importance of these aspects.

Important herb formulas that are first seen in Wang Tao's *Waitai Miyao* include *shigao tang* and *huang lian jie du tang*, although a very similar formula to this had appeared earlier in Sun Si-miao's writings under a different name.

Wang Bing

We know very little about the life of Wang Bing (aka Qi Xuan-zi) who worked in the imperial court in the middle of the Tang dynasty. He is believed to have had an interest in medicine from his youth but, like Huangfu Mi a few centuries earlier, he became frustrated about the very garbled state of the surviving editions of the *Neijing*. By Wang Bing's time some sections of the text had become repeated and the order of its passages had become disorganised. The chapters 'Ci Fa Lun' ('Essay on Needle Methods') and 'Ben Bing Lun' ('Essay on the Roots of Disease') were just titles with no surviving text. Determined to restore it, Wang first spent 12 years on a literature search, collecting and studying as many versions as he could find. One edition he obtained was one that had been compiled roughly a century earlier by Yang Shang-shan (c. 575–660), who had revised and annotated the version that had become known as *Tai Su* (Great Simplicity), which was an authentic but incomplete version of the *Neijing*. Yang Shang-shan had also produced an illustrated version called *Huangdi Neijing Mingtang* (The Illustrated *Huangdi Neijing*). Wang Bing said that he had also been fortunate to obtain a rare edition of the *Neijing* from his teacher to use as a benchmark for comparison with other editions. In re-constructing the text he tried to take care to distinguish the original parts of the text from his own commentaries and also from the parts he identified as later annotations to the original. These parts he highlighted by using red ink. In +762 he finished his *Buzhu Huangdi Neijing Suwen* (*buzhu* means annotated), a work that was especially valuable because of Wang Bing's characteristic knack of providing lucid explanations for many of the more abstruse passages.

Despite his apparent diligence, modern textual analysis has concluded that Wang Bing himself added Chapters 68–74 without highlighting this in any way; presumably this was because he was himself convinced of their authentic Han dynasty origins. For some reason Wang Bing missed the significance of the fact that these chapters were much longer than others, and written in a very different literary style to the more ancient original contents. The sections added by Wang Bing are the chapters that expound on the theory of *wuyun liuqi* (five movements six *qi*), the complex metaphysical method of practice that bases treatment on an understanding of the moment-by-moment changes in the energies of heaven and earth. These were charted using the ancient calendric system that used the 'ten stems' and 'twelve branches' to codify the changes underlying the climate and energetic state of the world at any point in time. The assumption was that these energetic changes in the heavens and on earth underlie health dysfunction in patients and the populace at large, either through a direct resonant linkage or indirectly through effects on the climatic conditions, and that this allowed predictions to be made about the consequences for human health. This system is sometimes referred to as 'chronobiology' or 'stems and branches' (*ziwu liuzhu*); the extent to which it was reliably predictive remains to be established.

Wang Bing's revision of the *Neijing* was important not only because it helped preserve the *Neijing* but because it also helped to foster a renewed interest in classical medicine in general. He is the first to refer to the Neijing's sister text as the Lingshu (Spiritual Pivot). This growth in interest in scholarly study of the earliest classics would later gather pace in the Song dynasty when chronobiology was further refined by important figures such as Shen Kuo and Liu Wan-su. Unaware that the chapters on which the system was based had been added just a few centuries earlier, they interpreted the extra length of these chapters to be an indication of their crucial importance rather than indicative of their more recent origins. So, Wang Bing's re-ordering and revision made the *Neijing* accessible again, but also imbued chronobiology with the authority of ancient Han scholarship. Whilst the original Han dynasty text did include medical doctrines based on seasonal and climatic factors, the chapters Wang Bing added took this aspect a step further and gave it greater emphasis.

My own view is that this new and elaborate style of practice came to the fore because it offered a way of aggrandising the power of the court officials and made

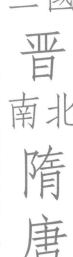

them more indispensable. It did this by enhancing the rulers' political power by predicting the illnesses and epidemics that might be expected to appear. Given that the security of the emperor, the alleged holder of the mandate of heaven, could be compromised by the occurrence of unforeseen natural and humanitarian disasters, the court 'scientists' were under pressure to find ways of demonstrating that the current imperial regime was indeed privy to the will of heaven. If they could accurately predict epidemics, and the particular nature of these epidemics, then the government could take preventative measures and thereby sidestep criticisms that might otherwise undermine the sense of the emperor's continued heavenly mandate when disasters did occur. Comparable in some ways to the modern-day promotion by governments of mass flu inoculation campaigns designed to give the impression of a knowing and benevolent government, they help public morale regardless of actual efficacy.

In the great scheme of medical 'systematic correspondence' it was always theoretically possible to correlate and codify events in the cosmos, changes in the climate and weather on earth, and so on, with changes in the human body. All kinds of statements and projections could be made, but without verification these would just remain speculative, relying simply on the belief that chronobiology rested on a medico-cosmological model that represented self-evident established truth. Robustly constructed, medical 'stems and branches' theory even provided get-out clauses to explain deviations from what was predicted, making it invulnerable to critical appraisal or refutation. As is well known in epidemiology today, there are indeed predictable cycles to many outbreaks of infectious and other diseases; some are indeed seasonal and some appear in longer cycles. Many illnesses do, in fact, correlate to changes in climate, so it is likely that the chronobiologists will sometimes have had their theories vindicated, also helping to make them less liable to refutation or obsolescence.

However, the scholars, mathematicians and court physicians who helped design this scheme seem to have downplayed a notion at the heart of classical medicine, the fundamental distinction between *xie* and *zheng*, between normal substance and pathogen in the body. In creating *wuyun liuqi* theory, medicine was seen as a balancing act where the aim was to help the energies of the body to be distributed in a pleasingly even and harmonious manner. The distinction, for example, between pathogenic *xie* fire and physiologic *zheng* fire were downplayed in this model, something that contrasted with classical medicine in which the aim was to locate and identify pathogens and expel them. Intellectually satisfying it may have been, but it was not necessarily an efficient or effective way to actually treat disease. Nevertheless, this strand of Chinese medicine theory survives as a style to the present day, especially in the West. Some advocates position chronobiology as the highest pinnacle of achievement in Chinese medicine, but it is an approach that has yet to benefit from much critical appraisal or research support in modern times.

In terms of the practical fulfilment of the mandate of heaven to please the populace, the persistence of chronobiology demonstrates its success as a tool of government. It reassured the people by allowing the court to issue warnings about impending epidemics, and to suggest that pharmacies stock up on suitable medicinals. The risk was, however, that if they continually got it wrong, the government would fall into disrepute – which, for different reasons, it did eventually anyway.

The work of other post-Han medical scholars

Through the 700 years or so following the Han dynasty, physicians became increasingly aware of the need for specialist areas of medical study. We see this in the appearance of surgical specialists mentioned earlier, and in the subjects included in the Tai Yi Shu curriculum. The rise of specialities is also reflected in the fact that well over a hundred specialist texts appeared in this period. In the Eastern Jin dynasty Chen Yan-zi wrote the earliest work specifically on gynaecology, his *Furen Fang* (Formulas for Women). Xu Zhi-cai (writing in +479–502) specialised in paediatrics and wrote *Xiaoer Fang* (Formulas for Children). Acupuncture specialist Zhan Quan (+540–643), together with his brother Zhen Li-yan, wrote an important work on the herbal treatment of parasitic diseases. Another physician called Xu Zhi-cai (+505–572) devised a more exacting and clinically useful way of classifying medicinals. Instead of the simple division into upper, middle and lower class substances that had been used in the *Shennong Bencao*, he sorted the substances into ten categories according to their main physiological effects.

Xu Zhi-cai's bencao schema

Xuan	Moving stasis
Tong	Diuretic
Bu	Tonic
Xie	Purgative
Se	Astringent
Hua	Transforming
Cao	Exterior releasing
Shi	Moistening
Jing	Pacifying
Chung	Sedative

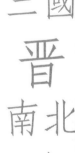

Subsequent medical thinkers revised this categorisation to include heat clearing and warming and other categories, and a thread was created that gradually led, over centuries, to a more satisfactory method of organising the substances in the *bencao* according to their main effect. This idea is picked up again when we get to the Ming dynasty and especially in discussing the Ming physician Zhang Jie-bin, and eventually culminated in the chapter on organisation system used in the modern *bencao* and *fangji* literature.

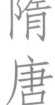

Lei Xiao (c. 5th century)

The processing of medicinals to alter their effects (*pao zhi*) had been part of the herb tradition at least since the Han dynasty. *Shennong Bencao* provides examples of this, especially in relation to processing intended to reduce the toxic effects of some herbs, but it was Lei Xiao who undertook to more fully systematise this area of therapeutics. Little is known about him, or even the exact period when he lived, except that the first mention of his text, the *Lei Gong Pao Zhi Lun* (Leigong's Essays on Herb Processing), appeared towards the end of the Tang dynasty. Lei Xiao describes the properties of about 300 herbs and details the appropriate methods of harvesting and processing of about 200 of them. The *pao zhi* methods he advocates include: steaming, baking, stir-frying, distilling, calcining, boiling in water and preparation with honey, vinegar, ginger or alcohol. The majority of these methods are still familiar in Chinese herb pharmacy practice today, and indeed, some modern pharmacology studies claim to have confirmed the value of many of Lei Xiao's techniques in detoxifying or in modifying herb effects. Lei Xiao's original work has been lost but its contents have survived, thanks to the many sections that were copied into later books, allowing the text to be re-constructed in the 20th century.

Acumoxa in the centuries following the Han

Acumoxa progressed greatly through the 2nd and 3rd centuries when it was widely used, and interest peaked with the appearance of Huangfu Mi's *Jiayi Jing* in +282. Then, as the empire disintegrated in the following centuries, most of the canonical texts were either lost or became very scarce, so little information on acumoxa practice survives from the end of the 3rd century to the start of the Tang in +618. It probably continued to be practised at this time, but perhaps slipping into the hands of wandering mendicants, very few of whom would be qualified in the classical style. Sun Si-miao's advocacy of acumoxa suggests that it continued to be used by scholar physicians in the first part of the Tang dynasty and, also around this time, we find acupuncture included as part of the imperial medical school curriculum. Besides Sun Si-miao's advocacy of acupuncture, another physician advocating this modality at the start of the Tang was Zhen Quan (+541–643). He and his brother Zhen Li-yan became renowned as acupuncturists as well as for their skill in the treatment of parasitic diseases using herbs. Zhen Quan is credited with writing *Zhen Fang* (Needling Formulas) and for creating the acumoxa charts *Mingtang Ren Xing Tu* (Illustrations of the Human Form for the Teaching Room). Derived mainly from Huangfu Mi's *Jiayi Jing*, these resources for practitioners helped to advance acumoxa practice, making it more accessible by presenting the information in a more convenient format. Later in the Tang dynasty, though, Wang Tao's compilation of treatments (*Waitai Miyao*) discussed treatment by moxibustion but did not advocate acupuncture; the likelihood is that accidents or infections may have made it less popular in high circles as the Tang progressed.

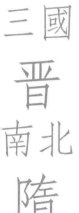

Progress of the Shang Han Lun

The *Shang Han Zhabing Lun* quickly sank into obscurity after the death of Zhang Zhong-jing in +220. Its ideas were probably not especially congruent with the mainstream medical doctrine prevailing at the time, and its transmission was hindered by the fact that its style was so terse and impenetrable that few could make sense of it. Luckily, on the command of the chief court physician, the *Shang Han Zhabing Lun* was reconstituted by the Wei dynasty (+220–265) pulse master Wang Shu-he. Wang expanded it and helped root it more strongly in previous Han dynasty classical literature by including some references to the *jing-luo* system and linking it to some more familiar ideas presented in the *Neijing* and *Nanjing*.

Zhang Zhong-jing is said to have derived the original schema used in his *Shang Han Lun* for describing febrile illness from a short paragraph of the *Neijing* (see below), but the *Shang Han Lun* text itself did not directly refer to the *Neijing* or offer any theoretical explanations. It is possible that Zhang Zhong-jing was the recipient of a specific lineage tradition, the origins of which are now lost.

[When asked about febrile diseases] Qibo answered:

When cold *xie* attacks the body, on the first day the *taiyang* is injured leading to symptoms of headache, dorsal neck pain and spinal stiffness; on the second day the *yangming* is affected with symptoms of hot body, eye pain, dry nose and an inability to lie down…on the third day the *shaoyang* becomes affected…hence the symptoms include chest and rib pain with deafness. When [only] the three *yang* channels are affected it has not yet entered the *zang* so it can be cured by inducing perspiration.

Taiyin is affected on the fourth day with symptoms such as abdominal fullness and dry throat…*shaoyin* will be affected on the fifth day…symptoms include dry mouth and tongue and thirst. On day six *jueyin* becomes affected…the symptoms include feeling miserable and congested with contraction of scrotum. (*Suwen*, Ch 31)

Wang Shu-he transferred some sections from the original text into his own book on pulse diagnosis, thereby supplying us with a useful glimpse of the original text prior to all the subsequent re-writes. Both the original *Shang Han Zabing Lun* and Wang Shu-he's editions then appear to have been almost completely ignored until the Sui dynasty began in +589, and even then it contributed little to medical theory or practice. Very few copies of Zhang's classic continued to be transmitted after Wang Shu-he, and it was barely ever mentioned amongst the texts transmitted in the master–disciple lineage system. A handful of physicians were aware of the basic *shang han* ideas before and during the Sui dynasty (+589–618), but references to its ideas remained very scant. On the occasions when the theory was referred to, writers failed to include mention of its originator. Chao Yuan-fang, for example, in his *Zhubing Yuanhou Lun* pathology text, discusses the subject of *shang han* but omits any specific mention of Zhang himself, suggesting that he was aware of some of its content but did not have access to the text itself.

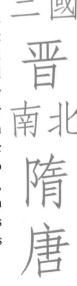

Apart from Sun Si-miao's discussions of his application of some *shang han* formulas in the Tang dynasty, there are then no substantive discussions of the text until the early decades of the subsequent Song dynasty in the 11th century. Sun Si-miao wrote that some of the teachers he knew owned copies of the *Shang Han Lun* but did not transmit (i.e. teach) the texts; by this he presumably meant that they were not in a position to explain it to their disciples. Sun said that he had heard of some physicians blindly applying *shang han* formulas without understanding the principles underlying them.

Even the endlessly talented Sun himself admitted that in the absence of any accompanying theoretical explanations the *Shang Han Lun* was hard to decipher. There is no mention of it in Sun's first book, *Qian Jin Yao Fang*, but by about +682 Sun evidently had managed to obtain a copy, seemingly without the *Jin Gui Yao Lue* portion. Sun Si-miao's interest in cold attack inspired a brief flurry of interest in it at the time, but this soon fizzled out. The fragments of text recorded for us in his *Qian Jin Yi Fang* have provided scholars with another glimpse of a version of the text before it was reconstituted and updated by the Song dynasty imperial medical academy.

It was Sun's respect for Zhang Zhong-jing's masterwork that may have helped secure a place for it in the official curriculum of the Tang dynasty Tai Yi Shu. In +758 the schedule for the state physicians licensing exam included questions on the *Shang Han Lun* as well as the *Shennong Bencao*, the *Mai Jing* pulse classic, the *Neijing* and other classics. So, as we will see in the next chapter, it was only much later when the Song emperors faced the problem of continual and calamitous epidemics that a new impetus arose to search for suitable treatments in the *Shang Han Lun*.

Other notable Tang texts

Xin Xiu Bencao

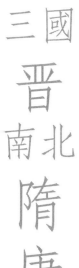

In +657 the court physician Su Jing proposed to the Tang dynasty rulers a project to further improve the *bencao* literature by a state-sponsored effort. A team of 20 leading scholars was convened to form a committee with the aim of surveying the medical herbs from all regions of China. Each district was required to submit to the capital (Xian) illustrated and detailed reports on the medical properties of the herbs and other medicinals used in their area for inclusion in a new text. Opinions about the efficacy of individual substances were gathered for possible inclusion, and those now considered to be of doubtful value that had appeared in earlier *bencao* texts were to be omitted from the new edition. Practical information such as data concerning the optimal conditions for growth and harvesting were also to be included.

After two years' work *Xin Xiu Bencao* (Newly Revised *Materia Medica*) was published in 54 volumes by the government and distributed across the country. Containing information on 844 substances, it departed from the upper-middle-lower classification system of the old *Shennong Bencao* and instead used a system based on the type of substance: mineral, herb, insect, bird, quadruped and so on. Later renamed *Tang Bencao*, this was the world's first state-sponsored official pharmacopia, published the best part of a millennium before the first equivalent text was produced in the West, the *Nuremberg Pharmacopia* of 1546. Unschuld, however, points out that the two texts are not comparable, and that the remit of the *Nuremberg Pharmacopia* is significantly stricter.

In +731 the Japanese physician Tanabe Fubito took a copy of the original *Tang Bencao* to Japan, where it survives today. Fragments of the original also survive in the British Museum and the Bibliotheque Nationale in Paris after their appropriation by European adventurers in the 19th century.

In the 8th century Cheng Cang-qi created a revised and improved version of *Tang Bencao* by writing *Bencao Shiyi* (Gleanings from the *Bencao*), but this has disappeared at some point in the last 400 years. Chen's work is known to be an attempt to bring a more practical clinical focus to medical practice; his particular innovation was to introduce a more practical ordering of the material by creating a ten-fold categorisation of formula types.

CHENG CANG-QI'S *BENCAO* CLASSIFICATION

Xuan	Disseminate
Tong	Open, unblock
Bu	Tonify
Xie	Drain
Qing	Clear excess
Zhong	Settle the heart *shen*
Se	Astringe
Zao	Dry
Shi	Moisten
Wen	Warm

Summarising Tang medicine

Right up to the end of the Tang dynasty there was virtually no tradition of keeping written records of case histories, so we are forced to speculate about the actual methodology of literate medical practice based on surviving theoretical and practical texts. Another difficulty encountered when trying to understand Tang medical practice is that the encyclopaedic style of most texts also offers little idea as to how literati physicians actually practised their medicine. It seems to suggest that medical practitioners often took short-cut routes to therapy, matching prescriptions to the main complaint, and if that didn't work, trying another formula. Many will have based their practice on chronobiology doctrine, so the classical ideal of treatment based on pattern differentiation probably slipped from the fore in this era.

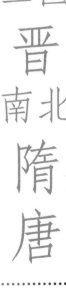
三國晉南北隋唐

Evidence for this emphasis on simple disease differentiation comes from the fact that the *Waitai Biyao* by Wang Tao is simply a large collection of herb formulas organised in a manner convenient for treating symptoms and diseases rather than underlying patterns of disharmony using simpler remedies. We also see from texts such as Wang Tao's that the formulas used in this period had departed from the skilfully focused prescriptions of Zhang Zhong-jing that typically incorporated between four and eight herbs, to formulas containing numerous ingredients. Although we might say that complex formulas are appropriate for complex illnesses, this approach can also be indicative of practice styles using poorly focused differentiation of the individual patient's condition. However, not *every* physician in this era was lazy or inept, as the quote by the early Tang physician Xu Yin-zong below indicates.

> People today are unable to use the pulses to make differentiations and thereby fail to identify the origins of disease. They make decisions on their feelings and use numerous ingredients. This is like hunting rabbits by sending out numerous men and horses in the hope that, by luck, one will stumble across the rabbit. This is negligent medicine. (Xu Yin-zong)

The apparent shift in the popularity of acupuncture in favour of moxibustion was probably due to an increased incidence of acupuncture-related accidents such as those from improper point location or adverse incidents due to infection.

The trendy new style based on the 'chronobiology' additions to the *Neijing* added by the imperial physician Wang Bing continued through the subsequent dynasties to the present day, where its elegant complexity is sometimes taken to be a measure of its profundity.

In addition, the Tang preoccupation with Buddhism and its Karmic explanations of causality, spirit medicine, chanting and so on led Chinese medicine on another path that deviated away from its more pragmatic and patient-centred classic roots. Nevertheless, benefits to medical practice from this foreign import came from the increased sense of kind, diligent and compassionate practice exemplified by Sun Si-miao with his statement of the ideal practitioner ethic. This outlook may have prompted an increasing impetus, not just to foster good healthcare to serve the elite ruling classes, but also for the wider population, an idea that was to gain more momentum through the Song.

Historians often characterise the Tang as the second golden age of Chinese civilisation after the Han dynasty. This perception is supported by the increased links with other cultures, flourishing cities and merchant activity bringing luxuries to market and all the trappings of an era of peace, poetry, art, music and beautiful pottery. From the point of view of classical Chinese medicine the Tang was, with some exceptions such as Chao Yuan-fang's pathology text, something of a period of stagnation, with comparatively little progress and innovation.

Tang dreams of high culture succumbed in the end to the usual corrupt political intrigues between court eunuchs and scholar officials, turning especially sour in +755 when the dissent of a military governor led to widespread troop revolts.

三 國

晋 北

南 隋

唐

Mercenaries who were recruited to resolve the situation instead compounded the problems, and the breakdown led to increasing famine and social disarray, to peasant unrest and eventually an uprising in +875. The dynastic rulers made themselves scarce, and in +906, the dynasty collapsed.

三國晉南北隋唐

5

SONG DYNASTY MEDICINE

The Tang dynasty declined into increasing strife before finally disintegrating in +907. After this, Southern China fragmented into ten separate kingdoms. In the north, with no predominant ruler for the next five decades, a pattern developed of brief and unstable rule by a succession of five local military commanders, each seizing power in turn, and then losing it through lack of ability to found a stable nation. One unifying thread running through this period was in the person of Feng Dao, who served as chief minister for four of the five rulers in this 'five dynasties' period. Feng flattered the second northern ruler by proposing that he would be more likely to be immortalised by posterity if he were to commission a grand project to have the famous classics re-edited and carved in stone. This grand scheme was rejected, but he later returned to his ruler with a cheaper option, saying that in Sichuan province he had seen a new technology whereby books could be printed using carved wooden blocks. Perhaps prestige could be gained instead by commissioning printed editions of the classics; to this the emperor agreed. Work was set in progress, and three very brief dynasties later the completed edition of annotated texts in 130 volumes was presented, albeit to an entirely different imperial court. Previous dynastic rulers had commissioned handwritten books and some woodblock printing had been used over the previous century, but the scale of Feng Dao's project set a new precedent.

In pressing for this publishing project in the run-up to the founding of the Song dynasty, Feng Dao introduced the notion that printing offered an opportunity to enhance the prestige and influence of the imperial court. He inadvertently helped to catalyse the first rumblings of a publishing revolution, initiating a completely new era in communications that would make a great contribution to medical and scholarly progress initially in China and later also to the whole world. In terms of political governance, the power of the printing press also gave the Song dynasty new possibilities for lending extra stability to the new regime, for instance, by using mass media to demonstrate government support of the welfare of the people and so reduce the tendency towards uprising and rebellion. For politics and government this increased focus on the needs of the people would contribute stability to the Song dynasty. For medicine the availability of mass publication would contribute significantly to medical progress.

In +960 Taizu declared himself first emperor of the Song dynasty. Being more skilful at statecraft than his 'five dynasties' predecessors, he succeeded in consolidating his position as ruler, and so found a lasting dynasty administered from Kaifeng in Henan province. As the Song dynasty got under way, innovative changes in the governance and structure of Chinese society began to exert a significant influence on the development of medicine. The increased imperial concern for the health of the wider population triggered a renewed spirit of investigation and the implementation of projects aimed at allowing ordinary people access to better healthcare. With the continued problem of epidemics, Emperor Taizu saw that more effective treatments were needed, and was wise enough to realise that showing concern for the populace would help instil confidence in his regime.

Taizu's Song dynasty progressed smoothly for well over 200 years before climate change, crop failures and the ever-troublesome northern barbarian tribes made life increasingly untenable in the north. In +1127 repeated skirmishes with the invading Jerchen northern tribes finally forced the government and the population to migrate south to create large settlements in the Yangzi river area such as the flagship new cities now called Hangzhou and Suzhou. This move south is the reason for the division of the Song dynasty into the Northern Song (+960–1127) and the Southern Song (+1127–1279). Other new cities were founded, and the previous system of feudalism and simple peasant self-sufficiency for the ordinary citizen began to evolve into a more intricate economy, with increased trade and interdependence between different professions.

Well before the move to the south the Song dynasty policies, such as agricultural reforms, brought a growth in commerce that in turn provided increased social mobility. The power and influence that previously came from admission to the Mandarin civil service had, in theory at least, always been accessible to all people through the state examinations system. In practice, government posts were filled almost exclusively by the aristocracy, or by the military through their family connections, and as a result of the fact that wealthy families were the only people able to afford the education needed to pass the crucial *jinshi* (mandarin doctorate) exams – the route to high official rank.

The Song dynasty changes softened class barriers such that it now became much more feasible to acquire wealth, status and influence by involvement in trade. The emergence of a new wealthy merchant class, combined with changes in the imperial attitude, allowed Song citizens better access to education, and so the doors to official positions opened wider than ever before, a situation that would have been unthinkable in previous centuries. New blood came into government circles, allowing more diverse influences on social policy to creep in; the new bureaucrats were now more likely to be connected to ordinary life than the previous grandees. The new Mandarins also had a more divergent intellectual outlook than those of previous generations, because of their origins and because the new civil service exams required study of a broader range of subjects than were on the curriculum before. As well as the traditional Confucian 'five classics' curriculum, scholars could now study law, medicine, finance and military strategy. Song officials were now more connected to the real world and the needs of the wider population than had ever been seen in China before, which meant that they brought to the administration concerns that had been of little interest to past Mandarins, subjects such as medicine, science and technology. Those who were attracted to these subjects were also better placed to develop their interests to a high level due to the fact that state service gave access to the rare and valuable imperial library facilities. In addition, the collegiate nature of the scholar system fostered intellectual exchange and debate amongst state-sponsored societies of scholars. These were all fertile conditions for a blossoming of intellectual achievement in medicine.

With the new wealth and stability came a surge in population that, with increased trade, greatly boosted taxation revenues and allowed the state to fund more benevolent ventures for the benefit of the population. New professional and craft guilds appeared, commerce was stimulated, and mass production industries such as porcelain and paper manufacture started. Out of all this a new social order began to take shape, leading to what has been seen by some as China's industrial revolution. This contributed to the formation of bigger medical industries and the mass production of medical products.

Buddhism remained popular at this time, partly because the second Song Emperor Taizong had been converted, but also because being a certified Buddhist gave tax exemptions. Daoism flourished too, and numerous Daoist hermits flocked to the mountains, attempting to subsist on little more than *lingzhi* (Ganoderma lucidum), mushrooms and fresh air. Since the Han dynasty the Daoists had been inclined to observe and classify nature and to carry out proto-scientific and alchemical experiments, but with the Song's new technological outlook, their work took on a renewed self-confident investigative vigour. New weapons for the military came from the alchemists' refinements to, and practical applications of, Sun Si-miao's discovery of an early form of gunpowder in the Tang dynasty. Innovations in ceramic manufacture led to very refined porcelain and the introduction of new and attractive glazes. The Song technology mindset was also applied to medicine, leading, for example, to the refinement of new drugs extracted from urine with active components that represent crude but potentially potent steroid hormone extracts.

USE OF STEROID HORMONES IN THE SONG

Extraction of the crystalline 'autumn mineral' drug from human urine had been mentioned by Han and Tang dynasty Daoists. Now, in the Song extraction of medicinals from urine began on an industrial scale, the detailed production process was published in +1025. From 600 litres of male urine an extract containing about 100g of relatively pure 'autumn mineral' – probably containing quite concentrated steroid and gonadotrophin hormones – could be refined using evaporation and careful sublimation. These extracts were used for medical purposes, especially in andrology.

Various other factors helped to create the conditions for medical advancement. The Song dynasty philosophy was neo-Confucianism, in which elements of the Buddhist and Daoist worldview were grafted onto the Confucian to form a philosophy that emphasised benevolence (*ren*) towards others. This humanitarian ethic became a driver for medical advancement. Neo-Confucianism also promoted the idea of understanding things by formal investigation, a factor that is also beneficial to the development of systematic and effective medicine. Intellectuals believing in the concept of *li* (理), a putative rational and understandable organising principle that was considered to underlie all phenomena, continued the age-old fight against beliefs of causality based on deities, demons and spirits. The new *zeitgeist* revitalised the work of those interested in science, technology and intellectual endeavour generally, leading to a renewed interest in the formal study of nature and man's relationship to it.

Also central to the Song ideal was a desire to create a cultured and peaceful way of life where innovations in technology, social order and government could benefit all. Mass production of porcelain was one benefit of this new refined lifestyle, a benefit that was poised to spread to the West during the mediaeval explosion of trade with the Middle East and Europe along the Silk Road. Historians often point to this period as the pivotal time, marking the transition from a mediaeval feudal country into the modern Chinese era. Indeed, along with the increasing transport of trade goods westward in the Song, Jin and Yuan dynasties came a transmission of some civilising ideas such as printing and possibly even the idea of universities. These issues are too much of a diversion to discuss here, except to note the similarity between the neo-Confucian scholar's distinctive clothing and that of European academia. The Western academic gown and cap, with its hanging tassels and square top, can be traced to mediaeval Italy, and it was merchants from Italy who were the first Europeans to trade extensively with China. The accidental unearthing of Italian gravestones built into the Nanjing city walls has provided evidence of Italians living in China in the late 12th century in the few decades prior to Marco Polo's famed travels. It may be that the graduate's gown and cap is actually a relic of the Song dynasty scholars' garb, and even the party spirit of mediaeval Europe was perhaps inspired by the frivolous atmosphere of 13th-century Hanzhou, with its jesters, jugglers, frivolity and fancy banquets.

The Tang dynasty imperial medical service existed primarily for the benefit of the court, and had little regard for the health of the general population. A complete change came with the first Northern Song emperors whose outlook had the explicit intent of benefiting ordinary citizens – a new community spirit that had a socialist character. In the centuries prior to the Song dynasty the health needs of the populace were met by a motley and diverse spectrum of folk and religious healers, wandering medical specialists and literate and semiliterate physicians. The well-heeled were physicians versed in the classical tradition that could be studied from one's peers and from the rare and ancient classical texts collected in imperial archives for the exclusive benefit of physicians to the nobility. In the Song dynasty the *wu* shamans, folk healers, religious healers and wandering bell doctors continued their work, but now the literati actively denounced such practices. This was pressure for better medicine in the community. Improved civilisation also meant that literacy rates increased too, and this, together with the availability of mass printed medical texts, allowed many more ordinary people to access formal medical knowledge. In this way many more people who were literate but not high-level scholars were now able to practise medicine using their own reading of the classical styles, a raising of standards that contributed to the marginalisation of folk and spirit healers. Inevitably, intellectual chauvinism remained, and the elite *jinshi* literati continued to criticise the more lowly scholar doctors for having insufficient depth of understanding of classic medical doctrine. In all probability, many ordinary physicians acquired skills and understanding that outclassed that of many elite physicians.

Medical publishing in the Song

From near the start of the Song dynasty professional medicine was propelled forward by the emergence of new and more efficient printing technologies, bringing great benefits of dissemination of knowledge first to China and later worldwide, as pioneers such as Gutenburg adapted the technology for use in Europe. Simple woodblock printing had been available in China since the publication of the Buddha's *Diamond Sutra* (+868), an original copy of which came to the British Museum thanks to the acquisitive activities of Lord McCarthy who effectively stole this and other texts from caves in Dunhuang.

In +1040 Bi Sheng invented the much more efficient moveable-type printing process, and in doing so he created the conditions for a big imperial publishing and distribution drive. Suddenly scholars at court could disseminate their writings much more efficiently and then, within just a few decades, even private individuals were able to reach a wide audience by the new publication industry. By the end of the Northern Song, at the beginning of the 12th century, a very significant boost to medicine had come from this new mass production publishing industry, leading eventually to print runs on a scale comparable to modern publishers.

Taizu, the first Song emperor, introduced some initial measures intended to begin the process of improving public health. Wishing to gather up more medical knowledge from the community, he offered cash rewards for the donation of privately held medical texts, and for those who could donate especially important texts he also made awards of official posts; such rewards tended to be better if the donor was already well placed in society. This was an important initiative because in the mayhem of the 'five dynasties' period, many of the books archived in the imperial library had disappeared. Taizu's new initiative would allow some to be regained.

Also very helpful to the development of medicine was the fact that Taizu himself took a personal interest in the subject. Even before he became emperor he had personally acquired a large library of herbal medicine and acumoxa texts, a collection that he later had published as an official compilation. By recognising medicine as an acceptable object of scholarship at the very highest levels of society, he did much to inspire official and public interest in the subject, and so helped raise the respectability of medical practice as a professional career path for scholars. Medicine had previously generally been viewed as a calling far beneath the dignity of most literati, or at least one suitable only for academic low flyers.

Fortunately this interest in medicine and public health continued with Taizu's successor Taizong, who also enjoyed personally dabbling in the subject. As his armies advanced south to bring more territory under imperial state control, he is said to have personally quizzed locals on the effects of herbs, and then to have tasked officials with the job of verifying these beliefs with a view to their adoption into medical orthodoxy.

NORTHERN SONG EMPERORS
Taizu, 960
Taizong, 976
Zhenzong, 998
Renzong, 1023
Yingzong, 1054
Shenzong, 1068
Zhezong, 1086
Huizong, 1101
Qinzong, 1126

Taiping Shenghui Fang (Imperial Grace Formulary)

In +978, Taizong commissioned a team headed by Wang Huai-yin to create the *Sheyi Puji Fang*, a vast medical compendium containing 10,000 formulas in 1000 chapters. This was not published and has since disappeared. Perhaps unhappy with this first compilation, in +982 Taizong ordered Wang Huai-yin to compile a new one. Completed in +992 this was the famed *Taiping Shenghui Fang* (Imperial Grace Formulary), the first important *fangji* (prescription) text of the Song dynasty. Its 100 chapters formed a compendium of a monumental 16,834 medicinal formulas, and so encompassed much of the entire *fangji* tradition. The inclusion of some chapters that presented *Shang Han Lun* prescriptions

TAIPING SHENGHUI FANG: CONTENTS OUTLINE
Chs 1–2 Diagnosis and prescription theory
Chs 3–7 *Zangfu* diseases
Chs 8–14 *Shang han* diseases
Chs 15–59 Throat, mouth, dental and eye diseases and miscellaneous internal illness
Chs 60–68 External medicine
Chs 69–81 Gynaecology
Chs 82–93 Paediatrics
Chs 94–95 Daoist alchemical medicine
Chs 96–98 Dietary medicine
Chs 99–100 Acumoxa therapy

raised awareness of this text and its potential in the fight against febrile epidemics.

The *Imperial Grace Formulary* devoted two chapters to acumoxa (*zhen-jiu*), mainly giving symptom indications for acupuncture points. The *qijing ba mai* (eight extraordinary channels) and their points were not discussed. The text covers *bu* and *xie* (supplementing and draining) needling techniques, the specific needling methods appropriate for individual points, and also some seasonal factors relevant to acumoxa practice. It also contains some illustrations of points and descriptions of the results that were to be expected following needling of specific points.

The 'Ming Tang' chapter of the *Imperial Grace Formulary* opens with a presentation of *san cai* (heaven-earth-man) theory; it then discusses acupoints and the use of moxa in paediatrics, and also defines the *cun* (proportional body inch) measurement system to aid point finding. Various acumoxa techniques and contraindications are given, but there is little detail on *jing-luo* theory or classical pattern differentiation theory. Later in the Song dynasty a seven-volume text appeared that gave a more pragmatic presentation of acumoxa practice; this was written by Wang Zhi-zhong, whose work is discussed later in this chapter.

Unfortunately, as it consisted of little more than a reworked compendium of previous flawed Tang dynasty writings, the *Taiping Shenghui Fang* was not sufficiently insightful or critical in its style to significantly advance medical theory or practice. Whilst it raised awareness of the *Shang Han Lun*, it offered little enlightenment on this classic's actual meaning, so its main value was as an encyclopaedia of medicine in use up until that time. Taizong's *Taiping Shenghui Fang* project was intended as a way to improve public health by the dissemination of detailed medical texts derived from the literate medical tradition, but its ability to achieve this objective was constrained from the start. Not the least of its limitations is seen in the fact that its distribution was limited to provincial government offices where it could be accessed by senior officials and not by the general public. This may reflect a tension between the altruistic policies of government that saw public benefit in greater access to medical information, and the instincts of the elite to keep access to valuable knowledge restricted to the right sort of people.

KAIBAO QINGDING BENCAO

Wishing also to revise the *bencao* tradition, Taizu commissioned nine top physicians from the imperial Han Lin academy (the inner sanctum of top government scholars and policy makers) to rewrite the main Tang dynasty *bencao*, the *Xin Xiu Bencao*. The lead authors for this project were Ma Zhi, a Daoist famed for his ability to compose highly effective herb prescriptions, and the Confucian gentleman scholar Liu Han, who came from a lineage of famous physicians. The work was published first as *Kaibao Bencao* (*Bencao* of the Kaibao Reign) in +973 but, not satisfied with the result, Taizu enlarged the team and demanded further revisions, leading to the publication of *Kaibao Qingding Bencao* in +974. On the plus side the *Kaibao Bencao* texts introduced many new substances into the *bencao* tradition, including *mo yao*, *shandou gen*, *gu sui bu* and *ying su ke*. Academically, though, both these *bencao* texts were weak – as uncritical re-writes of Tang texts, they included numerous mistakes, contradictions, repetitions and unsubstantiated opinions.

The continued reworking of old texts, predicated on a reverence for antiquity, was fast becoming a significant hindrance to progress – the unquestioning reverence for ancient information worked against the deletion of nonsense and promoted a stagnated mire of random information. Badly formatted and unwieldy, the re-writes of both of the *Kaibao Bencao* texts were impractical as clinical texts and obscured the presence of the material that was worthwhile. The original versions of both texts are now lost, but their contents are known from surviving later editions.

Founding of the bureau for revising medical texts

In terms of public health, a disadvantage of the greater mobility and creation of large urban areas was the increased incidence and more rapid spread of epidemics. Between +1045 and +1060 repeated epidemics, and their ineffectual treatment, triggered government initiatives to improve the treatment of these by re-examining current medical doctrine. With this in mind the government first published a formula text, *Wangshi Boji Fang* (Mr Wang's Formulas for Abundant Relief), in +1045, and the following year, *Qingli Shan Jiu Fang* (Qingli Reign Formulas for Public Relief) appeared. Unfortunately, the actual relief afforded by the availability of these works proved to be insignificant, so, in +1057, the newly founded Bureau for the Revision of Medical Texts was given the task of producing a new range of authoritative medical texts. The scholar Zhang Yu-xi headed a team that after three years' work published a new textbook, *Jiayou Buzhu Shennong Bencao* (Jiayou Period Supplemented and Annotated *Shennong Bencao*), containing 1083 entries. This, too, was built on the Kaibo Bencao that was compiled at the start of the Song dynasty, but now the authors attempted to plug gaps and improve the taxonomy (correct identification) aspects. Relaxing their reverence for ancient canons they abandoned the *Shennong Bencao*'s upper-middle-lower classification of the medicinals to create a more practical system based on the key indications and actions. The *Jiayou Buzhu Shennong Bencao* was not, however, updated to take into account recent advances in the refinement of Chinese medicine theory.

Over the next few decades the work of the Bureau for Revision of Medical Texts continued with the publication of new editions of the most important historic texts, including the *Suwen*, *Jin Gui Yao Lue* (sister text to the *Shang Han Lun*), Wang Shu-he's pulse classic *Mai Jing*, Huangfu Mi's *Jiayi Jing*, Chao Yuan-fang's aetiology and pathology text *Zhubing Yuanhou Lun* and Sun Si-miao's *Qian Jing Yao Fang*. In this way a library of newly revised classical core texts were published as official editions.

Tujing Bencao

The new more complex Song dynasty economy resulted in increased levels of trade in all sectors. In relation to medicine the result was that more peasant-collected folk herbs were adopted into professional medical practice, an idea that was a personal interest of Taizong. Expanded trade links with the provinces and other countries led to the importation of new medicinals such as cardamom from India and frankincense from the Arabian countries. Many of these new introductions were unfamiliar to practitioners; others were familiar herbs but which, in practice, were found to have different properties to those previously recorded. Such differences may have been due to local varietal differences or the different growing conditions in different regions. To tackle these new challenges Su Song was appointed in +1057 to head a group that went on to produce the *Tujing Bencao* (Illustrated *Bencao*), a work that specifically aimed to address the problems of identification, authentication, collection and preparation inherent in using both old and new medicinals. For this project regional governments were ordered to submit information on their local medicines along with samples and pictures. With a new-found intellectual rigour, the authors demanded verification of each medicinal's identity, indications, source and quality. Aiming to avoid hearsay and error, their process required that actual samples be studied for every substance so that the *bencao* information could be improved, and so that quality and authenticity could be better assured in future. There was probably a public health impetus to this work, as mis-identification must, with some regularity, have led to iatrogenesis or fatality.

Not content, either, to rely blindly on the authority of historical writings, the authors of *Tujing Bencao* also sought expert opinion from contemporary physicians about indications, actions, efficacy and identification of the medicinals. The aim was to standardise and reconcile what was previously a heterodox orthodoxy of information inherited from the historical literature. In +1062 *Tujing Bencao* was published, with its 933 illustrations and detailed information on the identification, collection, processing and indications of the medicinals. Some innovative prescriptions from the folk tradition were also included for the first time.

With the advent of this illustrated *bencao*, medicine was now becoming less blindly reliant on the ancient sources and more practical, reflective, systematic and safe. This was a major step forward and was a sufficient achievement to become the representative *bencao* for the next 500 years. Many more *bencao* texts were to appear later in the Song dynasty, but *Jiayou Bencao* and *Tujing Bencao* were the key writings that set a benchmark for professional herb practice. As we will see later, a similar benchmark was set for acumoxa practitioners with the casting of the bronze figure in +1020, which helped standardise basic practices of this branch of therapeutics. A weak aspect of *Tujing Bencao* was that, as a consequence of the early technology, the illustrations were very crude and distorted representations of the medicinals. They were insufficient for identification, but would have served as *aides memoires* to support learning gained on field trips. The first really high quality *bencao* illustrations appeared in *Lu Chanyan Bencao* (Steep Mountainsides *Bencao*), published in +1220 by Wang Jie, a text that presented 206 quite remarkable colour illustrations that are comparable in style and clarity to modern botanical illustrations.

Revival of Shang Han Lun

The Bureau for Revision of Medical Texts had succeeded in supplying a range of improved and revised core texts for general medicine. Continuing this effort Emperor Renzong, in +1048, commissioned a *fangji* text called *Effective Formulas of the Qingli Reign*, and then three years later, the *Imperial Grace Formulary* was abridged to create a general healthcare manual for popular use, the *Jianyao Jizhong Fang* (Concise

Formulary for Public Relief). Still the most pressing need was for better information on the treatment of epidemic disease.

Zhang Zhong-jing's Eastern Han dynasty classic *Shang Han Lun* was probably selected for analysis because it appeared to offer the promise of an answer for the unrelenting public health problem of epidemic disease. A few surviving versions of the *Shang Han Lun* had mouldered unnoticed on the shelves of the imperial libraries for 800 years; it had effectively been out of circulation and was yet to make any significant contribution to medical care. Tersely written and gracing the reader with little theoretical explanation, the few physicians who had accessed it over the centuries had struggled to make sense of this ancient classic, including the great Sun Si-miao who had briefly discussed the use of its formulas at the start of the Tang dynasty. Now some scholars in imperial medical circles suspected it might be important, so in +1057 the first Song edition was published by the Bureau for Revision of Medical Texts. This version was published as a woodblock edition under the editorship of Lin Yi. The editing and publication of a new edition of the *Shang Han Lun* did not necessarily go hand-in-hand with any understanding or proper interpretation of this classic – worthwhile interpretation only developed gradually over the next century or so. The original text was simply too sparse and too alien to the other medical teachings of the time to be easily assimilated into mainstream practice. Nevertheless, the imperial scholars had a sense that they were on to something important, and the excitement attached to the *Shang Han Lun* project is reflected in the fact that the majority of the next ten texts that were published by the Bureau after +1057 were versions of Zhang Jing's classic on cold attack.

Many famous physicians served on the editorial board for the Bureau for Revision of Medical Texts, but most influence lay in the hands of others. It was the non-medical bureaucrats who held most sway in deciding which texts were to be selected for review and publication. The first editions of these grand texts were very expensive, large character editions that were designated for distribution to imperial government offices, so, as Dr Asaf Goldschmidt pointed out in his PhD thesis, any educational benefit was confined to the handful of physicians who had access to these libraries. Elite physicians were inclined to resist access by lowly doctors to their state-of-the-art information, at least until their peers had first had a chance to assimilate the information. When subsequent editions appeared they were cheaper, small character versions (requiring less paper), produced in much larger print runs, fulfilling the imperial intent by mass dissemination of medical knowledge.

Cheng Wu-ji clarifies the Shang Han Lun

In the Song dynasty the texts that were officially selected for revision and commentary were biased towards those related to *shang han* study, even though very few physicians could actually understand that style. As well as being unable to make sense of its ideas and terminology, much of the time the patterns it described probably did not seem congruent with their own patients' clinical presentations. This is because the epidemics rampant at that time more often manifested as heat patterns rather than the cold attack patterns that are the central feature of *shang han* theory. Nevertheless, despite the difficulties and incongruities, by selecting this text for scholarly analysis and publication, the Song bureaucrats and physicians exerted a strong influence on the future direction of Chinese medicine. Had they ignored it, the path of Chinese medicine up until modern times is likely to have been significantly different. Some 20–30 per cent of the lead formulas in the Chinese medicine of today come from the *Shang Han Zhabing Lun*.

The early imperial Bureau editors of the *Shang Han Lun* corrected errors and polished the text to the best of their ability, but they themselves could offer little clarification of its meaning. Its ideas were too unfamiliar at first; then, as the text became better known, the problem became how to square this 'new' material with the existing classical theory base. A milestone in understanding and integration was achieved in +1140 with the publication of Cheng Wu-ji's clarified edition – his *Zhujie* (annotated) *Shang Han Lun*.

Living in Shandong around +1050–1140, Cheng Wu-ji had made a personal study of the *Shang Han Lun* for 40 years, and had gained extensive practical experience of its clinical application. He was the first to comprehensively explain it and integrate it with Han dynasty classical theory, and it now became clear that the keys to understanding Zhang Zhong-jing's text were extensions of the Han dynasty *yin-yang* thinking, especially hot-cold, internal-external, *shi-xu* and *xie-zheng*. As well as identifying that these were the keys to understanding the *Shang Han Lun*, Cheng was also able to reconcile the discrepancies between the various surviving versions of the text. In another book, his *Shang Han Mingli Lun* (Clarification of Cold Damage Principles), Cheng explains each individual symptom of *shang han* clinical discourse in detail, thereby creating a practical manual for its use with a new, much more insightful style of analysis. In a third text called *Yao Fang Lun* (On Medicinals and Formulas), Cheng described the strategies and practical application of 21 of the key formulas from the *Shang Han Lun*, and corrected misapprehensions he had come across in discussions with students and other physicians.

Cheng Wu-ji's work represents a significant turning point in Chinese medicine. He succeeded in bringing *shang han* theory and classical doctrine together in a lucid, comprehensive and practical way so that future clinicians could have clear guidance on its application. In addition, his work showed that it was actual practising clinicians rather than the rarified imperial scholars who were best placed to square the *Shang Han Lun* with clinical experience and classical theory. So now it was increasingly the practising physicians who took the lead from government officials in the exposition of theory and practice and in the integration of the classic explanatory model into medical literature.

THE PROBLEM OF INITIAL-STAGE HEAT DISEASES
As mentioned, a particular problem in understanding epidemics was that patients often presented with initial-stage heat disorders whereas the *Shang Han Lun* focused

much more on exterior cold patterns. Interpreting the apparent heat signs that appear in the course of an externally contracted epidemic illness presented difficulties, and so new investigation was called for to understand and reconcile these differences.

In +1186 Han Zhi-he, who had achieved great fame for his ability to successfully treat febrile diseases, produced a further commentary, his *Shang Han Weizhi Lun* (*Shang Han Lun*, Its Deeper Meaning). Han explained the appearance of exterior heat by saying that the presence of exterior cold constrained the *yang qi* and that this *yang qi* constraint transformed into heat – a situation that, with careful reading, is implicit in the original text. Presenting the text in plain contemporary medical Chinese, Han, for the first time, links the six *jing* channel pairs (*taiyang, yangming, shaoyang, taiyin, shaoyin* and *jueyin*) of the *Shang Han Lun* to the classic *jing-luo* channels of the *Neijing*. This link had previously not been clear. Later opinion four centuries later, however, was to reverse this view, with some claiming that the *shang han* system was referring to individual *zangfu* organs. Han also emphasised the key role of pulse diagnostics in distinguishing the *shang han* patterns; the original version of the *Shang Han Lun* is believed to have probably contained no information on pulses.

Another important *shang han* commentator was Pang An-shi (+1042–1099) who came from a long line of physicians and who had treated a great many *shang han* cases. Only one of his four texts survives, *Shang Han Zongbing Lun* (Discussion on Cold Damage and General Disorders). From his own studies and experience, Pang An-shi concluded that cold injury consisted of two distinct categories of disorder, and that this had been a source of confusion to earlier writers. He more clearly demarcated the *shang han* patterns, and distinguished the many possible forms of cold symptomatology that can arise, and suggested that the varied individual responses to attack were a product of both the prevailing climate and the patient's constitution. He aimed to reconcile some of the key problems that had arisen out of previous attempts to understand the text. Referring to a passage found in the *Suwen*, Pang said that in some patients the cold *xie*, which was generally contracted in the autumn or winter, remained dormant and unseen in the *ying-wei* system, only to manifest in spring, whilst in other patients the symptoms would be manifested immediately. The symptoms appeared identical but the underlying pathology was different. Pang wrote, 'When an illness transforms due to the warm *qi* of the spring we label it as a Warm disorder. When it changes due to the summer heat we call it Heat disorder', which presaged a gradually increasing interest in heat aspects of externally contracted illness.

My understanding of this retained *xie* possibility that was mentioned in the *Suwen* is that it happens because in the autumn and winter the body's *qi* is in the process of sinking inwards from the exterior. I believe the *Suwen* was saying that under these conditions cold *xie qi* can be drawn inwards from the climate without triggering the symptoms of an exterior defensive response. Months later, in the spring and summer, as the body's *zheng qi* moves back to the exterior, it exteriorises the latent *xie* and triggers a *yang* heat response in the form of a fever without the signs of an exterior cold attack. This, the *Suwen* calls 'spring warmth' illness.

Pang An-shi wrote, 'As for warm disorders that occur between the spring and the summer solstice, both the *Suwen* and the *Shang Han Lun* call them all cold damage – but the progress and outcomes of heat disorders, damp-heat disorders and warm wind disorders are not all the same. Symptoms for each differ and so the treatments [should also] differ.' So, this can be seen as the point at which physicians are beginning to realise that the ancient Han dynasty theories of acute illness attack need revision in the light of current clinical experience.

Another *shang han* commentator was Zhu Gong, author of *Text for Saving Lives*. Zhu integrated *shang han* theory with classical notions such as the *jing-luo* in a lucid manner and, like Cheng Wu-ji, applied what we nowadays identify as the classic *bagang* (eight-principle) differentiation scheme for his analysis. Later, three books by Xu Shu-wei (+1079–1154), of today's Jiangsu province, further developed Zhu Gong's work. In one of these, Xu presented a version of the *Shang Han Lun* in verse for easy memorisation, thereby helping to popularise its ideas. In his *Shang Han Fa Wei Lun* he annotated the official Song version of the text, stressing his view that the *bagang* was the crucial key to making sense of the *Shang Han Lun*. Here Xu analyses the ideas behind the *Shang Han Lun* and includes his own experience and views, including those on the application of acupuncture to febrile disease. His third text, *Shang Han Jiu Shi Lun* (90 Essays on Cold Attack), is even more innovative in that Xu integrates 90 case histories into his discussions. Apart from the value of Xu's insights gained from the meeting of his scholarship with his clinical work, this is also the first known occasion in Chinese medicine history when a physician published a compilation of detailed professional-level case histories specifically intended to educate other physicians.

These scholarly and practical efforts brought *shang han* study up to speed and rescued from oblivion the use of both its ideas and its formulas. Later we see how its initial promise of supplying an effective key to the ongoing problem of febrile epidemics was not realised, and the fact that most of the time physicians still failed to get reliable outcomes with these illnesses. Now, in addition to ongoing study of the *Shang Han Lun*, the focus of Song scholarly work in re-appraisal and publishing broadened to more general aspects of theory and practice.

Song Bencao literature

In 1092 Chen Cheng from Sichuan published his *Chuangguang Buzhu Shennong Bencao Tujing* (Expanded, Annotated and Illustrated *Shennong Bencao*), a text that discussed those medicinals he had personally found to be the most effective clinically. This work is now lost, but some fragments survive. As the focus of Chen's work was on his personal experience of practising medicine, reflecting on what worked and what was ineffective, he highlights the developing clash between those physicians whose work was based on unquestioning acceptance of classical teachings and those with a more pragmatic clinical outlook – a conflict that continued through the first half of the 12th century.

Tang Shenwei's Zhenglei Bencao

Innovative though it was, Chen's work on the *bencao* was soon to be surpassed by Tang Shenwei, a physician from Chengdu in Sechuan, one of China's richest areas for herb cultivation. Working independently between 1080 and 1098 he, too, cross-fertilised the data on the medicinals found in the *Jiayou Bencao* and Chen's *Bencao Tujing* with his own clinical observations to create an extremely practical clinical manual. He consulted a massive 243 textual sources on medical practice that had not previously been included in the *bencao* literature, including a range of Buddhist, Daoist and Confucian texts. Tang's personal character was recorded by a friend who described him as an exemplary physician who treated rich and poor with equal respect. When treating the scholar classes, Tang often asked for prescriptions or secret texts in lieu of a fee and, in gratitude, many of these patients continued afterwards to supply him with further useful information on herbs and formulas.

In around 1098 Tang completed his *Jingshi Zhenglei Beiji Bencao* (*Bencao* for Urgent Needs Classified and Verified from the Classics), a work that remained unsurpassed for 500 years. Today the name of this text is abbreviated to *Zhenglei Bencao* (Classified *Bencao*). This is the earliest complete bencao to survive intact to the modern era, and is notable for using a classification system that was more practical for working physicians. It lay unnoticed for a decade before two literati officials recognised its importance and had it published in 1108 as *Jingshi Zhenglei Daguan Bencao* (*Daguan Bencao*). Following its discovery it was then reprinted many times.

Kou Zong-shi's Bencao Yanyi

In +1116 another important privately written text, *Bencao Yanyi* (Expanded *Bencao*), was completed by Kou Zong-shi. Based on *Jiayou Bencao* and *Tujing Bencao*, it focused on fewer medicinals (472), but provided much more by way of detail and commentary. The excellence of Kou's contribution was widely recognised in the higher echelons of medicine and earned him a senior official post. This was the first text to fully integrate the classical doctrines such as *yin-yang*, *xu-shi*, hot-cold, internal-external and *wu xing* into the *bencao* literature. Also, the internal organisation of Kou's *Bencao Yanyi* reflected his clear insight into the importance of the traditional model; this shows in the fact that he arranges the herbs and formulas by classical diagnostic categories such as hot-cold, *shi-xu*, internal and external, and *xie* and *zheng*. These differentiations of principles Kou referred to as the eight necessities (*ba yao*, 八要). The publication of Kou's *Bencao Yanyi* was a crucial moment in the development of Chinese medicine as it represents the clearest re-discovery of the ancient differentiation framework that is today referred to as *bagang*, and functions as a key basis for navigating through the complexity of the clinical landscape. Whilst these distinctions in principles were an important part of the thinking of the *Neijing*, the *Shang Han Lun* and some Tang dynasty texts, it was only in the Song dynasty that they were explicitly identified as a central organising principle of classical medicine.

> In treating disease there are eight necessities [*ba yao*, 八要] that, if ignored, will prevent effective treatment... Careful regard to these is essential if mistakes are to be avoided. The first is *xu*...the second is *shi*...the third is cold...the fourth is heat... the fifth is *xie*, the sixth is *zheng*...the seventh is internal...the eighth is external.
> (Kou Zong-shi, *Bencao Yanyi*)

Within a few decades this *ba yao* idea was to be picked up and refined first by the famous Song paediatrician Qian Yi and then by the Jin-Yuan dynasty scholar Zhang Yuan-su to set the foundation for systematic practice right up to modern times. By emphasising the importance of the classical *bagang* ideas and the *si zhen* (four diagnostic methods), practitioners were urged to differentiate disease using classical principles rather than simply treating according to the disease. This has remained an important foundation of Chinese medical thought that has continued until modern times.

Kou Zong-shi's *Bencao Yanyi* was also the first text to begin to incorporate the idea of *gui jing* (channel affinity) into the *bencao*. It also improved the understanding of dosage questions. Previously physicians generally applied fixed textbook doses as if blindly following a recipe. Kou emphasised the tailoring of all aspects of treatment according to the disease state, its chronicity and the patient's age and body state. He strongly disapproved of the practice of unthinking copying of treatment protocols from textbooks without regard to the individual situation of the patient at hand. Kou is notable, too, for condemning the use of the mineral alchemical longevity drugs beloved of Daoists such as cinnabar (*zhu sha*, mercuric sulphide), saying they had been responsible for innumerable deaths. By setting a clear rational benchmark for physicians to work within and to evolve, Kou's work laid an important foundation stone for the future progress in Chinese pharmaceutics.

Kou Zong-shi's notably pragmatic and rational outlook may have been inspired by the work of the brilliant court polymath and pragmatist Shen Kuo (+1035–1095), who was working a few decades earlier. Shen Kuo, who counted medicine amongst his numerous interests, had contributed his own experience and observations on the effects and identification of medicinals above the blind acceptance of earlier literature. Kou Zong-shi's language, investigative style and willingness to challenge accepted truths followed on from and mirrored that of Shen Kuo. In earlier classics it had been agreed, for example, that cormorants give birth to their young by regurgitating them. Taking the trouble to observe the birds mating and hatching their eggs, Shen Kuo corrected this mistake and commented that facts were more reliable when they were derived from proper observation – an idea that was to re-emerge a few centuries later in Europe at the dawn of the scientific revolution.

Although not primarily a physician, Shen Kuo's writings include *Liang Fang* (Good Formulas, +1061). The original *Liang Fang* was lost in around +1500 but in +1126 it was combined with another work to create *Su Shen Liang Fang* (Fine Formulas from Su and Shen), thereby allowing it to be reconstituted. One notable inclusion here is the discussion on the preparation and use of refined extracts of child's urine for medical use. Shen's common-sense approach exemplified the emerging Song critical medical spirit. Perhaps his most profound impact came from a short passage in which he highlighted deficiencies in the way herbs were cultivated, harvested and supplied for use in the pharmacy. He campaigned for more systematic and sophisticated methodologies based on a better study of the individual species characteristics. Later in this chapter, when we discuss developments in anatomy at this time in history, we will see another example of Shen Kuo's brusque challenges to previous doctrine.

Zhenghe Shengji Zonglu (Holy Compilation for General Relief)

Emperor Huizong (ruled +1101–1126) was a refined scholar famed for his calligraphy who also gave active support to scholarly medicine. He seems to have possessed an understanding of the need to move away from symptomatic styles of practice and penned a medical text of his own, *Sheng Ji Jing* (Sagely Benefaction Classic), that continued the dynastic theme of bringing classic doctrine to the forefront of Song dynasty medicine. Emulating the *Suwen* canonical style, it mixed discussion of formulas with information on individual medicinal substances. Completed in +1118, Huizong's *Sheng Ji Jing* was annotated by the imperial physician Wu Ti, and was specifically intended as a teaching tool that integrated ancient classical theory with neo-Confucianist thought. Understandably, given that it was written by the emperor, it focused more on theory than on practice and encompassed *yin-yang, wu xing, san cai* (heaven-earth-man cosmology), *zangfu, jing-luo* and *wuyun liuqi* (phase energetics). Huizong also included discussions on diet, health regulation and herbal medicine.

As well as writing his own text, in +1111 Huizong also ordered the compilation by court scholars of a new encyclopaedic formulary text, *Zhenghe Shengji Zonglu* (Holy Compendium for General Relief), that, as the title implies, was intended to benefit the general population. Completed in +1117 this book too espoused the use of classical theories in clinical practice. It incorporated the full text of an important earlier acumoxa publication, *Zhenjiu Tujing*, that had appeared in +1026 and that is discussed in more detail later in this chapter. Covering herbal medicine, the *Holy Compendium for General Relief* presents meticulous discussions on some 20,000 formulas recommended for use in contemporary practice and gave detailed discussions on chronobiology (phase energetics, *yun qi*), which was a personal interest of Emperor Huizong. Encyclopaedic in style, it also emphasised diagnostic pattern differentiation and the understanding of *zangfu* functions. It presented detailed discussions of practical therapy, *wu xing* theory and the energetic effects of the formulas on the *zangfu* organs. Shortly after publication the Jin invaders, who were to succeed in displacing the Song court to south China, seized most of the copies that had been printed, so the text had to wait until +1162 before it could be re-published.

With the rapid expansion of printing in the last decades of the Northern Song dynasty (which ended in +1127), numerous texts appeared on many subjects; the majority of the medical publications were on popular medicine as distinct from the classical tradition. Many people, both lowly and literati, read these popular simplified books and practised medicine without any real understanding of diagnostics or theory. This is understandable because the great complexity and expansive extent of the classical medical literature made it very challenging to see the wood for the trees. A significant difficulty for medical study, both in the Tang and early Song dynasties, was the fact that so much of the literature consisted of immense and unwieldy compilations composed simply of symptom indications and innumerable possible treatments for these. Classical medicine, written in abstruse language, was not easy to understand or to translate into coherent practice; it was far easier simply to look up a remedy for a particular symptom, something that was unhelpful for the progress of the high-level classical tradition. Fighting against this, with their higher level of criticality and their ongoing clarifications of the classical tradition, the best Song medical scholars began to reconcile the received tradition with actual clinical practice and endeavoured to make the classical medicine more transparent. In this work they helped to unite in more practical ways the *bencao*, the *fang shi* literature and the classical doctrines. This clarification and rationalisation process was to further mature in the subsequent dynasties and help classical-style practice survive and progress in the face of competition from more simplistic medical styles.

Establishment of the Song imperial pharmacy service

One of the most senior and influential ministers working between +1068 and +1076 was the renowned political and social reformer Wang Anshi, who championed many of the Song economic and cultural reforms aimed at improving life for the ordinary citizen. These reforms included measures to improve the lot of peasants, to counter fraud, to improve education and to reduce inequality. In modern terms we could see Wang Anshi's politics as socialist in nature – the ideals he fought for were humanitarian and egalitarian. Included amongst the many reforms he championed were innovations specifically intended to ensure that professional healthcare was no longer restricted to the ruling and wealthy classes. As we have seen, these were ideals that influenced even those at the very apex of power.

In +1069 the implementation of some of Wang's new social reforms began; one of these was the stipulation that the buying and selling of medicines would now fall under state regulation. This offered the dual benefits of improved public health as well as a new source of government revenue. In theory a new state medicine service would allow ordinary citizens access to something approaching the level of healthcare enjoyed by the upper echelons of society, and by +1076 imperial bureaucrats had set up China's first government-run pharmaceutical service in the capital (now Kai Feng in Henan province). Known as He Ji Ju (Universal Benefit Service), this fell under the jurisdiction of the Imperial Medical Bureau, Tai Yi Ju. Officially the actual pharmacy outlets were called Taiyi Ju Shuyao Su (Imperial Physicians Bureau for Prepared Medicines), but they soon became popularly known as Mai Yao Suo (Selling Medicine Places). He Ji Ju founded its own imperial drug factory with quality standards that were officially regulated and enforced.

Government-approved ready-made medicines were manufactured for general use; some were intended for mass distribution during epidemics or for preventative use when epidemics were anticipated. Previously, medicinal formulas were most often supplied fresh and ready for decoction, but He Ji Ju promoted the increased use of herbs that had been preserved by methods such as drying, powdering or forming into pills to ensure year-round availability. These methods of dispensing herbal medicines were cheaper and more efficient.

For its first 25 years the influence of the imperial pharmacy was mainly in the capital. A second factory was opened in +1103, and soon there were seven retail outlets. At first most were called Shu Yao Suo (Prepared Medicine Shop), but in +1114 they were renamed Yiyao Huimin Ju (Medicines for the People's Welfare) and Yiyao Heji Ju (Medicines of Unified Standards). The imperial pharmacy became an established part of life in the capital and then gradually spread throughout the country, eventually reaching small towns, villages and border areas. In +1136 the new Southern Song government, now based in Lin An (today's Hangzhou), re-established five pharmaceutical bureaus in the capital named Taiping Huimin Ju (Great Peace to Benefit the People).

One division of the imperial pharmacy service, the Zhangxiu Heliang Yao (Medicines Quality Regulation Administration Committee), aimed to protect public health with various official measures. They introduced quality control systems that were designed to counter the sale of fake or poor quality medicines and, in addition, a wide range of new standardised over-the-counter medicines were made available for over-the-counter sales. This soon became a very profitable enterprise; it developed rapidly and began to contribute significantly to government revenues.

The prepared medicines manufactured and sold by the imperial pharmacy were supplied in patient-friendly formats such as pills and powders. Apart from convenience for the patient, the idea of powdering herb formulas gave more efficient extraction of active components so that lower quantities of expensive and rare substances could be used for the same effect. Powdered formulas could also be formed into pills and tablets by mixing with honey or starch, and many of the medicine formats that we see in use today originate from the He Ji Ju pharmacy days. Costs were kept to a minimum by reducing the wastage that inevitably occurs with decoction methods, and wastage was also reduced by the fact that pills had a longer shelf life than loose herbs. The changed format is reflected in the fact that many formulas originating in the Song dynasty end in the words *san* (散, powder) or *wan* (丸, pill), rather than *tang* (汤, decoction).

Imperial pharmacy products were recognisable by their official seals, and their authenticity was ensured by the threat of fixed punishments for anyone caught marketing counterfeit products. Expiry dates and formal policies for the destruction of old stock were introduced, and officials could also be punished if lax management allowed stocks to dwindle; in this way the government set new higher regulatory standards for medical practice and dispensing. New techniques were developed to improve shelf life, and prices were controlled so that better regulated and more affordable medicine was widely available. Because these ready-made medicines could be stored for long periods and their quality was reliable, the service was a great success, both with doctors and their patients.

The He Ji Ju service was especially valuable in times of crisis, such as floods and epidemics, when private pharmacies might struggle to continue to provide a service. It also gave ordinary people easier and cheaper access to classically inspired medicine, an approach later summed up in a slogan:

> Choose a formula according to your symptoms, use the [ready-made] prescription. There is no need to go to doctors and no need to prepare and process. Seek your relief in the prepared pills or powder and the illness will be cured.

Many aspects of the official imperial pharmacy were remarkable and innovative. It was a vast, very complete and wide-ranging organisation that employed numerous officials of various ranks to supervise the complex procedures of procurement of medicinals, quality control, production and sale of the products. Quality controls were in place during the purchasing process and, in relation to monitoring stock procedures, ensured that any stale or degraded materials were dealt with immediately. Detailed regulations specified exact production methods and stipulated, too, that manufacturing processes should be carried out by properly trained staff and that quality control procedures such as the use of expiry dates be adhered to. The regulations ensured that medicines were constantly available day and night, even during floods, drought and epidemics. Employees who committed breaches of duty, such as the mis-selling of medicines, could be punished with lashings.

He Ji Ju officials were engaged in research and development of a sort; experts were sent on search missions for new formulas and trading links were set up with distant countries leading to the introduction of new substances for the *bencao*. The bureau also assigned specific people to carry out research into improved herb processing (*pao zhi*); methods developed included: water grinding, calcining, quenching in vinegar, preparation with alcohol, ginger or honey, roasting and burning and dry frying. This, for instance, was the time when the *yin* blood-nourishing medicinal *shu di huang* (cooked Rehmannia glutinosa root) was distinguished from *sheng di huang* (the relatively uncooked form) by cooking it with wine and digestion-aiding herbs such as *chen pi* (citrus reticulata peel) and *sha ren* (cardamom pods). Preparation in this way was found to make *di huang* less indigestible, to reduce its cooling properties and increase its *yin* blood-nourishing effects.

Improvements were made in the technology of medicine manufacture; commonly used formats included water pills, vinegar pills, alcohol pills and honey pills as well as refined preparations such as *gancao gao* (liquorice syrup) and *e jiao* (gelatine). Some special pills, such as those used in gynaecology or those intended to affect the mental state, were coated with gold or silver leaf, with the powdered *qing dai* (indigo) or the mineral *zhu sha* (cinnabar) to improve their preservation or effect.

The 'socialist' mindset behind the imperial pharmacy had medico-political implications. As more prepared and over-the-counter medicines became available, some aspects of classical medicine that were previously reserved for people with access to high-level physicians now became more freely available to the public. The ordinary person who had previously been reliant mostly on folk medicine, temple medicine and on wandering bell doctors now had more choice. The more modestly educated local physicians had easier access to a good range of classical formulas and, because of imperial medical publishing initiatives, practitioners could better themselves educationally. In addition, the ordinary person also had more opportunity to either self-medicate or, more likely, to seek the advice of the pharmacy staff. This situation obviously represented a threat to the literati physicians who may also have felt a sense of the erosion of classical medicine because their professed more expert diagnostic skill and their crucial formula tailoring arts were bypassed by the ready supply of off-the-peg medicines. This is an issue we return to in the next section.

It was not only the high-level classical physicians who were made uncomfortable by Prime Minister Wang Anshi's reforms; in +1076 he was ousted from his post by conspirators whose own interests were threatened by his innovations. Despite this, Wang Anshi's medical reforms were such a popular success that they endured long after his demise.

Taiping Huimin Heji Ju Fang

In +1110 the imperial pharmacy, under a team headed by Chen Shiwei, published a compendium of all the formulas that were routinely supplied by the state pharmacy – *Taiping Huimin Heji Ju Fang* (People's Benevolent Pharmacy of the Taiping Era). This was effectively the standard catalogue of the range of products available and their uses – a state pharmacopia.

The *Taiping Huimin Heji Ju Fang* formulary collection soon became a popular reference text for the many new literate ordinary physicians, but the elite physicians were less enthusiastic. It allowed a new profession to fill the gap between expensive medical scholar care and folk medicine. As mentioned, many saw this as a threat to their position as it facilitated cheap over-the-counter medicine prescribing that bypassed their services. It also meant that people without a rigorous training could set up as doctors, and so the classically trained physicians countered the rise of the He Ji Ju by taking every opportunity to emphasise the superiority of those who had been through

> **SOME *TAIPING HUIMIN HEJI JU FANG* FORMULAS**
>
> *Ba zheng san*
> *Chuan-xiong cha tiao san*
> *Er chen tang*
> *Huo-xiang zheng qi san*
> *Liang ge san*
> *Mu-li san*
> *Ping wei san*
> *San ao tang*
> *Shen ling bai-zhu san*
> *Shen su yin*
> *Shi quan da bu tang*
> *Shi xiao san*
> *Si jun-zi tang*
> *Si wu tang*
> *Su-zi jiang qi tang*
> *Xiang ru tang*
> *Xiang su san*
> *Xiao huo luo dan*
> *Xiao yao san*
> *Zhen ren yang zang tang*

arduous and expensive training in the classical doctrines at the imperial medical academies.

The literati physicians argued that patients' symptoms and illnesses may appear similar, but the underlying causes and individual body conditions may be very different. A formula that successfully cured a headache in the past could not be relied on to cure this individual's headache now, and only a scholarly physician trained in classical theory and diagnostics could provide reliable medicine. Later, the last of the 'four masters' of the Song–Jin-Yuan dynasties, Zhu Dan-xi, parodied this error, comparing the patient to someone who had dropped his sword in the middle of a lake and, intending to come back the next day to find it, marked the place it was lost by putting a notch on his boat.

As with so many grand benevolent ventures, ancient and modern, the imperial pharmacy idea gradually slipped from its founding idealistic principles into profiteering, fraud and corruption, eventually petering out in the Yuan dynasty. The massive funds that were needed to underwrite the endeavour in the face of such fraud were ultimately rooted in the emperor's private treasury and so, now riddled with embezzlement, the drain on resources became untenable. Ever-greater quantities of stock were stolen from the factories and pharmacies, rare and costly products were appropriated, and fake substances were substituted so that the charitable supply of medicines to the needy dried up and state-regulated medicine dwindled away.

THE RISE OF LITERATI PHYSICIANS

Around +1127 the centre of Song government moved south to what is today Hangzhou to begin the Nan Song (Southern Song) where, as a consequence of imperial approval, medicine remained a well-regarded career. Consequently the numbers of classically trained physicians grew, and the growth of medical scholarship meant that classical medical terminology increasingly became a standard part of professional medical practice. The increased academic ethos and access to publishing meant that many more physicians were in a position to disseminate their own thoughts and experiences, and so a much larger class of trained literati physicians was able to advance their skills and to communicate with their peers using a common specialist language and the printed word.

The new esteem that medicine enjoyed reached a high point in the Yuan dynasty (+1260–1368) when medical graduate status was officially considered equal to that of legal and warfare specialists. Medicine remained a rather less popular option, though, because medical graduates had fewer career openings in official government service, and so those recruited into medical training tended not to be the highest academic flyers. With this recruitment problem in mind Emperor Huizong, the penultimate Northern Song emperor, in +1103 established a new and highly prestigious medical school that was specifically designed to attract greater numbers of the most elite scholars. To support this change the term *ru yi* (literati physician) was coined as a distinguished label to indicate the high status of its graduates, and thereby increase the attractiveness of a career in medicine. Huizong's strategy worked well, and the policy continued to exert an influence through the subsequent Southern Song and Yuan dynasties. As well as the rigorous teaching of classical medical theory there was extensive clinical experience built into the training; this required students to write up case histories for marking. By the end of the Song dynasty a medical degree was recognised as the equal of other subjects in the imperial university. The next section details progress to this point.

Medical education in the Song

Right at the start of the Northern Song in +960 the government allowed Tai Yi Shu (Imperial Medical Office), that had been inherited from the preceding Tang dynasty, to continue. For a few decades it remained poorly regulated, but in +992 it was renamed Tai Yi Ju (Imperial Medical Bureau) and its status upgraded somewhat. Emperor Zhen Zong (+998–1022) introduced blind marking of all official exams and drastically expanded the education system, but medical educational reform continued to lag behind at this time, even given the support of the first Emperors Taizu and Taizong.

Social pressures worked against reform. In the Tang dynasty, official posts had usually passed along aristocratic family or military lineages; entry to imperial medical training was through the exam system that had been initiated in the Sui dynasty (+589–618), and this required a level of education that was accessible only to the aristocracy. The new Song regime, espousing peace, prosperity and benevolence, led to greater meritocracy and wider access to learning generally, but such a change could not occur overnight. Eventually, though, a new entrance system offered a fairer route to influence and, over the space of a few decades, the open access education policy allowed new blood into the system. The admission process for Tai Yi Ju was formidable, requiring references, family history and evidence of prior learning. Students had to complete a year of foundation studies before entry to the medical school, where they studied general medicine and accessed nine specialist departments.

Early in the 12th century, as Tai Yi Ju's rise to respectability gained momentum, it emulated the imperial university with its 'three hall method' (*san she fa*), which was an academic ladder system, the first rung of which was success in the entrance exam. Students then progressed stepwise according to exam success using a system called *sheng she* (ascending halls) which divided them into three grades: *wai she* (the outside hall), *nei she* (the inside hall) and *shang she* (the upper hall). The very talented could skip a grade or even graduate ahead of schedule. Exams were divided into public and private exams, with monthly private exams and an annual public exam. To gain clinical experience the student clinic provided treatment for military personnel and students from the other imperial colleges, and each student kept a printed case book that was used to record their cases and the treatment outcomes. The curriculum was regulated in every detail, and medical education now emulated the standards of the most prestigious state university, Tai Xue, so that for the first time a medical school was subsumed fully into the official state education system at the highest level.

Various measures were put in place to ensure fairness and to prevent cheating by candidates or unfair marking by examiners. Candidate anonymity was ensured by blind marking of exam scripts, with the candidate's name obscured. This method had already been used in Tang dynasty education but now, for an even more secure process, scribes were employed to copy scripts so that individual candidates could not be identified by their handwriting.

Student intake was initially capped at 120; then, in the decades following Wang Anshi's political reforms, student numbers stood at about 300 and, as medicine became an ever more popular academic pathway, numbers rose into the thousands. Early on, acumoxa study was included in the curriculum and, once it became established, the new imperial pharmacy service was given control of Tai Yi Ju.

Medical education continued to mature through the Song dynasty, and the success of Tai Yi Ju meant that edicts were then issued for a network of new local medical colleges to be founded, modelled on Tai Yi Ju. The intent was to generate even more classical physicians to serve the whole country, but the response from provincial centres to this initiative was lacklustre. Keen young scholars preferred to study in the capital and were reluctant to relocate to remote provinces to study.

> **SET TEXTS STUDIED IN THE TAI YI JU**
> *Suwen*
> *Nanjing*
> *Mai Jing*
> *Shang Han Lun*
> *Zhenjiu Jiayi Jing*
> *Qianjin Yao Fang*
> *Qianjin Yi Fang*
> *Zhubing Yuanhou Lun*
> *Taiping Sheng Hui Fang*
> *Shennong Bencao Jing*
> *Buzhu Bencao*
> *Longmu Lun* (Dragon-wood Essays)

Textual sources on acumoxa

The practice of acumoxa, and especially acupuncture, had declined considerably through the Tang dynasty. Even with active support for acupuncture from the first Song emperors much more publishing emphasis was placed on herbal medicine such that in the Northern Song in excess of 100 herbal texts were published by the Imperial Medical Bureau compared to just 18 on acumoxa – although many of the herb texts did include sections on acumoxa. *Taiping Shenghui Fang* (Imperial Grace Formulas), published in 992, devoted Chapters 99 and 100 to acumoxa using material copied from *Zhen Jing* (Acupuncture Classic) and two other late Tang writings which were the main surviving acumoxa texts. However, as a result of official support, acumoxa gradually re-established itself as the Song dynasty progressed.

Taizu, the first Song emperor, liked to dabble in acumoxa, and the fourth emperor Renzong also took a personal interest in this therapy. It is said that when his headache cleared after needling himself at Du 16, Renzong is said to have been so delighted he exclaimed '*xing xing!*' ('clearheaded!'), thereby giving the point a new alternative name. On another occasion Renzong is known to have received acupuncture treatment from a court official called Li Gong.

In 1034 Emperor Renzong was suffering a bout of illness that had failed to respond to the herbal prescriptions given by his court physicians, so an outsider called Xu Xi was summoned to help. To the dismay of the court physicians, Xu Xi proposed applying acupuncture treatment to the emperor's chest, just below the heart, so it was felt prudent to have the treatment demonstrated first on some volunteers. Renzong was then successfully treated, and Xu Xi was financially rewarded and given an official post at Tai Yi Ju. This is one incident that probably helped raise the status of acupuncture because shortly afterwards Renzong demonstrated his support by commissioning a text intended to standardise the acupoints and the *jing-luo* system. He also ordered new revisions of important acumoxa texts. All these events suggest that acupuncture had now become reinstated as a respected and accepted therapy in the highest circles of Song dynasty society.

Just prior to Renzong's rule, Emperor Zhenzong (ruled 997–1022) had also shown his support for acupuncture by ordering the revision of two acumoxa classics and the publication of a text on acumoxa points; this was published as *Tongren Shuxue Zhenjiu Tujing* (Chart of the Bronze Figure Acumoxa Points) in 1026 under the editorship of Wang Wei-yi. This meticulously researched book clarified disagreement about point locations and gave indications and methods of needling for 354 acupoints, and stressed the importance of proper anatomical knowledge in point location. It also presented an extensive discussion of the *jing-luo* system and its associated symptomatology, pathology and pattern differentiations. One section discusses *zangfu* patterns and their treatment in terms of acupoint formulae. Moxa, needle manipulation and other techniques employed in acumoxa practice are discussed and, besides acumoxa, *Zhenjiu Tujing* includes some information on the *bencao*, herb formulas (*fangji*) as well as diet, *shang han* studies and health exercises.

Straight after publication, the full text of Wang's acupoint chart was carved on stone tablets totalling two metres high by seven metres in length, placed in the capital Kaifeng so that practitioners could duplicate the text for study by taking rubbings. In 1971 some of the original tablets were excavated from parts of the Beijing city walls that had been built in 1445.

To accompany Wang Wei-yi's text the casting of life-size bronze acumoxa statues was ordered as a teaching tool to represent the newly standardised acupoint information. Casting of these bronze figures was completed in 1027; one was installed in the medical academy (called Yi Guan Yuan at this time) and the other in the Hall of Benevolent Assistance (Ren Jia Dian). The original versions were cast in separate pieces that could be detached to reveal the internal organs. They were pierced with the 354 points described in the *Zhenjiu Tujing* (acumoxa chart), and with the point names inlaid in gold.

As part of their examinations in acumoxa, students at the medical academies were required to diagnose a case and then apply acupuncture needles to the water-filled figure, which had been dipped in opaque yellow wax to hide the holes. Success in locating and needling the points was thus instantly apparent. To stand a chance of passing this exam students had to have learned to very accurately find the acupoints as the holes were only two or three millimetres in diameter; this represented a demanding test of knowledge and skill.

Further copies of the bronze figures were also cast and distributed, and one of the two originals was sent on tour around the provinces with the intention that local craftsmen would copy them locally for use in local medical institutes and so spread medical knowledge more widely. A few of these copies survive today, although none of them include the internal organs that are believed to have been a feature of the originals which are now lost.

These bronze acupuncture models were a significant innovation. Previously, acupoint locations were described in words with occasional sketchy illustrations supported by mentor tuition of variable quality. There was much disagreement and confusion between sources about the location and application of acupoints. We might call this situation a 'health and safety issue' today, and it must have sometimes led to injury and fatality. The mentor system allowed mistakes to accumulate and be passed on so that the quality of medical practice was degraded through a process akin to Chinese whispers. The bronze figures, together with the associated scholarship needed for their design, forced the number of points on each channel to be standardised and the number of main channels to be fixed at 12 main ones as well as the *ren mai* and *du mai* channels running up and down the midline of the front and back respectively – a standard that continues today.

In addition to safety and standardisation, the work on *Zhenjiu Tujing* also helped acumoxa move away from simple symptomatic practice to incorporate classical *jing-luo* and diagnostic theory. Its drawings were also much more accurate and anatomical than before, so the study of anatomy began to progress as a result of Wang's work. Other Song developments in relation to anatomy are outlined later in this chapter.

Zhenjiu Tujing and its accompanying bronze statues were the first attempt in the Song to provide a systematic, standardised acumoxa practice and to help integrate theory and practice for teaching purposes. It also served to counter poor practice and reduce injury by improving knowledge as patients were easily harmed by incorrect point location.

The fact that acupuncture was now, once again, accepted by the top literati physicians is reflected in the fact that many, such as Zhang Cong-zheng (aka Zhang Zi-he) and Li Gao (Li Dong-yuan), used it alongside acupuncture. These Jin-Yuan dynasty physicians are discussed in the next chapter. Next we outline the prominent Song physician Wang Zhi-zhong's perception of acupuncture and moxibustion.

WANG ZHI-ZHONG'S ZHENJIU ZI SHENG JING,
A NOTABLE SONG AUTHOR

Wang Zhi-zhong, also called Shu Quan, lived in Zhejiang province during the Southern Song and wrote his seven-volume *Zhenjiu Zi Sheng Jing* (Acumoxa Life-giving Classic) in 1165. Although this work focused on acumoxa, Wang believed that a good physician should have a range of skills: 'Good doctors are not those who practise only acupuncture without using moxa nor those who just use moxa and neglect acupuncture. Just applying acumoxa but lacking [the ability to prescribe] herbs does not make a good doctor either.'

Wang Zhi-zhong's work gave detailed instruction on the various methods of selecting, locating and treating acupoints including discussion on contraindications for acumoxa. In his practically orientated clinical manual, Wang describes the application of acumoxa in about 200 illnesses, including *shang han*, jaundice, wasting diseases, abdominal fullness, masses (*zheng jia*) and accumulations (*jiju*), oedema, ulcers and sores. In addition he introduces various extra points such as *mei chong, ming tang, dang yang* and *bai lao*. Wang offers details for the first time on the application of *du shu* (Bl 16), *qihai shu* (Bl 24), *guanyuan shu* (Bl 26) and *feng shi* (GB 31).

The practical value of Wang Zhi-zhong's text is further enhanced by the inclusion of 46 illustrations and various handy clinical tricks such as his systematic approach to the proportional body inch (*tong sheng cun*) system, traditionally used as an aid to locating acupoints. He wrote, '[Take the] inner side of the second section of the [patient's] middle finger, the left hand for males and the right for females; the distance between these two lines is one inch.' This remains today a basic rule of thumb for locating points, and is one of many examples of Wang's innovations that survive into modern practice. Wang, like Sun Si-miao in the Tang dynasty, emphasised the central place of *ahshi* (tender) points in acupuncture, and also discussed the importance of the patient's position during treatment for optimal effect. In relation to the *ahshi* concept he advocated palpating for the best points: '[When we] press it with a hand the patient feels better.' A strong advocate of moxibustion, Wang Zhi-zhong's *Zhenjiu Zi Sheng Jing* includes a detailed review of the history, development and methods of this treatment. He describes special techniques for treating wasting diseases such as pulmonary tuberculosis, moxibustion of haemorrhoids, the use of the acupoint *gaohuang shu* (Bl 43) and the use of moxa-partitioning agents such as garlic and aconite. His writings also include discussions of special needle techniques, many of which are included in modern practice.

Wang noted that some practitioners were unthinking and reckless in their use of moxa; he especially condemned the habit of blindly mimicking moxa protocols in found old texts whilst taking no account of the patient's actual illness. He did advocate the use of regular moxibustion for health maintenance using points such as *qihai* (CV 6), *guan yuan* (CV 4) and *zu san li* (St 36). He said: '*Qihai* is the place where man's primal *qi* is generated; for this reason [the famously sprightly but very aged] Liu Gong-du said: "I have no particular secret for supporting my health, just not allowing the *yuan qi* to assist my joy and anger and always keeping *qihai* warm."' On the same subject Wang also quoted a pre-Song acumoxa text which said that 'if you wish to remain in harmony do not allow *dan tian* (Ren 4), *san li* (St 36) and *qihai* (Ren 6) to become dry', referring to the practice of causing a blister or small suppurative sore to form at these places. In the treatment of some illnesses he wrote that suppurative moxibustion was essential to therapeutic success: 'After moxa treatment if a sore forms the illness will be cured; if it does not then the illness won't be healed.'

Wang included a personal dimension to his writings, and related some of his experiences of practising acupuncture on himself. When discussing the acupoint *xin hui* (Du 22), he said: 'In my youth I studied very hard [which is perhaps why] in my older years I developed a cold head. If I drink too much I get a hangover that feels like I have fractured my skull. Then I treated the point *xin hui* and not only does the head not feel cold any more but only the other day I got very drunk and suffered no head soreness at all!'

Song dynasty specialisms

From the Han dynasty and before, medical practice had always had its specialists, midwives, prescription gentlemen (*fang shi*), battlefield traumatologists and sores and ulcers specialists. For most of Chinese history medical craftspeople have wandered from town to town, applying specialist skills in treating ailments such as haemorrhoids. Zhang Zhong-jing could be said to have specialised in acute epidemic infections and Sun Si-miao in the Tang divided his textbooks into specialist areas such as midwifery, dietary medicine and so on. The fact that the Tang imperial medical school was divided into specialist departments also points to a tradition of specialisms, but it was in the Song that highly educated medical scholar doctors began to formalise specialist study and to take it to a new standard. Notable amongst these was Qian Yi, who is seen as the founder of pre-modern paediatric medicine in China.

QIAN YI (1032–1113)

Qian Yi (style name Zhong Yang) came from Yun Zhou in Shandong province. His father, although a skilled acupuncturist, was a wandering alcoholic and a wastrel who eventually embarked on an overseas adventure from which he failed to return. When Qian Yi was three years old his mother died and he was adopted by an uncle from whom he learned medicine and gained specialist knowledge about paediatric medicine. When he was 20 his aunt told Qian Yi about the disappearance of his father and he felt compelled to embark on a quest to find him. Over a period of ten years he made five journeys across the eastern seas searching for him, and eventually found him in a foreign fishing village and brought him back home to Shandong.

Qian Yi went on to become the most famous Song dynasty paediatrician and a significant contributor to the wider field of medicine. His surviving masterwork is the three-volume *Xiaoer Yaozheng Zhi Jue* (Knack of Paediatric Patterns) that was compiled and edited by his student Yan Xiao-zhong. This was published in 1119. A major Qing dynasty library inventory (*Si Ku Quan Shu*, Complete Books of the Four Libraries) described this book as 'the ultimate [paediatric text] – unrivalled for generations'. His other books, including *Shang Han Lun Zhi Wei* and *Ying Ru Lun*, have unfortunately been lost.

Specialising in paediatrics for over 40 years, Qian Yi gained significant experience, leading him to become a very famous Shandong physician. When he was 50 he

宋

successfully treated a highly placed princess and was then awarded membership of that inner sanctum of China's intellectual elite, the Hanlin Academy. Later he cured Prince Chi Zong's muscle spasms using *huang tu tang* (yellow earth decoction), and Qian's success in this case led to his appointment as imperial physician. With this highest-level stamp of approval numerous imperial officials and nobles sought consultations with Qian Yi, thereby adding even more to his fame.

Qian Yi based his style equally on his study of the *Neijing* and of the various historical styles, which he reconciled with his own astute clinical observation. His approach to understanding paediatric physiology, pathology, diagnosis and treatment was innovative. Children's physiology and pathology, Qian taught, was different to that of adults: 'Their *zangfu* are formed but are delicate and are not yet fully mature, their *qi* and blood are as yet insufficient so they are rather unstable and apt to suddenly become *xu* and *shi*; they are also quick to become hot or cold.' He developed specialist inspection-based diagnostic methods he called 'patterns manifested on the face', and 'patterns seen in the eyes' to identify internal patterns of disharmony. The *Song Dynasty History* describes some examples of Qian Yi's inspection skills: 'After examining a young prince he concluded immediately that he could be cured without recourse to medicine; on another occasion he correctly predicted that a child, although well at the time, would progress to develop epilepsy.'

An early proponent of differentiation using the eight-principle patterns (today called *bagang*), Qian Yi was the first to apply *zang* pattern diagnosis to paediatrics. Based on his descriptions of *xu* and *shi* conditions of the five *zang*, he devised appropriate treatment strategies for supplementation or drainage. In doing this he laid a foundation stone for modern *bian zheng lun zhi* diagnosis and treatment. Qian Yi taught that in paediatrics one should use mild-acting medicinals and treat children cautiously, avoiding drastic attacking or strong purging methods as well as thoughtless supplementation. Through a lifetime's study he established a relatively complete paediatric system of treatment according to pattern identification.

Qian Yi gave detailed and lucid descriptions of many children's diseases such as measles, whooping cough, acute and chronic 'fright wind', speech impediments, non-closure of the fontanels, rickets, weakness and emaciation. Another notable contribution was his introduction of a set of standards and methods for paediatric nursing. His influence was not confined to paediatrics, and many of his ideas benefited general medicine, surgery and gynaecology. It was Qian Yi's introduction of the method of 'pattern identification of the five *zang*' that was soon to inspire Zhang Yuan-su to more firmly promulgate pattern diagnosis by differentiating *zangfu* conditions of *xie-zheng*, *biao-ben*, *han-re* and *xu-shi*.

The important *yin*-nourishing formula, *liu wei di huang wan*, was Qian Yi's inspired modification of the ancient *Shang Han Lun* prescription *jingui shenqi wan* in which he removed *fu zi* and *rou gui* to convert it into a formula suitable for the treatment of diabetes in children. *Liu wei di huang wan* is of particular historical significance because it became an emblematic formula for the *yin*-nourishing and kidney-strengthening schools that developed in the subsequent Jin-Yuan and Ming dynasties.

Qian Yi's *liu wei di huang wan* was to be the inspiration for numerous variant formulas introduced later, such as:

- Zhu Dan-xi's *zi yin da bu wan* (yin-nourishing great tonification pill) created by combining *liu wei di huang wan* with *huan shao dan* (return to youth tablet)
- Li Dong-yuan's *zi yin shen qi wan* (yin-nourishing kidney *qi* pill)
- Wang Hao-gu's *du qi wan* and *xie shen wan*.

In the Ming dynasty, Zhang Jie-bin's kidney tonic formulas such as *zuo gui wan*, *you gui wan* and *da yuan yin* were also derived from *liu wei di huang wan*.

Qian Yi invented many other formulas that have contributed to modern practice, including: *dao chi san, xie bai san, yi gong san, xie huang san, bu fei e jiao tang, ren shen bai du san* and *shengmai gegen tang*. Many of Qian Yi's formulas function to remove heat, an observation that may reflect the fact that heat illnesses were becoming more prevalent or more recognised in his time.

INNOVATIONS IN ANATOMY DURING THE SONG

Although it is sometimes said that Chinese medicine is characterised by its lack of study of anatomy, there are Song dynasty records of the dissection of two prisoners and, in this period, two anatomical texts appeared. Also, as we saw earlier, the bronze acupuncture figures cast for teaching purposes originally included a set of internal organs. Physicians in China have long recognised the importance of human anatomy, and anatomical terms frequently appear in the *Neijing* where there is evidence of meticulous end-to-end recording of the dimensions of the gastrointestinal tract in the Han dynasty. At no point in history, though, did Chinese medicine develop the fascination with or precision in the study of morbid anatomy shown by the Italian anatomists of the 16th century or the fad for anatomy as a form of popular entertainment that appeared in early 19th-century England. Chinese physicians generally put function above structure in their quest for medical know-how. Anatomical knowledge was information possessed by butchers, bonesetters, trauma specialists and, to some degree, by midwives. The surviving Chinese records of forensic post-mortem procedures themselves also presuppose human dissection and its associated knowledge, so it is clear that anatomy was not quite as neglected as is often suggested. It seems that traditional classical physicians were satisfied with a relatively sketchy outline of anatomy, at least until the Qing dynasty, when this issue was singled out by Westerners as evidence of the great superiority of medicine from the West, leading to increased study of anatomy by Chinese medicine physicians such as the rather amateur efforts of Wang Qing-ren (1810). A focus on the relative sophistication, safety and effectiveness of actual treatment methods at that time might have been more telling when properly reconciling the cross-cultural medical balance sheet; the relative merits of treatment East–West 200 years ago would, I believe, come out firmly in favour of Chinese medicine.

As part of the desire in the Song to advance medical knowledge some efforts were made to develop anatomical knowledge with the production of new charts. Notable is the *Ou Xi Fan Wu Zang Tu* (Chart of the Organs of Mr Ou Xi-fan) that appeared in 1045, and also the *Cun Zhen Tu* (Collected Truths Chart) by Wu Jian, based on dissections conducted between 1041 and 1048. These publications were based on the morbid anatomy of a total of 56 people (including Mr Ou Xi-fan) who had been executed by the Song government and the cadavers made available for dissection. The original charts have been lost, but their contents and details of the way in which they were prepared are recorded in Zhao Yu-shi's *Bin Tui Lu* and Ye Meng-de's *Yan Xia Fang Yan*. They mainly depict visceral anatomy in both text and diagram format, and give reasonably accurate descriptions of the anatomy and locations of the internal organs. They do, however, lack the great precision of the European anatomists working five centuries later.

> Below the lungs there are heart, liver, gallbladder and spleen, below the stomach there is the small intestine, below the small intestine there is the large intestine; the small intestine is clean, clear and empty, while the large intestine there is debris and waste; alongside the large intestine there is the bladder.
>
> Kidneys: there is one slightly to the right below the liver, the other is slightly to the left above the spleen; spleen is on the right-hand side of the heart.
>
> There was widespread yellowish stuff that was fat. (Wu Jian, *Cun Zhen Tu*)

The descriptions included observations of pathological phenomena such as 'Mr Meng Gan had suffered much from coughing so his lungs and gallbladder were blackened'; with modern eyes, however, we can identify some basic errors. It was said, for instance, that there are three openings in the throat, one for food, one for water and one for gases. This mistake in *Cun Zhen Tu* was identified and corrected by the renowned Song dynasty polymath Shen Kua.

A successor to *Cun Zhen Tu*, *Cun Zhen Huan Zhong Tu* (Chart of Collected Truths Encompassing the Inside), was compiled by Yang Jie between 1102 and 1106 and published in 1113. This was based on the dissection of people in Sizhou; the original chart included graphic representations of the viscera together with the 12 channels and collaterals of acumoxa theory. Again, the original has been lost, but some of its contents have survived, this time in Sun Huan's *Xuan Menmai Nei Zhao Tu* (Chart of the Pulse Gate Reflecting the Profound Mysteries), which was published in the Yuan dynasty.

Yang Jie's anatomical diagrams consist of 'human body – anterior view' and 'human body – posterior view', and depict the internal organs in the chest and abdomen cavity. There are also separate diagrams of all the systems including a right lateral chart of the internal organs in the thorax. The 'heart *qi* chart' illustrates the main blood vessels in the right part of chest and abdomen. The 'sea of *qi* diaphragm chart' describes the diaphragm and the shape of the main vessels and oesophagus. The 'systemic chart of the spleen and stomach pouch' describes the digestive system. The 'water-separating gate chart' describes the urological system, and the 'systemic chart of the life gate, the large and small intestine and bladder' describes the reproductive system. All the charts are attached with detailed textual explanation.

In general the anatomical descriptions in Yang Jie's text are accurate, and correct some of the mistakes in Wu Jian's *Ou Xi Fan Wuzang Tu*, so his work represents a milestone not only for Chinese medicine, but also for the history of medicine generally. Naturally the work contains some misapprehensions; for example, it was stated that the small intestine had a connection with the bladder, a mistake that probably arose because classical doctrine indicated an energetic connection between these viscera. It is a human trait to see what we expect to see; indeed, it was only in the 1990s that anatomists in the West realised that the clitoris is very much larger and more extensive than had previously been recognised. Authors in the subsequent Ming dynasty, such as Gao Wu in his *Zhenjiu Ju Ying* (Acumoxa's Assembled Heroes) and Yang Ji-zhou's *Zhenjiu Dacheng* (Acumoxa's Great Successes), often quoted the anatomic material of *Cun Zhen Tu* which tells us that anatomy was taking an increasing part in Chinese medicine writings following the investigations of the Song dynasty.

Anatomical knowledge also underpinned the Yuan dynasty forensic manual *Xi Yuan Zhi Lu* of 1247, which is discussed in the next chapter.

In sum

Imperial patronage and the appearance of a mass publication industry, combined with a benevolent appreciation of public needs, drove a Song revolution in medicine and medical education, raising the status of medicine as a profession. The *Medical Encyclopaedia* provided a pinnacle of Song writing on formulas and contemporary best practice generally, whilst the *Illustrated Bencao* brought the study of individual herbs to a new level. The founding of the imperial pharmacy enabled reliable supplies of authentic, quality-controlled medicinals and gave wider access to medicine far superior to folk treatment. There was integration, exploration and development of *bencao* and *fang ji xue* writing traditions, and classical doctrines became more fully integrated into practice. The *Shang Han Lun* was re-discovered, interpreted and brought to physicians' attention after eight centuries of neglect. Acumoxa was rescued from its decline in the Tang dynasty and re-instated into literati mainstream medicine; it was also standardised and developed by royal patronage, by increased formal investigation and by the production of the bronze acumoxa statues.

State-organised medical schools also helped create new generations of rational and scholarly physicians with a commonly agreed and coherent theory base. Large numbers of popular self-taught healers appeared accompanied by a flourishing of both state and private publishing – linked to the growth of printing technology. Qualified physicians' dominance was threatened and they responded by stressing the importance of classic notions and good education in medical practice. Having updated and standardised the classical tradition, the scene was set for some new innovations to develop through the Jin and Yuan eras.

6

SOUTHERN SONG AND JIN-YUAN MEDICINE

A perpetual source of irritation through much of China's history has come from the various militaristic 'barbarian' cultures in the far north such as the Mongols, the Liao and the Jin, who were constantly fighting the Han Chinese. Generally these people were struggling to escape from the marginal lifestyle provided by the harsh terrain in these northern parts. At the time of Huizong, the art and culture-loving last emperor of the Northern Song, the main threat came from the Jin tribes originating in Manchuria. Huizong's administration had first persuaded the Jin people to collaborate with him in subduing the aggression of the Liao people, but as soon as this had been achieved, the Jin then turned on China itself, invading the capital Kaifeng in 1127, and imprisoning Huizong and his entire court of 3000 or so people. In a very short time the whole of northern China was under Jin control, forcing the Han Chinese civilisation to retreat en masse 1000 kilometres south to found a new capital in Hangzhou (then called Lin An), leaving control of the north to the Jin barbarians based in Beijing (then called Ta Tu). As part of the peace negotiations the conquerors demanded the original Song dynasty cast bronze acupuncture figures, which were subsequently lost. The mass migration southward marked the start of the Southern Song dynasty, a period that became a flourishing and prosperous cultural highpoint involving fine dining, boating on the lake, poetry and dancing. Eventually, the Mongols were to overthrow the Jin dynasty in the north before then invading southwards to bring the Southern Song dynasty to an end, and then in 1369, the Mongol Yuan dynasty itself was overthrown.

As we have seen, the Northern Song government had made considerable efforts to reappraise and develop the classical medical tradition, actively supporting the dissemination of medical knowledge and the altruistic ethos of making better healthcare accessible to the populace. Now, in the Southern Song capital of Hangzhou, high culture and civilisation reigned, the intellectual respectability of medicine continued, and the impetus to see it improved remained intact. The loss of life from epidemics remained an important concern for both people and government, and so medical scholars carried on their quest for more effective treatments for febrile illnesses.

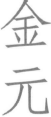

The public welfare ideal that had stumbled in the Tang dynasty was revived by the early Northern Song emperors who also took an active personal interest in medicine, some even going so far as to learn some classical medicine themselves. With stronger imperatives from the very top, the previously ineffectual Tang healthcare initiatives could be actualised. The founding of the Song dynasty Imperial Medical Bureau gave an institutional embodiment to the emperor's active support for medical scholarship. As well as feeding innovation, it also gave much greater status to physicians and to medical study generally. The Song dynasty advances in printing technology meant that imperial medical officials were now much better placed to foster real medical and public health advances and to put them in a position to disseminate the benefits more effectively. As a result of all this imperial patronage there was an exponential growth in the numbers and quality of literate physicians with a neo-Confucian ethic (*ruyi*). The ground was now more fertile for medical innovation to continue in the following Jin and Yuan dynasties.

In the last chapter we saw, too, how Kou Zong-shi's *Bencao Yanyi* began the progress toward a more explicit introduction of what we now call the eight principles (*bagang*: hot-cold, internal-external, excess-deficiency, *yin-yang*). I say 'more explicit' because the *bagang* ideas appeared frequently in the *Suwen* and had been an important developing theme in the classical tradition since then in key texts such as the *Shang Han Lun*. Kou Zong-shi's own distillation and re-packaging of this idea differed slightly from the modern version in that it incorporated *xie* and *zheng* in place of *yin* and *yang*. As Song scholarly medical influence progressed into the Jin and Yuan dynasties, the increased clarity of this simple scheme designed to facilitate clinical orientation helped guide medical practice away from its ever-present tendency to slide into either symptomatic therapy on the one hand, or medicine based on abstruse metaphysical speculation on the other.

Medical education in the Jin-Yuan dynasties

Jin dynasty medical education continued the Song system of state-regulated medical training, and the Yuan dynasty also supported medical education, leading to the founding of new medical schools across the country. A specific government department was set up to regulate medical education and to oversee the testing and selection of doctors everywhere. The imperial Medical Publishing Bureau continued for the ongoing editing and dissemination of medical books, and official regulation of the activities of the medicinal herb supply industry remained. The Yuan dynasty imperial medical school included many specialist departments, and at this time the study of orthopaedic treatment received a lot of attention. Carrying on the Tai Yi Shu (medical academy) tradition, students of medicine were subjected to rigorous examination and assessment procedures, and systems of reward and punishment were in place for teachers.

The Southern Song and the Jin-Yuan dynasties were a time of much medical innovation. Especially famous are the contributions made by the 'four masters' of this period: Liu Wan-su, Zhang Cong-zheng, Li Dong-yuan and Zhu Dan-xi. In line with convention, these four are the main focus of this chapter, although discussion of their work should not be allowed to completely overshadow the brilliance of contributions made by other figures, especially that of Zhang Yuan-su who directly or indirectly influenced three of the four famed masters. We later review some of the other important developments in this period, such as the writing of specialist texts on specialities such as paediatrics, gynaecology and improvements in pulse and tongue diagnostics, and the maturation of forensic medicine in China. First, though, it is useful to examine the work of Chen Yan.

Prominent Jin-Yuan physicians

Chen Yan

Chen Yan (aka He Xi and Chen Wu-ze) was a native of Qing Tian in today's Zhejiang province. Considered exceptionally bright, he became renowned for his skill in pulse diagnostics, prescription writing and for his ability to accurately predict the course of his patients' illnesses. He is best known for the contribution he made to Chinese medicine aetiology in his *Sanyin Jiyi Bing Zheng Fang Lun* (Formulas for the Three Categories of Pathology) or *San Yin Fang* (Three Causes Formulas) written between 1161 and 1174.

As a Confucian physician, or *ruyi*, Chen rooted his thesis largely in his study of classical Han dynasty medical doctrine; in particular his *San Yin* idea was derived from statements found in Zhang Zhong-jing's classic, *Shang Han Zhabing Lun*. Chen Yan's work aimed to systematise disease aetiology; this was needed because existing writings on this subject, such as the Tang dynasty classic *Zhubing Yuanhou Lun* (Chao Yuan-fang's *On the Origin and Symptoms of Disease*), lacked clarity and coherence. In the process of his attempts to systematise the bewildering complexity of disease causation, Chen Yan realised that all aetiology could, in the first instance, be subsumed under three main categories:

- *Nei* – internal causes

- *Wai* – external environmental causes

- *Bu nei-bu wai* – 'not internal, not external'.

Gaining a clear understanding of the causes of a patient's illness is an important aspect of professional medicine for various reasons: it leads to meaningful preventative medicine, it allows ongoing causative factors that might hinder therapeutic progress to be identified and corrected through lifestyle advice, and it allows clearer analysis of the ways that pathogenesis from multiple contributory causalities can conspire together to create illness.

In his *San Yin Fang* Chen summarises his argument that 'at the crux of medicine there is nothing outside these three causes'. Essentially quite simple, his scheme

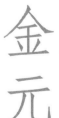

offered greater clarity in guiding practitioners towards an understanding of aetiology by reducing some of the mire of complexity of previous work on the subject.

Chen's reference to internal causes of disease primarily meant the traditional *qi qing* (seven emotional excesses), whilst his external factors meant the *liu yin* (six environmental excesses) as well as the then still-puzzling epidemic disease pathogens. His 'not-external, not-internal' factors referred to miscellaneous aetiologies: dietary causes such as starvation, over-eating and eating unhealthy foods, injury by animals or insects, lacerations and injuries, overwork or indolence, poisoning and illnesses contracted through unsuitable sexual activity.

The injurious effects of excessive emotions were, he said, considered internal aetiologies because although they may manifest themselves on the body exterior, they all first arose internally from *qi* constraint of the *zangfu*. By contrast, the *liu yin* or exterior pathogens initially invaded the *jing-luo*, but once inside the body they could affect the *zangfu*, so they were considered to be external causes. Any of the three causality categories may induce illness singly or in combination, so, although the various factors could not be separated completely, they helped guide physicians in untangling aetiologies when examining patients. Chen considered that it was of crucial importance to trace the causes of the energetic patterns of disharmony underlying a patient's illness before applying treatment.

> In treating diseases we must know causes; without knowing causes there is no way to understand the origins of pathology…ignorance of causes leads to the application of wrong treatments. In the proper treatment of illness we should examine its three possible causes; when the relative contributions of the three causes are clear, then there is no treatment that fails to hit the mark. (Chen Yan)

Chen Yan's contribution was more than simply delineating these three broad categories; he also specified the typical aetiologic mechanisms underlying the classical disease patterns, and explained the causal links between the two. Making this linkage explicit provided a crucial reminder for physicians of the systematic nature of professional medical discourse. For future literati physicians Chen's clarification of the classical medicine principle of 'in diagnosis seek the cause' became a distinctive, more concrete and now more achievable ideal of professional medicine. This is a characteristic that represents a point of contrast between literati physicians and their competitors, the less educated dilettante physicians and pharmacy dispensary specialists who had come to the fore in the Song dynasty.

Chen offered the issue of dizziness as an instance of his *san yin* theory in action, and as an example of the greater clinical precision that could be expected from a professional physician. Compared to the often rather opaque literate medical writings of others, Chen Yan was plain speaking; reading this relatively lucid account helps us to appreciate Chen Yan's contribution to modern standard clinical practice.

> Dizziness may involve any of the three causes, it is not simply due to just wind attacking the head. It may be triggered by external attack to the three *yang* channels

[of the head] which can all induce dizziness, heavy head, stiff neck. With wind there will be sweating, with cold there is sharp pain, with summer-heat there is hot and stifling sensation and with dampness there is sticky heaviness, vomiting and faintness. These are all external factors. [On the other hand] joy, anger, sadness and worry all can stagnate the *qi* of the *zang*; in this way, constraint is generated and saliva clumps to form thin mucus and ascends together with any rebellious *qi* lingering in *yang* meridians. This makes people dizzy and nauseous with pain around the eyebrows and eyes and an inability to open the eyes properly. These are classed as internal disease factors. Furthermore, starvation and overeating, injury resulting from sweet and greasy food or excessive sex can all cause excess above and deficiency below. Furthermore, tooth extraction, lacerations, vomiting, diarrhoea, blood loss and heavy uterine bleeding, all can cause dizziness, blurred vision, room rotating or passing out when trying to get up. These belong to not-internal, not-external aetiology. Thus each of these types should be treated with different methods. (Chen Yan, *San Yin Fang*)

As well as outlining his 'three causes' theory Chen's *San Yin Fang* also provided discussions of many common illnesses in internal medicine, surgery, gynaecology and paediatrics. Alongside this he included some 1500 formulas, many of which had not been recorded prior to the Song dynasty, an important example of which is the commonly used phlegm-dispelling formula *wen dan tang* which appears first in Chen's text. The text is clearly laid out and uses a lucid, concise analysis that is supported by discussions of clinical evidence, rationale, treatment methods and prescriptions. The great importance of the *San Yin Fang* was recognised at the time, earning it a summary in the inventory of the imperial library that said it presented 'high-grade theory – quite simply essential and not to be compared with other coarsely written and verbose material'.

In addition to this, his most famous contribution, Chen Yan compiled a *bencao* text, and in 1161 also completed a text called *Yi Yuan Zhi Zhi* (Treatment Based on Aetiology), a six-volume herb formula text. This remained unpublished.

Four masters of the Jin-Yuan

The mood of the Song-Jin and Yuan dynasties involved a public-spirited impetus to make the benefits of the learned medical tradition more widely available, both socially and geographically, by promoting medical scholarship and by the introduction of a state-run pharmacy service. With the new higher regard for medical scholarship, numerous great medical thinkers flourished at this time. As mentioned earlier, traditional accounts of the Jin-Yuan era identify four famous scholar physicians – Liu Wan-su, Zhang Cong-zheng, Li Dong-yuan and Zhu Dan-xi – who are each credited with founding a particular school or current of practice with its own following. These styles continued to evolve in the subsequent Ming dynasty, and each has contributed something to modern thinking and practice,

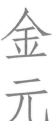

especially in relation to Chinese herb practice, although this should not be taken to obscure the fact that each of the four masters also made use of acumoxa treatment.

Liu Wan-su (1120–1200)

Alive roughly from 1120 to 1200, the first of the four great Jin-Yuan doctors was Liu Wan-su (official title Tong Xuan Chu Shi) from Hejian in Hebei province. Later in life, as his fame grew, he was given the nickname Liu Hejian (Liu from Hejian), which is why the style of practice he developed is often referred to as the Hejian school.

Fascinated with medicine from childhood, Liu is said to have obsessively studied the *Neijing* and to be rarely seen without a book in hand. Like most scholar physicians of his time Liu believed that the fundamental rules (*fa*) and methods (*shu*) of medicine should be rooted in the wisdom of the earliest classics. He was especially interested in combining these fundamental ideas with the then popular *wuyun liuqi* (five movements, six *qi*) medical cosmology doctrine, and probably knew the writings on this subject that had been published in 1099 by the similarly named Liu Wen-shu.

Inevitably, Liu Wan-su's clinical work involved the challenge of treating febrile patients and so, along with most physicians of the time, he would have been frequently witness to the premature deaths of friends and loved ones. Many of his contemporaries attached great value to the *wuyun liuqi* calendric ideas and its associated *san cai* (heaven, man, earth) philosophy, and so Liu believed that medicine should take more account of these. Intrigued by medical *wuyun liuqi* doctrine, he was almost certainly unaware that most of the *Neijing* discussions on this subject (*Suwen*, Chs 66–74) had been added to the text only four centuries previously by Wang Bing and were not part of the original Han dynasty text. To Liu Wan-su the fact that these sections were so complex and so much longer than the others served only to emphasise their importance. For Liu and his contemporaries, support for the validity of the medical cosmology theories was provided by the fact that epidemics do indeed occur in regular cycles and at particular times of year. So, taking his clinical experience in treating high fevers together with *wuyun liuqi* theory, and his own reading of the *Neijing*, Liu Wan-su introduced new ideas on heat and fire diseases that became the basis of his heat-clearing style. This may be an instance of the paradoxical and not uncommon occurrence in Chinese medicine for erroneous ideas to generate useful and effective new avenues of theory and therapeutics.

Liu wrote that 'distinguishing *yin* and *yang*, *xu* and *shi* is most important…[but] the way to [fully] understand an illness should involve matching its illness *qi* (*bing qi*) to the transformations of *wuyun liuqi*'. In order to achieve its internal mathematical symmetry the *wuyun liuqi* system needed to reconcile the five-phase scheme with the six-part and twelve-part calendar cosmology. This was achieved by splitting the fire phase into two aspects, namely into ministerial and princely fire corresponding to the *sanjiao* and pericardium respectively. Liu interpreted this doubling of the fire phase as an indication of an extra emphasis that ancient physicians accorded to fire as an aetiological agent. So, before moving on to outline Liu's *wuyun liuqi* ideas, we first examine the founding of his heat and fire school of practice.

With the frequent failure of Song dynasty medicine to successfully treat febrile epidemics in mind, medical scholars in the early part of the Song dynasty had worked hard to make sense of *shang han* theory in the hope that the answers lay in that ancient and sagely text. Now, unfortunately, despite all the scholarly work in deciphering the *Shang Han Lun*, febrile epidemics continued to devastate communities, and so physicians began to realise that the promise of the *shang han* study had not been fulfilled and that a different approach was needed. They noticed that manifestations of heat predominated over cold in most acute infections of the time. To Liu Wan-su it made more sense to investigate the importance of pathogenic heat in acute disease than cold, and in doing so he eventually founded the heat clearing school (*liang re pai*), also known as the Hejian doctrine after Liu's home province. Liu appears to have been the first to take account of the fact that the warm pungent herbs and prescriptions appropriate for *wind-cold* acute exterior invasion were, more often than not, ineffective in treating current febrile disease. As we will see later in this chapter, Liu was to gain some personal experience of this issue.

Through his dedicated study Liu Wan-su is reputed to have reached a very high level of scholarship. He achieved considerable respect from his peers as well as gaining considerable fame amongst the local population for his success in treating the dreaded epidemics of the time. Liu's reputation reached the attention of Emperor Jin Zong (Wan Yuan-Jing) who offered Liu high-status government posts on three occasions, but each time Liu declined, saying he preferred to practise among ordinary people – although it is possible to think of other reasons why he might have wished to avoid service as a court physician. To this day Liu remains a folk hero in the modern Hejian region, where his name survives as a local legend and tourist attraction.

Liu is likely to have been exposed to the work of the very eminent and innovative Song dynasty paediatrician Qian Yi who, in the course of making pioneering developments to *zangfu* differentiation, designed formulas intended to clear *zangfu* heat such as *xie huang san* and *xie bai tang*. Qian Yi's work may have helped inspire Liu to develop his own heat clearage style.

'Fire-heat theory' (*huo re lun*) was Liu Wan-su's main thesis – the proposition that fire and heat are the cause of many illnesses. He justified this in the standard classical manner by citing evidence from the *Neijing* and *Shang Han Lun*. Based on his own clinical experience, Liu described over 50 types of fire disease that he had derived from the ten categories of heat and fire disease that appear in Chapter 18 of the *Suwen*. An especially notable innovation included here was his delineation of an exterior wind-heat pattern for the first time in Chinese medicine, an idea that was later to be adopted and embellished as one of the strands of the Qing dynasty warm febrile school discussed later in Chapter 8. Prior to Liu's work the concept of wind-heat exterior invasion did not exist.

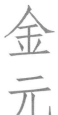

Liu saw that the devastating epidemic fevers generally involved more heat signs from their onset than fitted with the cold progression patterns of the *Shang Han Lun*. It seems likely that Liu's theories, although justified with classical quotes, really arose from clinical facts and the evident gap between what the *Shang Han Lun* said that clinicians should see, and what was actually observed in febrile patients in the Song–Jin-Yuan dynasties. Throughout history physicians can be divided into those who simply learn and apply doctrine, and those who are sufficiently unsettled by disparities between what the textbooks say and what they see in practice to begin to question current practice. Liu Wan-su belongs in this latter group. The tendency for Chinese scholars to overly revere the orthodoxy of early classical texts is sometimes taken as evidence of a backward-looking and innovation-weak approach; the physicians who do most to advance the medicine are often those who take a critical stance and are prepared to revise their opinions in light of new information.

Part of Liu Wan-su's thinking came from his study of the *wuyun liuqi* medical cosmology theories that employed the 'guest-host' concept to describe the relationship between the influences of heaven, earth and mankind. With this in mind he reasoned that man was warm blooded and activated by *qi*, so the basic host *qi* of our bodies could be seen as warm and *yang*. When a *guest* pathogen entered the body, following good Confucian behaviour, it assumed the qualities and behaviours of the host, so in terms of medicine pathogens all tended to become hot. This contribution to Chinese medicine thought is known as 'similar transformation' theory, an idea that was the start of a new way of seeing acute heat disease. Further accumulation of interior heat added to this effect.

Based on his similar transformation theory, Liu concluded that any of the six environmental *qi* (*liu qi*) could transform into heat or fire. He believed, too, that when any of the emotions became extreme, they could also generate heat or fire patterns that built up on the interior. In other words, heat and fire may be generated either as a consequence of exterior pathogen invasion or as a result of internally generated disease factors. Such heat or fire pathologies might develop in a variety of ways. Especially relevant in relation to fevers was Liu's realisation that a hot clinical presentation could develop as a consequence of *yang qi* constraint, which was itself due to cold invasion: 'Take cold and heat,' he wrote, 'although these two are very different; still, a cold pathogen may stagnate inside such that *yang qi* becomes constrained and turns to heat.' This was the first time that this possibility had been explicitly recognised in the classical writings, although, again, it was already implicit in the *Shang Han Lun*, for example, in the application of the formula *ma xing shi gan tang* in lung heat wheezing following a wind-cold invasion.

We get a glimpse of Liu's rationale when we look at his discussion of the pathogenesis of febrile convulsions: 'In the case of wind-heat, wind corresponds to wood, wood is able to generate fire so wind is able to generate fire. Conversely extreme fire is able to generate wind…so wind is born from heat; the *ben*-root is heat but the *biao* is wind so [extrapolating this] we can say that wind is heat.' The practical clinical implication of this is that to treat or prevent febrile convulsions, which has the characteristics of wind, we should focus on heat clearage because this, in Liu's view, represents the *ben*-root of the problem.

Other classical physicians of the time were applying general treatment principles taken from the *Shang Han Lun* which had been summarised as a medical epithet: 'Use warm medicine to relieve the exterior, treat the exterior first and then the interior; it's never too late to purge.' Liu's writings helped to introduce new perspectives. He became skilled in the application of cold medicinals and introduced the novel idea of releasing exterior conditions using cold and pungent substances. He also believed that it was often necessary to simultaneously regulate both the exterior and interior – releasing the exterior whilst also clearing heat and nourishing *yin* on the interior. He devised new formulas to do this, and so laid some of the important early foundations for the Qing dynasty *wen bing* (warm febrile disease) style of practice that emerged over the following centuries. Liu divided febrile illness into three types: exterior patterns, simultaneously exterior and interior patterns and interior patterns. In treating exterior illness he most often used cold-pungent or sweet-cold formulas and especially interesting was his use of *gan cao*, *hua shi* and *cong shi*.

Febrile illnesses can change hour by hour, and these changes provide important clues as to the success or otherwise of the treatment, and highlight the need to adapt treatment to changing conditions. This, for example, is the situation where it is necessary to check the pulse and other signs frequently. If exterior signs had not been relieved after the patient had sweated and there was no change of the original symptoms, Liu used *liang ge san* to bring down the fever. If the fever had improved but not completely gone following diaphoretic treatment, then he advised *tian shui san*, *huang lian jie du tang* or *liang ge san* to regulate *yin* and *yang* and drain *zangfu* heat. If the exterior fever pattern remained unrelieved and the patient's condition was not suitable for purging, for example, because of weakness, then Liu advocated *bai hu tang* to clear it.

Liu Wan-su's core approach is summarised in the following table:

Illness	Principle	Formula
Simultaneous exterior *xie* and interior heat (*tong bing*)	Heat clearing and heat stasis removal according to depth of *xie* and severity of illness	*Fang feng tong sheng san* or *liang ge san* plus *yi yuan san*
Heat illness at *shaoyang* stage	Harmonise *shaoyang* and clear heat	*Xiao chaohu tang*
Strong heat in *shaoyang*	Clear fire in *shaoyang*	*Da chai hu tang*
Severe internal heat	Purge heat from *yang ming*	*Xiao cheng qi tang, da cheng qi tang* or *tiao wei cheng qi tang*
Heat penetrated to blood level	Purge heat, clear fire and cool the blood	*Cheng qi tang* plus *huang lian jie du tang*
Fever remaining after purge or damp heat diarrhoea remains	Clear heat and damp	*Liang ge san* or a low dose of *huang lian jie du tang*

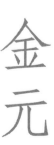

金元

In this way Liu's treatment of heat illness addressed some important aspects of acute illness that had generally been missed by previous physicians, which is why his style later became known as the 'cold and cooling school'. Although he invented 'heat and fire theory' and was skilled in the use of cold herbs and formulas, he did not neglect pattern differentiation to match the treatment to the patient's diagnosis and condition, applying cold, hot, warm and cooling methods as appropriate.

> ...if the pathogenic *qi* is hot then clear the heat, if it is cold then expel the coldness; the same basic principles apply to all six *qi* – reduce the excess and supplement deficiency, remove the pathogens and support the *zheng qi*. That is the way of medicine. (Liu Wan-su, *Suwen Xuanji Yuan Bing Shi*)

These very clear principles shine through in all of Liu's writings and are fundamental to modern practice, but were not always self-evident to Liu's contemporaries. Of the 348 formulas written in his *Huangdi Suwen Xuan Ming Lun Fang*, we find 39 cooling formulas, 44 warm ones and the rest that combine herbs with cold and warm and neutral qualities. So, although Liu Wan-su is remembered as the founder of the heat clearing school, it is important to note that he was not doctrinaire about this style, and in practice used a broad range of approaches.

Various aspects of the modern style of Chinese medicine come from Liu's Hejian style; for example, when discussing *damp-heat* he writes:

> ...when dampness is retained without being dispersed it can generate fire-heat which we call *accumulated damp generates heat*. Furthermore, damp is earth *qi* and fire generates earth, damp illnesses stagnate and stew internally which affects water flow and so the production of water is inhibited.

For another instance of the way that Liu's style has informed modern thinking, Liu describes the tendency of the various heat and fire pathogens to injure *yin* fluids when he wrote, 'There's nothing worse than fire to dry 1000 things.' This idea is so ingrained in modern practice that it requires a stretch of the imagination to appreciate the fact that most early physicians could have neglected its importance.

LIU WAN-SU AND INTERNAL HEAT

Up until Liu's time the usual understanding of the adverse effects of excessive or unregulated emotional changes was simply that they injured the function of the corresponding *zang* organs. This aspect of aetiology theory was based on the correspondences found in the *Suwen*, 'sadness injures the lungs, anger injures the liver...' and so on, but the actual nature of such injury was rather poorly defined. Liu's insight helped characterise the effects: 'All harm from injury due to the five emotions', he said, 'results from fire or heat.' More specifically, he understood that such heat also has a tendency then to exhaust *yin* leading to *xu* restlessness. In his *Suwen Xuanji Yuan Bing Shi* text, Liu lists various emotional states such as fear, restlessness, anxiety, *dian-kuang* (mania-withdrawal) and *yu* (constraint-depression), and contends that all of these illnesses may be classified as fire-heat issues. He postulated a vicious circle that may arise such that fear, for example, harms the kidneys, leading to water becoming deficient, allowing heart fire to flare up. When this happens, he said, the person becomes even more easily frightened so that further damage can occur to the *yin* aspect of the kidneys. Restless-agitation (*fanzao*), a symptom often seen in febrile conditions, is thereby taken by Liu to point to a fire diagnosis. When such patients have *shi* excess fire such that their kidney water is reduced, they may lose their emotional stability and become mentally agitated. Furthermore, Liu said that internal heat manifests itself on the exterior of the body: 'Excess heat obstructs the pores of the skin which leads to internal stagnation.' Again, although familiar to practitioners today, these insights were novel in Liu's time.

'Strokes,' Liu said, 'occur when a person's lifestyle is out of order such that heart fire flares up and kidney water that has been exhausted is not able to control it, a state of *yin xu* and *yang shi* causes heat stasis, the heart *shen* becomes disturbed, the tendons and bones disabled and the person collapses unconscious.' This can develop when the five emotions are extreme; Liu emphasised the water-fire and heart-kidney relationships, saying that 'nothing exceeds the ability of water to moisten things', which translated into the treatment principle 'nourish kidney water to control the heart fire'. This basic principle formed the basis of medical thinking on the subject for numerous later physicians.

Liu carefully studied his patients to better understand the way that heat and fire develop and act in the body, which led to his development of the idea of heat or fire transformation, the ways that external pathogens and internal emotional disharmony can intermingle and transform into patterns involving heat or fire. Again, these ideas were implicit in the Han dynasty classics, but Liu felt that this understanding had not been emphasised sufficiently in the teachings of his era; consequently he advocated the use of treatment with a cooling nature to treat these conditions. Having specifically identified the possibility of heat invasion of the body's exterior levels, he specialised in using cool-pungent herbs such as *bo he* and *ju hua* to clear exterior wind heat, and herbs such as *cong bai* and *dan dou chi* to disperse constraint at the exterior, and so allow heat constrained internally to be released. This was a novel and significant departure from the main thrust of the *shang han* style that routinely applied warm pungent herbs such as *ma huang, gui zhi* and *xi xin* in acute exterior illness. Prescriptions for heat illnesses, such as *zhizi dou chi tang* and *ma xing shi gan tang*, were used in the *Shang Han Lun*, but their importance as heat-clearing formulas appears to have been under-recognised prior to Liu's time. Much later, in the 17th and 18th centuries, Liu's work was to influence the *wen bing* or epidemic febrile diseases, which correspond to (and preceded) the Western concept of contagious disease.

As suggested above, as well as addressing the issue of acute illness due to exterior heat patterns, Liu also emphasised the importance of recognising interior heat and the need for its removal. This helped found the idea of similar transformation – the tendency of interior heat patterns to predispose to exterior heat invasion.

Alongside his many important innovations in herbal medical practice Liu also used acupuncture, focusing especially on the use of the *wu shu xue* (the five 'transport' points distal to the elbows and knees).

In sum, Liu's great contribution was to increase understanding of heat and fire as pathological factors, the way that there can be both external and internal contributory aspects and that the consequence of heat disease was generally injury to *yin* and fluids. The treatment style he developed therefore tended to include combinations of heat clearage and *yin* nourishment.

LIU WAN-SU'S CONTRIBUTION TO CHRONOBIOLOGY

As part of his attempt to understand *wuyun liuqi* theory, Liu Wan-su reconciled the 19 categories of pathogenesis taken from Chapter 74 of the *Suwen* ('Zhi Zhen Yao Da Lun') with the *wuyun liuqi* categories of disease development. This involved improving the congruence between illnesses of the five *zang* organs with those predicted in *wuyun* (five movements) theory, and taking into account the illnesses associated with the *xu* and *shi* of the *zangfu* and the pathological influences of the six *qi* – cold, summer-heat, dryness, dampness, wind and fire. By doing this work Liu formulated a new doctrine of *zangfu* six *qi* pathogenesis; he said that 'when organs and channels become diseased they do so with no regard to whether the original *qi* is excessive or deficient; the six *qi* interact with each other and this itself can cause illnesses'. This was a novel derivation of the original *yunqi* doctrine.

Liu also re-evaluated the traditional *yunqi* belief in *kang ze hai, cheng ze zhi* (harm is avoided by restraining the excess). Liu Wan-su's style of *wuyun liuqi* aimed to correct the tendency of practitioners to apply *yunqi* doctrine in a mechanical way without regard to the patient at hand. He opposed the previous idea of a fixed energetic influence whereby each year in the 60-year cycle governed a particular *qi* that was allegedly associated with specific illnesses. Liu also challenged the prevailing view that illnesses were entirely governed by *wuyun liuqi*, and wrote that 'it is people themselves who govern their lives… Practising Buddhism or Daoism is a personal choice and so is the choice to live a short life and die young. People make these choices themselves.' This more flexible and pragmatic approach clearly makes more sense to the modern mind than a mechanical application of chronobiology.

LIU WAN-SU AND THE XUAN FU

As well as the work just described, Liu Wan-su was also interested in reviving the *Neijing* idea of an anatomical and functional entity referred to as the *xuan fu* – *xuan* means dark, profound and abstruse, and *fu* is the same *fu* as *zangfu*, so it suggests a functioning hollow organ able to 'receive and discharge'; *fu* also means palace. Generally, mentions of the *xuan fu* in the Han classics is taken to mean the pores of the skin and, in this context, *xuan* may be taken to refer to the fact that these organs exist at the limits of visual perception. Liu Wan-su's interest in this subject would have arisen as a consequence of his study of the disease mechanisms involved in exterior attack as these patterns typically manifested as alterations in sweating which is a function of the skin pores, and it was the derangement of sweating in febrile conditions suggested to Han dynasty physicians that this was the location of the pathogenic process. A parallel concept, the *cou li*, appearing, for example, in Zhang Zhong-jing's *Jin Gui Yao Lue*, referred generally to the superficial tissues that provide structure and integrity to the skin. Liu believed that the function of the *xuan fu* overlapped with that of the *cou li*, that together could be described as the pores and the interstitial tissues found at the body surface.

> The sweat pores on skin are the orifices that vent *qi* and fluids; they are called the '*qi* gates' because they act as gates for venting *qi*; they are also called *cou li*, which means the route and texture for *qi* and liquid to come in and out; another name for these is *gui men* – 'ghost gates', meaning they may be seen as the gate of the nether world; yet another name is *xuan fu*, meaning the deep and mysterious mansions. But in relation to the *xuan fu* [concept more widely] there is nothing in the body that doesn't have this function; including man's *zangfu*, skin and hair, muscle, tendon and membrane, bone and marrow, nails and teeth. Indeed even everything [living?] in the world has this aspect, [the *xuan fu*] being the gates through which *qi* can ascend, descend, enter and exit. (Liu Wan-su, *Suwen Xuanji Yuan Bing Shi*)

Liu developed this new theory about the channels through which *qi* and fluids could disperse and permeate through the body using the idea of the *qiji* or *qi* mechanism derived from the *Neijing* passage that asserts:

> …if there is no entering and leaving there will be no growing and getting stronger; if there is no ascent and descent there will be no transformation and storage. So [even] with ascent and descent, entering and leaving, without qi there is no being. ('Liu Wei Zhi Da Lun', *Suwen*)

In essence, this *qiji* idea proposes that life depends on the movement of *qi* – that in essence, this movement involves the dynamics of entering and leaving, ascent and descent, and storage and transformation. Liu claimed that it was the *xuan fu* that were the routes for these activities, and linked his new interpretation of the *xuan fu* idea with his emphasis on fire aetiology, saying that fire, as well as other pathogens and emotional changes, could obstruct and block *xuan fu* function.

> Man's eyes, ears, nose, body, consciousness and *shen* work properly when [*qi*] ascent, descent, entry and exit is free and facilitated. If there is blockage the sense organs will not function. If the eyes can't see, the ears can't hear, the nose can't smell, the tongue can't taste, the sinews are weakened and the bones are painful, the teeth are decayed, the hair falls, the skin is numb, the intestines cannot leach and drain, this is all because hot *qi* is indignant and constrained, the *xuan fu* are closed so that *qi* and fluid, blood vessels, the *ying*, *wei* and *shen* are unable to ascend and descend, enter and leave. The severity of the constraint and blockage determines the severity of the illness. (Liu Wan-su)

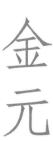

Later, the *xuan fu* concept was to become further extended by Qing dynasty medical scholars to refer to the extensive communication channels between all parts of the body through which the *qi* mechanism (*qiji*) operates, thereby positing a structural ground for the *sanjiao qi* dynamic. One step smaller than the *sun luo* (grandson vessels, capillaries), the *xuan fu* are today seen as the smallest functional entity in Chinese medicine physiology. Some modern theorists have now taken this idea further by comparing the *xuan fu* functions with biochemical intercellular transport and communication systems.

Liu's main publications are listed in Appendix 2.

Distinctive formulas in Liu Wan-su's style include:

- *Fang feng tong sheng san*, a firm statement of Liu's belief that internal heat should be cleared in some cases of exterior wind-heat. This formula briskly clears heat from all levels by simultaneous purgation, urination and exterior release alongside *zheng qi* protection using qi and blood supplementation.
- *Liu yi san*, which treats summer-heat-damp with fever, sweating and thirst.
- *Dihuang yin-zi*, for windstroke (*zhong feng*) with loss of speech due to both *yin xu* fire and *yang xu*, leading to phlegm formation that obstructs the heart orifices with consequent inability to coordinate the tongue.
- *Gui ling gan lu yin*, for summer-heat obstructing the *qi* mechanism, leading to fever, headache, fluid stasis, obstructed urination and diarrhoea.

Next it is timely to discuss the very influential physician scholar Zhang Yuan-su, who, although not included as one of the four masters of the Jin-Yuan, was at least as influential as they were, and taught directly or indirectly three of them. It is perhaps Zhang who comes closest to being the founder of the modern style of systematic differentiation of *zangfu* patterns underlying illness in each individual.

Zhang Yuan-su (1151–1234)

Zhang Yuan-su (style name Zhang Jie-gu) lived in the Jin dynasty in Yi Zhou, which is now Yi Xian in Hebei province. He took the imperial youth scholarship examination when he was eight, and at 27 he succeeded in passing the *jing yi* (meaning of the classics) exam that allowed inauguration as a scholar official. Later, though, his progress was interrupted when he was downgraded for 'offending a taboo'; this probably involved him inadvertently causing offence by using a word belonging to the emperor in the intricate imperial snakes and ladders power game. This fall from grace prompted him to abandon his career as a bureaucrat and switch his attention to medicine. Zhang quickly learned the Han dynasty medical classics, a study he considered was an essential prerequisite before being able to claim any professional ability in medicine.

Zhang Yuan-su's style also drew on his study of Wang Shu-he, Sun Si-miao and the Song paediatrician Qian Yi, and from these influences he distilled his own doctrine that became known as the *Yi Shui* School, named in honour of his home province. This style took Qian Yi's relatively new *zangfu* differentiation approach and refined it into a more detailed system that is recognisable as the foundation of modern Chinese medicine's *zangfu* differentiation. Zhang deserves a place as one of the great medical thinkers of the Jin-Yuan dynasties.

According to records in *Jin Shi* (Golden History), Liu Wan-su, the founder of the heat clearage school, was at first very disdainful toward Zhang Yuan-su, but the tables were turned when Liu himself contracted a fever which failed to resolve. After eight days of illness Liu remained very unwell, suffering headaches, vomiting, an inability to eat and delirium. Finally, Zhang Yuan-su was called to attend to his colleague, but Liu Wan-su just faced the wall, refusing to meet Zhang's gaze. 'Why are you so rude to me?' Zhang asked. Taking his pulse he asked Liu what medication he had taken and then said, 'That is a mistake, that is a cold and descending prescription; if you continue to take it you will continue to get worse.' Liu, it is said, agreed to take the warm formula prescribed by Zhang, and then quickly recovered. After this encounter they allegedly became good friends and colleagues, and Zhang's reputation benefited by association, as did his academic outlook. He himself now came to be influenced by Liu's Hejian school, and incorporated this into the styles he had previously acquired.

A prolific medical author, Zhang Yuan-su's most important writings were:

- *Yi Xue Qi Yuan* (Medicine Explained), a general text on medicine
- *Zhen Zhu Nang* (Pouch of Pearls), in which Zhang proposes his new approach to the classification of medicinals
- *Zangfu Biaoben Hanre Xushi Yong Yao Shi* (Use of Medicinals Based on *Zangfu*, Root-Branch, Cold-Hot, *Xu-Shi*)
- *Suwen Bingji Qi Yi Bao Ming Ji* (Protecting Life by *SuWen* Pathophysiology, 1186), a critical re-appraisal of the *Suwen* theories.

He is also said to have composed texts entitled *Yi Fang*, *Yao Zhu Nan Jing* and *Jie Gu Ben Cao* and some other writings, but only fragments of these survive.

In his *Yi Xue Qi Yuan* Zhang condemned the common practice of blind reliance on ancient formulas such as those from the *Shang Han Lun*; instead, he insisted, treatment must match the individual, the time and the place. He integrated his mastery of *Neijing* theory with the subsequent historical tradition and his own clinical experience to found the *zangfu bian zheng pai* (*zangfu* pattern differentiation school). His writings provided detailed discussions of the physiology and pathology of the *zangfu* and described their illness patterns in relation to *xu-shi*, *han-re* and *biao-ben*, and described the progress and prognosis of disease from a *zangfu* perspective.

> Today's *yunqi* is not the same [as that of the Han dynasty]; ancient and contemporary follow different tracks and so the old formulas are inappropriate for modern illness. (Zhang Yuan-su)

Writing on liver disease, for example, Zhang begins with a presentation of Chinese medicine's account of the normal physiology of the liver before giving a detailed listing of the clinical changes that can be observed in those parts of the body that manifest liver patterns (i.e. the liver channel, eyes, hypochondrium and so on) in various pathological situations. He then outlines a standardised therapy for each of these conditions; a very systematic approach was applied in the same way to the other *zangfu* such that both theoretical concerns and practical clinical experience were factored into his method. Zhang explicitly advocated a lucid medical practice style based on *zangfu* differentiation and laid the foundation for the further development of *zangfu* pattern differentiation theory (*zangfu bian zheng lunzhi*) in subsequent practice. Once again this innovation was not entirely new – understanding of *zangfu* pathology and its analysis using schemes such as hot-cold and *xu-shi* had been implicit in the classical tradition since the *Neijing*, but Zhang Yuan-su's work was needed to formulate the knowledge into a properly coherent and compact doctrine.

When discussing *zangfu* physiology and pathology, Zhang Yuan-su emphasised the central role of spleen and stomach function in providing the body with nourishment:

> …the spleen corresponds to earth…digesting and grinding the five grains it is located in the chest and supports the four sides…the stomach is the spleen's *fu*…the root of man, a strong stomach *qi* allows the five *zang* and six *fu* all to be strong. ['Four sides' refers to the idea that all the other *zangfu* take their nourishment from the middle *jiao* and that the spleen and stomach take a pivotal middle position between the other *zangfu*. In modern times we now understand the functions attributed to the spleen to also include those of the pancreas.]

Zhang routinely used *qi* and blood-increasing medicinals to support weak spleen function, an approach that was to influence many future physicians starting with his student Li Dong-yuan (Li Gao, another of the four masters), discussed later. Li Dong-yuan especially admired Zhang's formula *zhi zhu wan*, that paired *zhi ke* and *bai zhu* in a deceptively simple formula, and Li's very successful stomach and spleen style was largely a development of Zhang's ideas. In this way Zhang Yuan-su's insights were transmitted to Li Dong-yuan and then on to Luo Tian-yi and Wang Hao-gu, and from them to form a lineage that continued through the Ming and Qing dynasties to modern times. So, whilst he is credited as the creator of the *Yi Shui* School, Zhang Yuan-su can also be seen as the original inspiration for the ongoing 'strengthen earth school'.

Another great contribution of Zhang Yuan-su was his advocacy of more clear-minded and orderly methods of understanding the contents of the *bencao* and their application in constructing prescriptions. He wrote detailed essays describing the *bencao* substances in terms of their flavour, temperature characteristics, channel affinity and ascending-descending-floating-sinking nature. By characterising the energetics of the standard medicinals in a systematic and detailed way, he not only helped divert physicians' thinking away from symptomatic therapeutics, but he also allowed formula construction to become significantly more refined, ordered and flexible. Zhang Yuan-su believed that the nature and flavour, richness and lightness of the substances were all different, and that better practice would result from improved clarification of these distinctions.

An example of this in action can be seen in Zhang's channel attributions of the herbs that drain fire: *huang lian*, he said, drains heart fire, *huang qin* drains lung fire, *bai shao* drains liver fire, *zhi mu* drains kidney fire, *shi gao* drains stomach fire, and so on. Attributions such as these had been implicit rather than explicit in previous literature, but now they were clearly delineated for a future, more sophisticated pharmacognosy model. This advance offered greater precision and coherence for more exact practice of Chinese medicine; less reliance was to be placed on symptom indications and more on the medicinals' *qi*, flavour and energetic dynamic effects. In another innovation Zhang also divided herbs and prescription methodologies into five overarching types – those substances used to treat wind, damp, summer-heat, dryness and cold. His desire was to promote a more exact system that matched medicines with the correct properties needed to treat specific syndromes rather than just diseases and symptoms, an approach that also included the use of the *wu xing* relationships of engendering and restraining to explain the logistics of treatment.

Today, when reflecting on the formulas of Zhang Zhong-jing, it is quite easy for us to recognise a precision of understanding of herbs and their functions in the prescription. This is largely because we now have access to the analytical tools sharpened for us by Zhang and countless subsequent scholarly physicians. Without this we would struggle to understand the way the formulas work. Looking at the *shang han* formula *xiao qing long tang* (small green dragon decoction), for example, we can appreciate its skilful dynamic balance of herbs that move with those that constrain, herbs that float with those that sink and for its use of herbs that enter the lung domain and perfectly match the pattern of dysfunction in the lungs. Its Han dynasty author Zhang Zhong-jing clearly had an understanding of the manner in which herbs could descend *qi* or float to release the exterior even if his terse style omitted discussion of such matters. Somehow this sublime energetic use of medicinals and understanding of the *zangfu* pathology in disease, evident in the Han classical tradition, had become obfuscated in later centuries. Zhang Yuan-su was insightful enough to be able to identify, define and reclaim the essence of classical practice using innovations that remained true to the spirit of classical medical thought.

> …the method of selecting appropriate medicinals to match the patient's clinical diagnostic pattern involves identifying substances with the correct *qi*, taste, *yin* and *yang*, thick and thin as well as the *xie qi* and channel affected. (Zhang Yuan-su)

Like Liu Wan-su, Zhang Yuan-su also studied *wuyun liuqi* doctrine and incorporated the cosmologies into his own theories and prescribing style. He suggested that herbs could be categorised according to the *wuyun* (five movements) and formulas according to the six *qi* (environmental *qi*); this was a unique innovation that influenced Li Dong-yuan and many other subsequent doctors.

In sum, Zhang's contributions can be seen as organisational; his *bagang*-based *zangfu* differentiation offered a systematic framework for understanding and tying together diagnosis and internal medicine practice. His classification of herb properties, such as channel affinity, directionality, taste and so forth, helped to better organise Chinese medicine's understanding of the various medicinals and their function in prescriptions. As Li Dong-yuan's teacher, he

> **SOME IMPORTANT ZHANG YUAN-SU FORMULAS**
>
> *Zhi zhu wan*
>
> *Jiu wei qiang huo tang*
>
> *Men dong yin zi*
>
> *Tian ma wan*
>
> *Jin ling zi san*
>
> *Shao yao tang*
>
> *Nei shu huang lian tang*

is also acknowledged as the inspiration for the founding of the stomach-spleen school, and all of his contributions are central to the modern interpretation of the tradition.

Zhang Cong-zheng (1156–1228)

Like Liu Wan-su, Zhang Cong-zheng (aka Zhang Zi-he) believed that an essential key to understanding pathology lay in the study of the climatic *qi* of heaven and earth, and its ability to induce pathogenic *qi* processes in the body. Professor Paul Unschuld notes that Liu's ideas were rooted in the idea of balancing heat and cold and other qualities of *qi* without necessarily taking full account of the distinctions between *xie qi* and *zheng qi*. As we saw earlier, though, Liu Wan-su did consider the *qi* of the *zangfu*, and did use medicinals to expel exterior pathogens and herbs such as *da huang* to drain internal heat from the body as well as using tonics to support the body's *zheng qi*. However, Zhang Cong-zheng perhaps had a better understanding of the *xie–zheng* dichotomy implicit in the *Shang Han Lun*, and could make these distinctions more clearly. Spending a lifetime studying pathogen expulsion, he took a more vigorous approach, one that he justified with the *Neijing* passage 'disease is due to the presence of *xie qi*; combating pathogens ceases illness'. Zhang realised that more specific attention was needed on the study of the ways in which *xie qi* could be expelled from the body – not simply countering its energetic effects by, for example, applying coldness to heat. Both the *Neijing* and *Shang Han Lun* had outlined the three appropriate routes by which to expel pathogens, but Zhang Cong-zheng realised there was room for improvement in this aspect of treatment.

Like many other Confucian scholar physicians (*ruyi*), Zhang had made a detailed study of the early foundation classic texts. His conclusion was first that a main thrust of the Han literature taught that pathogens should be expelled from the body to prevent continuing damage, and second that there were essentially only three routes out of the body through which pathogenic *qi* could be persuaded to leave. These were through the 'exterior' (skin), through the 'lower orifices' and through the 'upper orifices' in the head. With this orientation in mind he believed that the primary aim of diagnosis should be to identify the nature and location of pathogenic

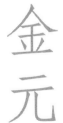

qi in the body, and that once done, treatment should be aimed at expulsion via the appropriate route. Zhang thereby became the founder of the *gong xie pai* (attack and drain school), sometimes slightly inaccurately referred to as the purgative school.

As a youth Zhang had studied and learned the major medical classics, focusing initially on the *Neijing* and *Shang Han Lun*. He passed the various state scholarship examinations, but then chose to follow a medical career path rather than a life in imperial service. Later in life, aged around 60, Zhang had achieved such renown as a physician that he was summoned to the court to serve as an imperial physician. After only two or three years of service he resigned from his official post, it is said, because he preferred to make his skills available to the common people. This he did by becoming an itinerant doctor, an absurdly humble choice for such a high-ranking and venerable *ruyi* scholar, a calling that was more usually taken up by relatively uneducated folk medicine practitioners or bell doctors. For Zhang, the humbleness thing did not work out quite as intended as he soon attracted a retinue of *ruyi* followers. A bell doctor arriving in town accompanied by finely dressed scholars writing down his every word would certainly have drawn attention to his high status. It was one of these disciples, Ma Zhi-ji, who recorded Zhang's ideas, cases and prescriptions and published them after his death in the classic *Shiqin Rumen* (A Scholar's Duty to His Parents). In this book Zhang emphasised the need for practitioners to keep in mind a clear distinction between the body's own *zheng qi* constituents and pathogenic (*xie*) *qi*.

Zhang saw that the imperative to identify the nature and location of *xie qi* in the body had been neglected through the Tang dynasty when there had been a blurring of the *zheng–xie* axis in medicine as scholars focused more on medical chronobiology, *jing-luo* and *wu xing* balancing ideas – all models of patho-physiology that tend to downplay the *xie–zheng* dichotomy. This omission may also be seen as a consequence of the fact that the *Shang Han Lun, the* classic manual on the effects and treatment of *xie qi*, was largely neglected until roughly a century before Zhang Cong-zheng's birth.

In his *History of Ideas* Unschuld summarises the key difference in Zhang's approach compared with his contemporaries. Liu Wan-su and others believed in:

> the organic homogeneity of qi inside and outside the body, a conception which defined illness solely as an imbalance in the distribution of these *qi* among the various *zang-fu*. Zhang Cong-zheng, therefore, directed his therapeutic efforts not to the establishment of a state of equilibrium, but to the decisive expulsion of harmful influences.

Zhang's campaign was against the simple balancing of *qi* without regard to differentiation of *zheng* and *xie* such as is seen in some present-day acupuncture styles. The fact that some of these balancing styles are common in Japan may reflect the fact that the initial importation of Chinese medicine into Japan occurred during the Tang dynasty. The different styles may also reflect the prevalence of different medical needs at different times, and in the face of different healthcare needs. When

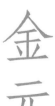

pathogens abound, pathogen removal is a prime concern; when emotional causalities abound, then energetic balancing acts may be more suitable.

This *xie–zheng* distinction is crucial in much of Chinese medicine practice. The body's *zheng qi* is what carries out proper body function, physiological fire gives the middle *jiao* the ability to carry out *yunhua* (transformation and transportation) so we can absorb nutrients, and *jinye* fluids moisten the body and (for example) lubricate joints. By contrast, *xie* heat in the stomach and spleen is not able to carry out the proper energetic transformation of food, but merely makes food rot and fester, leading to foul eructation and inflammation that hinders the digestive process and injures *yin*. Similarly, *xie* dampness cannot provide proper moisture to lubricate the joints and, on the contrary, obstructs the free movement of *qi*, for example making joints stiff and sore.

> The origins of *xie qi* are inexhaustible. We may be confronted by suffering due to the six excesses: wind, cold, summer heat, damp, dryness and fire…but none of these are inherent bodily constituents; therefore in treatment we should apply attacking methods to expel the pathogens, rapid expulsion of *xie qi* should be the main objective and when *xie qi* is expelled, *yuan qi* recovers.
>
> …treating disease requires emphasis on expelling pathogenic *qi*; by doing this we allow *zheng qi* to be stable. We should not be afraid to use therapeutic attacking methods…first treat the *shi*, later treat the *xu*. (Zhang Cong-zheng, *Rumen Shi Qin*)

Zhang Cong-zheng became the inspiration for the *gong xie pai* (attack and drain school) that employs formulas mainly intended to remove pathogenic *qi* from the body – most famously using purgative herbs such as *da huang*. Discussions of this style often reduce Zhang's influence down to this aspect, but a closer examination reveals that Zhang's methodology involved more than simple purgation, and included all of the three methods seen at the root of *Shang Han Lun* medicine – diaphoresis, emesis and purgation. By the term 'diaphoresis' Zhang meant more than just sweating induced with diaphoretic herbs such as *ma huang*. He used many methods that serve to eliminate *xie qi* from the exterior, including acupuncture, moxibustion, massage and hot compresses. Also, Zhang's use of the term 'emetic' meant more than simply induced vomiting; it included any technique intended to expel *xie qi* via the upper orifices such as induced sneezing and even therapeutic lachrymation. Likewise, purgation can be taken to mean any technique intended to expel *xie qi* through the lower orifices. Substances that do this are not necessarily purgatives but may simply have a pronounced downward-moving effect on *qi*, such as diuretics or herbs that guide *zhuo qi* (turbid *qi*) to descend. Often, though, Zhang did employ frank purgation as an initial step in therapy. It may be that his apparent success in treating a wide range of diseases with bowel purgation is partly a testament to the broad therapeutic range of the famous purgative herb *da huang* (see the box on the next page).

DA HUANG AND THE SILK ROUTE TRADE

From early mediaeval times valuable and exotic items of trade came to the European market along the Silk Road. The quintessential purgative *da huang* (Rheum palmatum root) was the prime medical substance of trade as it was seen as a cleansing health panacea, a kind of ginseng in reverse, able to remove toxicity from the body. Its reputation may well have its roots in the *gong xie pai* style of Zhang Cong-zheng. European apothecaries used to send runners to the Middle Eastern markets to collect this turkey rhubarb that had been brought from China. British physicians, irritated by the high cost of imported *da huang*, sent an industrial spy to China to collect seeds, but this first mission failed when it was realised he had returned with seeds from the wrong plant. Later, a second mission was more successful, and many acres of *da huang* crops were grown in Kent, but the endeavour gradually died out when it became clear that the home-grown crop was much inferior to the imported product. Modern studies have shown that *da huang* has distinctive and varied pharmacologic properties over and above its purgative qualities, including antibiotic, antifungal and anti-inflammatory properties, that may help explain its reputation as a panacea.

Zhang's style stood in contrast to that of his contemporary, the tonics advocate Li Dong-yuan. Zhang claimed that physicians too easily resort to tonics and that for many illnesses this was a serious disservice to patients. Many subsequent physicians agreed, and so the attack and drain school continued.

Zhang Cong-zheng tended to use existing classic formulas and only very few of his own invention; examples are *mu xiang bing lang wan*, a formula for severe, chronic food stagnation, and *yu nu jian*.

In short, Zhang Cong-zheng explored in some detail the question of how *xie qi* can be identified, located and expelled appropriately, and his straightforward approach influenced many physicians in the subsequent two dynasties.

Li Dong-yuan (1180–1251)

Li Dong-yuan (Li Gao, aka Ming Zhi) was born into a wealthy family in Zhen Ding in Hebei province. When he was a child his mother became ill and died following treatment from a poorly skilled doctor who was unable to make a diagnosis. Driven by helplessness and frustration, and at great expense, he apprenticed himself for many years under the famed Zhang Yuan-su from whom he learned Zhang's *zangfu* differentiation methodology and the use of formulas aimed at regulating digestive function. From this Li developed his spleen and stomach doctrine that specialised in strengthening and regulating spleen function with sweet and warm substances to treat illnesses due to internal damage. Later generations came to call this style the earth reinforcing school.

The main tenet of Li Dong-yuan's style was his belief that 'numerous illnesses can arise from spleen and stomach dysfunction', an idea that had been derived from the *Neijing* statement 'as long as the stomach *qi* remains there will be life; absence of stomach *qi* leads to death'. Li saw the digestive system, the spleen and stomach, or middle burner in Chinese medicine shorthand, as the foundation of life.

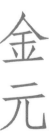

'*Yuan qi* is the essential *qi* pre-natally, but the sole source of our nourishment after birth is the stomach', so all the other forms of *qi* in the body he considered were ultimately derived from the absorptive power of stomach *qi*. Injury to the spleen and stomach injury therefore weakens *yuan qi*, and this then leads to numerous kinds of ill health because 'the earth is the mother of everything'. With this argument he aimed to promote the primacy of the idea of middle *jiao* dysfunction in medical therapeutics, even including the idea that some febrile diseases should be treated by strenghtening the spleen, and, in Li's view, even some fevers were attributable to spleen and stomach illness.

Thinking more deeply about properly regulated *yuan qi* activities in the body, Li (inspired largely by his teacher Zhang Yuan-su) considered that it had four movements – ascending, descending, floating and sinking – and that these *qi* activities were interconnected and interdependent. This *qi* dynamic (*qiji*) idea, too, had existed in the Han dynasty classics. Li said, 'When ascent ends descent begins; when descent ends ascent begins; *yuan qi* works like an endless loop to nourish everything.' He saw the spleen and stomach as pivotal in the ascent and descent of *yuan qi* in the body from the kidney domain in the lower *jiao*, reaching upward to the rest of the body before descending downward again. The middle *jiao* was also seen as responsible for transporting the nutrients from food to irrigate the organs and to nourish the whole body and at the same time to eliminate waste products.

So, according to Li Dong-yuan, the key to health maintenance was to promote the rise and fall of the essential *qi* of the *zangfu*, circulating *qi* to transform and generate. Li's emphasis was on promoting spleen *qi* ascent because his experience suggested that it was this *qi* movement that was most easily lost when the middle *jiao* function declined; he considered that once ascent was strong, descent would recover. When the essential *qi* from food was raised by the upward action of spleen *qi*, then *yuan qi* would be sufficient to support other functions in the body. Conversely, when spleen *qi* ascent weakened, the consequences were widespread and many health problems developed: 'If the stomach is *xu*, neither the *zangfu* nor the *jing-luo* are properly nourished by *qi* and so all aspects will become ill.' He also said that 'spleen and stomach *xu* causes blockage of the nine orifices'.

Li Dong-yuan's yin fire theory

Discussing illnesses due to internal injury, Li explained pathology largely in terms of what he called *yin fire*. This was a refinement of his ideas on middle *jiao* function and its relation to *yuan qi* generation and distribution. To most of those trained in the current version of standard Chinese medicine, the term *yin fire* suggests an internal heat pattern arising from a decline of *yin*, but Li Dong-yuan's use of the term had wider and rather more complex connotations. These included the idea that heat symptomatology may arise from spleen *qi xu* patterns. So, *yin fire* was mainly the development of pathogenic heat from a range of clinical possibilities consequent on middle *jiao qi* mechanism failure.

Some quotes from his writings offer insights into Li Dong-yuan's thinking:

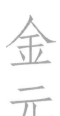

When spleen and stomach *qi* descends this will cause the essential *qi* of food to fail to ascend…such that cold and heat will be generated. [By this Li meant that when the *yang qi* of the spleen fails to ascend and is instead constrained and retained, the *yang xu* may manifest as coldness and the constraint may begin to transform into fire.]

Spontaneous sweat and frequent urination causes *yin fire* to subjugate earth [and] as the consumption of *ying*-blood becomes significant the *ying* (nutrient *qi*) *qi* hides in the earth, so *yin fire* becomes abundant. [These are all situations of *yin*-fluid consumption and blood *xu* leading to internal dryness and consequent transformation into fire.]

When damp *qi* in the spleen and stomach descends to the kidneys and becomes obstructed inside, the consequence is that *yin fire* rushes upwards. [In this situation, Li was saying that the essential *qi* of food could flow downwards and contribute to damp stagnation that mixes with ministerial fire and heat from stagnation, leading to upward rebellion of *yin fire*.]

Stagnation in the heart causes the seven *shen* (spirits) to lose their proper form; [we find] there is only fire in the pulse. [Here Li was highlighting his view that emotional states could also contribute to fire symptomatology; in this instance, he outlined a situation of heart restlessness that transformed into fire. The 'clear pathogens' advocate Zhang Cong-zheng, roughly contemporary with Li Dong-yuan, would probably have objected to this line of reasoning, saying that the febrile symptoms were the result of an external pathogen invasion that should be expelled.]

In sum, the prime signs of *yin fire* in Li's doctrine include feverishness of flushing on exertion, restlessness, signs of heat above and cold below, and other indicators of a fundamental *yin-yang* disharmony.

In his *Pi Wei Lun* (Essays on the Spleen and Stomach), Li Dong-yuan sets out what he saw as the three main mechanisms behind the weakening of the middle *jiao* and stirring up of *yin fire*:

- Improper diet: 'Stomach injury can be due to unregulated eating habits; the resulting illness causes insufficient *qi* and a decline in *shen* (spirit) which can culminate in high fever.'

- Over-work: 'Exhaustion of the muscles and the whole body leads to spleen injury; spleen illness causes laziness and a desire to lie in bed, slack and weak limbs and loose bowels.'

- Emotional injury: 'Joy, anger, worry and fear all consume *yuan qi*. They feed heart fire such that fire then subjugates earth and the person becomes ill.'

He taught that inappropriate diet, fatigue and emotional excesses interweave with each other to cause illness, but Li believed that the emotion aspect was the primary trigger. Usually, Li said, 'illnesses are caused by the five emotional excesses: joy, anger, sadness, worry and fear that prevent stomach *qi* from flowing freely; this

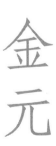

is then compounded by improper diet and imbalances between work and rest. Eventually *yuan qi* is damaged.'

Li Dong-yuan's treatment approach focused especially on assisting the spleen *qi* ascending function, most often using warm reinforcement of the spleen and stomach along with strengthening *qi* and ascending the *yang qi* of the spleen. When he identified *yin fire* due to a pattern of *qi xu* in the middle *jiao*, Li used his celebrated method of removing heat using sweet and warm substances to benefit the spleen and stomach whilst also lifting the *yang qi* and at the same time reducing fire and heat. This is exactly the approach seen in his famous prescription *bu zhong yi qi tang* (supplement the middle lift *qi* decoction). In his view, 'If an illness is due to internal damage and insufficiency is mistakenly interpreted as an exterior excess invasion and thereby drained, the patient will become even more deficient'; Li said that instead we 'should use sweet and warm substances to reinforce the middle and raise *yang*; use sweet and cold medicines to reduce the fire and it will be cured'. In a sense, Li was pointing out that not all fevers and heat patterns were due to attack by exterior pathogens; such symptoms could also arise from internal dysfunction. It is likely that Li's views sprang out of his particular patient load that may have included many patients who fitted this picture, such as pulmonary tuberculosis and brucellosis.

One other aspect of Li Dong-yuan's thinking concerns the relationship between *yin fire* retained in the body and *yuan qi*, including its implied link with the ministerial fire of the kidneys. His view was that as the middle *jiao* became weakened, with consequent descent of spleen *qi* and constraint due to dampness accumulation, then pathogenic *yin fire* built up, and that this began to displace and usurp the body's ministerial fire and its *yuan qi*. These two forms of *qi* – the pathogenic *yin fire* and upright ministerial fire at the root of all body function – he said, were fundamentally incompatible with each other. They could not, he claimed, co-exist in the same place, and so *zheng* (upright) fire was displaced or replaced by *yin fire*, which itself was unable to drive proper body function. For this reason one of his famous aphorisms was '*yin fire* is thief of *yuan qi*' or, as Li says elsewhere, 'fire and *yuan qi* cannot co-exist simultaneously... When one wins the other will lose.' Conversely, he believed that when the stomach and spleen *qi* were robust and properly regulated, then the tendency to *yin fire* was inhibited, and *yuan qi* remained strong and effective in maintaining health.

Of course the possibilities for pathogenesis due to internal damage are far more extensive than those emphasised by Li Dong-yuan. Also, his theories should not obscure the fact that many fevers and heat conditions are indeed externally contracted and require external release and not spleen regulation. Li's outlook was doubtless conditioned not only by his training but also by the context of his time. As detailed a little more later on, some modern commentators say that war, social stresses, epidemics and crop failures must often have created an environment that included fear and anxiety, excessive work and starvation. Others point out that Li Dong-yuan lived amid the wealthy and privileged classes; well fed and insulated from harsh realities, they could more easily indulge in emotionality, sedentary indolence and injure their digestion with dietary excesses. Others, such as Zhang Cong-zheng, may well have experienced a very different patient demographic, leading to different perspectives on appropriate treatment. Later commentators pointed out that Li's well-heeled elite patients were more averse to the harsher pathogen expulsion treatments such as purgation, sweating or emesis, preferring instead expensive and pleasant-tasting tonic prescriptions.

Modern advocates of his style point out that the clinical pictures described by Li Dong-yuan parallel those of many modern Western patients, and that some modern illness epidemics, such as allergies, immune disorders and emotional disturbances, can be analysed using *yin fire* theory and treated using his prescription principles.

Li Dong-yuan's treatment style

Believing in nurturing the spleen and stomach and regulating their ascending function, Li Dong-yuan's main treatment principles therefore involved warming and reinforcing the spleen and stomach, benefiting *qi* and ascending clear *yang*. On top of this basic idea he made further adjustments based on his *yin fire* idea. Famously this involved the notion of clearing heat using sweet and warm medicinals to tonify the spleen and stomach, lifting the *yang qi* and reducing fire and heat by removing constraint.

Warming and boosting the spleen might be considered inappropriate when feverish illnesses were the consequence of exterior attack, but Li's perspective was just the reverse. He claimed that mistakenly treating internal *xu* damage as an exterior excess pathogen would worsen the *xu*. For internal *xu* fevers he said, 'The use of sweet-warm medicines to reinforce the middle and lift the *yang* and the use of sweet-cold substances to reduce the fire will result in cure.' His flagship formula *bu zhong yi qi tang* is a classic exemplar for the use of sweet and warm medicinals to remove heat. It aims to treat internal damage heat patterns manifested as heavy breathing and wheezing, hot body and restless, forceful and big pulse and headache, or constant thirst, and aversion to wind-cold with mixed cold and heat signs. Contemporary practice considers that, used in this circumstance, it is remarkably effective.

Li used reinforcing *qi* and lifting *yang* as a main method, but when there was obvious *yin fire*, he also included bitter-cold medicines such as *huang bai* to treat accordingly. So he did not abandon the use of fire clearing with bitter and cold herbs, or the use of substances to release the exterior to expel fire. These two methods he also felt were also protective of *yuan qi*, compared with the method of lifting *yang* to reduce fire; they worked in opposite ways but ultimately helped to achieve the same aim.

In addition, Li used his rather complex *sheng yang tang* formula to treat a symptom pattern of 'discomfort in the throat and diaphragm, *qi*-counterflow, urgent feelings inside, no bowel movement', an entirely novel approach to the treatment of *qi* deficiency constipation. In treating numerous other types of illnesses, Li also focused on spleen and stomach tonification, lifting *yuan qi* and descending and holding *yin fire*. For example, in surgery, he used *sheng yu tang* to treat a patient with blood injury

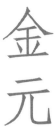

and malignant sores. He used *huangqi rougui chaihu jiu tang* (an alcohol decoction) to treat swollen and hard *yin* cellulitis. In gynaecology, he treated metorrhagia using *huangqi danggui renshen tang*. In paediatrics, he employed *huangqi tang* to treat chronic infantile convulsion. In ophthalmology he used *yuanming nei zhang shengma tang* to treat cataracts and used *danggui longdan tang* to treat white nebula in the eye. Study of the way Li used these formulas for these conditions helps to reveal the character of Li's style of treatment.

In his writings Li Dong-yuan focuses on illnesses due to internal damage and their relation to inappropriate eating habits injuring the stomach and exhaustion damaging the spleen, and on the ways that some illnesses can mimic exterior attack. He said that when such misdiagnosis led the practitioner to the use of formulas such as *da xian xiong tang, xiao cheng qi tang* or *yin chen hao tang* (all formulas that are aimed at attacking *xie* pathogens) then, in his view, the patient's condition would definitely worsen. His book *Nei Wai Shang Bian Huo Lun* (Essays on Differentiating Interior and Exterior Attack) aimed to address this issue by discussing the ways that internal or external damage could be distinguished using careful clinical assessment. Here he describes methods such as pulse palpation, distinguishing cold and heat symptoms, examination of the palm, mouth and nose and distinguishing weakened or excessive *qi*, differentiation of headache, examination of tendons and limbs, appetite and so on. These writings inspired many later physicians to use a meticulous clinical style.

When designing his formulas Li used Zhang Yuan-su's approach, taking into account the actions of each of the medicinals in terms of the new detailed understandings developed by his teacher, namely their:

- ascending, descending, floating and sinking actions

- emissary functions (*bao shi*)

- strength or weakness of each medicinal's flavour

- channel affinities.

Li often advised patients on eating habits, advice that emphasised eating warm food, avoiding over-eating and having a balanced diet. A favourite approach was to prescribe modifications of Zhang Yuan-su's *zhi zhu wan* (consisting of *bai zhu* and *ju pi*), making many formulas based on this kernel to treat patterns of spleen and stomach deficiency with stagnation. Sometimes, when he needed to treat excessive patterns of spleen and stomach, he was known to use strong attacking medicines to purge. So, although Li Dong-yuan was known for using sweet-warm spleen-reinforcing methods, he didn't reject other methods, and did not stand entirely in opposition to the attack and drain style of Zhang Cong-zheng.

The *Pi Wei Lun* style Li founded had a big influence on subsequent medicine, with a prominent stomach and spleen-strengthening style continuing through the Ming dynasty and up to modern times. One admirer, Xu Lu-zhai, said: 'Dong Yuan's medicine is the dao of medicine. Those who have committed themselves to study medicine should read all of Dong Yuan's books; only then are they properly placed to talk about medicine.'

These days Li Dong-yuan's emphasis on middle *jiao* injury due to emotional stresses, overwork and dietary irregularity, although very useful, is generally also seen as rather too restrictive. Consideration of internal damage aetiologies has to involve other possibilities. Li's outlook here can in part be explained by the fact that when he was formulating the ideas in his *Pi Wei Lun*, the country was at war. Life was hard for the many who were living in fear of the Mongol invaders, experiencing food shortages, famine and cold conditions, and having to work hard, and these factors may well have been especially damaging to the spleen and stomach *yuan qi* system. Furthermore, Li's emphasis on internal causes for heat and febrile conditions may also have been an

> Li Dong-yuan contributed many formulas to modern practice:
> - *Bu zhong yi qi tang*
> - *Dang-gui bu xue tang*
> - *Dang-gui liu huang tang*
> - *Fu yuan huo xue tang*
> - *Hou-po wen zhong tang*
> - *Qiang-huo sheng shi tang*
> - *Qing wei san*
> - *Sheng mai san*
> - *Sheng yang yi wei tang*
> - *Tian-tai wu-yao san*
> - *Zhong man fen xiao wan*
> - *Zhi-shi xiao pi wan*
> - *Zhi zhu wan*
> - *Zhu-sha an shen wan*

inappropriate distraction. As we have seen previously, the ineffective treatment of febrile epidemics was a key concern for Song–Jin-Yuan physicians. Li Dong-yuan's primarily internal aetiological explanations for fevers, and their treatment using middle *jiao* strengthening and regulation, may well have been erroneous in many cases, and the application of *Pi Wei Lun* theory to epidemic febrile conditions may have involved some element of over-enthusiastic application of doctrinal belief.

Before moving on to discuss the fourth of the famous Yuan masters, we divert to another influential physician of the time, Wang Hao-gu.

Wang Hao-gu (c. 1200–1264)

Styled Jin Zhi, and given the nickname Hai Zang Lao Ren (Venerable Ocean-Concealing Man), Wang Hao-gu was a leading Yuan dynasty physician of Hebei province. As a *jin shi* scholar (graduate of the highest imperial examinations), he was already fluent in the historical classics before turning his attention to medical study. Struggling to make sense of some of these, he was fortunate to be in a position to be able to study with two of the most celebrated Jin-Yuan masters – Zhang Yuan-su and Li Dong-yuan.

Wang Hao-gu served for a while as an army physician and presented his experiences from this time in his 12-volume *Yi Lei Yuan Rong* (Medicine from the Army Base). In these writings he introduced a novel differentiation system according to the identification of heat or cold in the various sectors of the *sanjiao* system, and discussed the differentiation of heat and cold in the *qi* and blood levels. His formulas

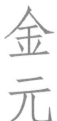

金
元

were directed at clearing heat or warming cold illness conditions in the locations he described – an innovation that much later contributed to the Qing dynasty *wen bing* school that used *sanjiao* and four-level (*wei, qi, ying, xue*) pattern differentiation as a basis for understanding and treating febrile disease.

Recognising the importance of the *Shang Han Lun* Wang Hao-gu made a special study of the *yin* stages, which had been neglected in favour of the more exterior patterns, and published this work in his *Yin Zheng Lue Lie*. In these writings he elaborated on the causes, patterns, diagnosis and treatment of the *yin* (internal) syndromes described in the *Shang Han Lun* and added many of his own ideas. For instance, where Zhang Zhong-jing had presented the *yin* stages of *shang han* as a progression of an external attack to the interior, Wang believed that *yin* syndromes could also appear as a consequence of other aetiologies such as consuming cold food and drinks, inappropriate use of cooling medicines or by adverse environmental conditions – 'frost and dew, mountain mist, rain dampness and fog'. He proposed the idea that the strength and harmony of the interior of the body determines our ability to resist external attack – 'As long as the inside is at peace any exterior [adverse climatic factor] has no way to enter.' He also expanded the clinical uses of *shang han* six channel theory by introducing many other diseases into the system, for example internal phlegm and thin mucus accumulation, and internal injury of fluids by fire that he considered could be associated with *yang ming* dysfunction.

As a follower of Zhang Yuan-su and Li Dong-yuan, Wang Hao-gu's treatment style is seen as part of the *Yi Shui* School that used new approaches to formula construction, emphasised warm-tonification of the spleen and stomach, as well as focusing on the ascent-descent body dynamic and on the channel affinities (*gui xing*) of the medicinals. Wang was not, however, such a prisoner of doctrine as to exclude other treatments where appropriate. He is credited with formulating various *xie qi* removal formulas such as the wonderfully dynamic *jiu wei qiang huo tang* – for cold-damp channel invasion with body stiffness and headaches – and *da qiang huo tang* – for wind-damp headaches. (*Jiu wei qiang huo tang* has also been attributed to Wang's teacher, Zhang Yuan-su.) Wang Hao-gu's favourite medicinals included *liu huang, fu zi, wu tou, rou gui* and *gan jiang* (sulphur, aconite, cinnamon and dried ginger), and formulas such as *hui yang dan* (return the *yang* tablet), *huo yan san* (firebolt powder) and *fu zi san*.

Wang Hao-gu also used his interpretation of the *Shang Han Lun Liujing* six channel patterns to treat paediatric skin rashes. In his *Ban Zhen Cui Lun* he advised practitioners to 'treat the external patterns with external medicine [and] treat internal patterns with internal medicine; thus the middle and the exterior can both be harmonised and the rash will be led out'. He advocated the use of a range of different treatment principles in paediatric fevers such as '*fa* (to vent or emit), *duo* (to seize), *qing* (clear), *xia* (purge), *li* (facilitate), *an* (calm) and *fen* (to separate)'.

The formulas he most often used for these treatment principles included *bai hu tang, xi jiao di huang tang, gan lu yin zi* and *xie bai san*. This focus on heat-clearing formulas provides further evidence of Wang Hao-gu's flexible style, which was not confined to the doctrinaire use of warm-tonification but was rooted in pattern differentiation.

Wang Hao-gu's writings include:
- *Yin Zheng Lue Lie* (On the *Yin* Syndromes) in one volume
- three volumes of the *Tang Ye Ben Cao* (*Bencao* for Decoctions)
- two volumes of *Ci Shi Nan Zhi* (Hard-won Knowledge), in which he discouraged the use of purgatives and the incorrect use of tonics
- one volume of *Ban Zhen Cui Lun*, which focused on paediatric febrile rashes.

Zhu Dan-xi (1281–1358)

A native of Yi Wu in Zhejiang province, Zhu Zhen Heng lived his life by the River Danxi from which he got his nickname Dan-xi Wong (Old Man Dan Xi). Zhu began studying medicine at the age of 30 because he wanted to find a cure for his mother's recurrent sufferings with abdominal pains, and after some research he was able to acquire sufficient knowledge to successfully restore her health. In the following years his father, two uncles, his brother and his wife all died due to medical errors, and this prompted him to recommence his medical studies at the age of 40. In his early forties he travelled widely to study with various medical mentors in Jiangsu and Anhui. Then, after persistently waiting at his door for three months, he eventually persuaded the renowned Hanzhou physician Luo Zhi-di, a follower of Liu Wan-su, to help him continue his studies. After two years Zhu is said to have acquired Luo's medical knowledge, and in this time he had also absorbed the teachings of the other two Jin-Yuan masters – Zhang Cong-zheng and Li Dong-yuan.

Both scholarly and clinically adept, Zhu soon became a very renowned physician in Jiangsu and Zhejiang provinces. Uncorrupted by fame he continued to give his full attention to his patients; his noble generous spirit was legendary amongst locals who said that 'even when wind and snow is imminent Zhu still comes out'.

Zhu Dan-xi's most notable writings are:
- *Ge Zhi Yu Lun*
- *Ju Fang Fa Hui*.

He also wrote:
- *Shang Han Bian Yi*
- *Bencao Yanyi Buyi*
- *Waike Jing Yao Fa Hui*.

Zhu's work compiled by later followers:
- *Dan Xi Xin Fa*
- *Jin Gui Gou Yuan*.

ZHU DAN-XI'S YIN NOURISHING AND HEAT CLEARING SCHOOL

Based on his interpretation of the ideas of ministerial fire that had been mentioned in the Han dynasty classics, Zhu's central thesis was that '*yang* always tends towards excess and *yin* to insufficiency'. In addition he was inspired by the notion that the *yang* functions of movement and transformation were a fundamental characteristic of everything in nature. He concluded that in relation to body function, the root source of such movement and activity in the human body was ministerial fire – *xiang huo*.

> Heaven masters everything [and is permanent], so permanence is due to activity and movement; man's longevity also depends on activity as well; so endurance exists in moving which is the result of ministerial fire. (Zhu Dan-xi)

Xiang huo consists of two aspects: constancy and change. It normally resides in the *jing* essence and *xue* blood of the liver and kidney, and these are functionally linked to the gallbladder, bladder, pericardium and *sanjiao*. *Xiang huo* therefore works by activating the functions of these *zangfu* as the basis for proper body function or, in Zhu's words, 'for fortuitous benefit and enduring vitality'.

In disease, by contrast, when *xiang huo* fails to properly fulfil its activating function, then 'the harm can be big, change and transformation can be quick, the situation can become severe, and death can come suddenly'. In other words, Zhu believed that this was the main factor underlying pathogenesis, the reversal of health and even death, and so he often stressed the importance of actively conserving *xiang huo*.

The main factors causing unregulated and aberrant *xiang huo*, in Zhu's understanding, were extreme emotional disturbances, unregulated and excessive sexual cravings and rich diet. He wrote that 'the five *zang* all have their own [inherent latent] fire which builds up when irritated by five emotions… With excess anger fire arises in the liver; with drunkenness and excessive indulgence in food fire arises in the stomach; with sexual draining fire arises in the kidney; with sadness fire arises in the lungs; when the heart suffers from princely fire this can cause scorching and then death.' Zhu Dan-xi thought the adverse effect of rampant *xiang fire* in causing illness came from 'the consumption of true *yin* by grilling and boiling; *yin* deficiency causes illness, and when *yin* reaches the point of exhaustion death results'. From this we can see that Zhu's *xiang huo* theory was derived from both Liu Wan-su's 'fire and heat' thesis and from Li Gao's *yin fire* ideas.

Linking the movement and changes of heaven and earth, sun and moon, and *yin* and *yang* in nature, together with the human life cycle of birth, growing, strengthening, ageing and decline, he promoted the idea that is summed up as '*yang* gets excessive and *yin* gets insufficient'. Evidence of this natural law, to précis Zhu's rationale, was to be found in the wider universe. The heavens and the sun are *yang* whilst the earth and moon are *yin*; the heavens extend beyond the earth's limits and so the heavens are much greater in dimension than the earth; the sun is *yang* and is virtually always full whilst the moon is *yin* and much of the time is empty; the sun is brighter than the moon. Whilst human beings are alive they are nourished by the contrasting *qi* of heaven and earth, the *yang qi* from the skies is *qi*, the *yin qi* of the earth is akin to blood. *Qi*, Zhu taught, tends to become excessive whilst blood is usually insufficient. 'The growing and declining of the *yin qi* in the body depends on the moon's fullness and emptiness, so we can see *yang* is usually excessive [and] blood is usually insufficient.'

Furthermore, Zhu argued, the natural progression of man's growth, development and strengthening as well as his sensory functions of vision, hearing and speech were all *yang* activities that needed to be supported and balanced by sufficient *yin*. *Yin qi*, he said, was generally difficult to generate and prone to insufficiency, such that *yang excess* and *yin deficiency* was a given in human physiology.

Turning to human nature, Zhu noted that 'the human mind is easily tempted by materialistic cravings for pleasant sounds and sexual pleasure; the heart is often touched in such a way that *xiang huo* acts rashly, thereby consuming more *yin* and leading to problems of *yin*-essence deficiency'. In everyday life, Zhu said, 'it's easy to move around but much harder to be quiet... All activity is fire', so unregulated *xiang fire* was harmful, consuming true *yin*, so that *yang* was excessive and *yin* was insufficient. With these ideas underlying his clinical practice, Zhu advocated treatment to nourish *yin* and reduce fire. He taught that by nourishing *yin* fire diminishes by itself, and that by reducing fire we can indirectly replenish *yin*. So Zhu's style became known as the *yin* nourishing school (*zi yin pai*), a style epitomised by the formula *da bu yin wan* (great *yin* supplementation formula).

So for Zhu, the preservation of good health meant controlling the rashness of *xiang huo* by conserving and nourishing *yin* essence. In his *Ge Zhi Yu Lun* (Prescriptions to Keep up Your Sleeve) he included chapters offering lifestyle guidance for longevity that included advice on sexual restraint and diet, including advice on vegetarianism. He taught that people should avoid living an indulgent life with dietary excesses, and that people should avoid marrying too young in order to allow their *yin qi* to fully mature, and that once married, sexual activity should be moderate. To avoid excessive and uncontrolled stirring of *xiang huo*, lustfulness should be kept at bay, and the consumption of rich and fatty foods, alcohol, meat, fried pastry and grilled, roasted, spicy, sweet and greasy foods should all be avoided. He claimed that 'craving foods and an excess indulgence in the five flavours' often caused illnesses, so he advocated a light and vegetarian diet. Zhu said, 'The naturally harmonious flavours of grains, vegetables and fruit are able to nourish *yin*.' He also advocated a lifestyle that balanced activity and stillness with the emphasis on the latter: 'stillness is the main thing' – people should keep calm minds and curb cravings so as to protect and support the *yin qi* and to maintain the body's *yin-yang* balance.

OTHER CONTRIBUTIONS TO CLINICAL PRACTICE

Although Zhu's core orientation, summed up in his *yang excessive–yin insufficient* dictum, meant that his clinical style was rooted in the use of a *yin*-supplementing medicinal, he often combined this with fire clearing. He also emphasised individualised syndrome differentiation as opposed to a blind doctrinaire treatment. The *yang excess–yin deficient* label attached to Zhu's style somewhat understates his contribution. For example, he recognised that the route of *yin* nourishment was through the stomach and spleen, and so he aimed to ensure that the middle *jiao* function was properly regulated. Various other innovations and insights came out of his clinical experience, and these have since joined the main body of Chinese

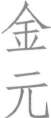

medicine theory. One example is his view that 'when lifestyle [work and rest] are disordered, then water fails to control fire', which, he said, contributed to the development of windstroke.

During the Jin-Yuan period there were new advances in phlegm-fluid and blood stasis theory. Zhang Cong-zheng, the attack and drain Jin-Yuan master, contributed to phlegm theory, and his ideas on this were then further elaborated by Zhu Dan-xi, for example by adding the idea that retained and accumulated thin mucus (*yin*) could result from the body's failure to properly eliminate dampness.

It was Zhu who originated the idea that excessive phlegm heat could lead to the stirring up of internal wind. He believed that most people from southeast China had constitutional damp earth (i.e. spleen dampness) that led to the production of phlegm. This phlegm, according to Zhu, could then generate excessive heat, which then transformed into wind. So, he said, we should treat the phlegm first and, as a secondary treatment principle, nourish and activate blood to prevent the generation of wind. In his discussions on the mechanism of phlegm disease he wrote, 'Phlegm ascends and descends with the *qi*; there is nowhere it cannot go', and this led to 'coughing, vomiting and diarrhoea, dizziness and heartburn, palpitation and panic attacks, cold and heat swellings, pain, obstruction in the gastric area and diaphragm, or there is rumbling noise in the chest and hypochondria, or cold feeling on the back and chest, [and] numbness of the limbs'. His basic approach for such phlegm disorders was to 'reinforce the spleen earth and dry spleen dampness'. This has become a standard part of modern practice.

Zhu's saying '10,000 illnesses all start with *yu*' provides an example of another of his contributions, and summarises his belief that stagnation syndromes (*yu*, sometimes misrepresented in English texts by the word 'depression') lie at the root of many illnesses. He examined the complex interrelationships between stagnation of *qi*, damp, heat, phlegm, blood and food that he called the six *yu*. Zhu taught that although each of these could cause illness on its own, very often they intermingled and combined together. In this conception, the start of any illness often (or even always) involved *qi* stagnation, and if this remained unresolved, it usually transformed into heat and fire. The more prolonged or severe the *qi* stasis, the more rapidly and severely the fire developed, and so, according to this perspective, it was often just as important to regulate *qi* as it was to disperse stagnation as well as including interventions to clear fire.

Once established, more complex *yu* stagnation disorders might take hold that combined *qi* stasis with stasis of fire, damp, food, phlegm and blood. This complex of stasis patterns was, Zhu believed, self-generating and self-sustaining, and could not be treated without the comprehensive strategy epitomised in his formula *yue ju wan*. Focusing on only one or two of the contributory stagnation elements left the conditions for the stasis to quickly return. This was a very important contribution as it offered new insights for understanding and treating common complex disorders.

Zhu Dan-xi lived at a time when many literate medical practitioners still routinely treated patients simply by prescribing formulas for main disease symptoms that were taken straight from the *He Ji Ju Fang* (People's Universal Benefit Formulary). A disease-orientated approach that de-emphasised individual pattern discrimination could be especially inappropriate during epidemics when failure to carefully examine the patient, guesswork and formulaic medicine could have damaging or fatal consequences. Zhu Dan-xi, due to his *yang excess–yin deficient* belief, was especially concerned about the misuse of pungent, warm and fragrant herbs that tend to dry and consume *yin*. He singled out the herb *chai hu* as a prime example of a medicinal that was often recklessly prescribed at the expense of patients' *yin*. Zhu claimed that its overuse 'plunders the *yin*'. Opinion today is that Zhu may have overstated his case in relation to *chai hu*, and that some other substances are worse if misused. The impact of Zhu's, perhaps excessive, concerns about *chai hu* have carried through to modern practice, something that serves to emphasise the strength of his influence in the last eight centuries.

In developing the understanding of internal heat, its clinical aetiology and role in the patho-physiology of *yin xu*, Zhu's contribution to Chinese medicine was significant. In the few centuries following his death he was remembered as 'the embodiment of medical greatness'; his fame spread widely across China and to 15th-century Japan where admirers founded the Dan Xi Scholars Society to study and promote his work.

Zhu Dan-xi formulas

The following brief survey of the formulas introduced in Zhu Dan-xi's writings reveals a broader range of approaches than suggested by the outline representation of his style as *yang excessive–yin weak* and 'numerous illnesses caused by *qi* stasis'.

Formula	Function
Da bu yin wan	*Yin* tonification
Zuo jin wan	*Yin* tonification
Bao he wan	Food stagnation
Ge hua jie cheng tang	Damp heat food stasis due to alcohol excess
Bei xie fen qing wan	Remove damp obstruction in bladder
Er miao san	Clear damp heat in legs and lower *jiao*
Gun tan wan	Drain phlegm heat from lungs
Hu qian wan	For wasting and paralysis from deficiency
Ke xue fang	For blood-streaked phlegm expectoration
Yu ping feng san	To consolidate *wei qi* on the exterior
Yue ju wan	To resolve the six *yu*

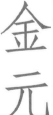

Medical cosmology in the Jin-Yuan period

Wang Bing's Tang dynasty edition of the *Suwen* added the seven chapters that formed the first detailed discussion on *wu yun liu qi* (five movements six *qi* or chronobiology) which sparked ongoing interest in chronobiology study through the Song, Jin and Yuan dynasties.

CHAPTERS ON *WU YUN LIU QI* IN WANG BING'S *SUWEN*

Ch 66 'Tian Yuan Ji Da Lun' ('Noting Heavenly Origins')

Ch 67 'Wu Yun Xing Da Lun' ('Five Movements')

Ch 68 'Liu Wei Zhi Da Lun' ('Six Energies Subtle Theory')

Ch 69 'Qi Jiao Bian Da Lun' ('Changes of the Six *Qi* Intersections')

Ch 70 'Wu Chang Zheng Da Lun' ('Five Normal Patterns')

Ch 71 'Liu Yuan Zheng Ji Da Lun' ('Records of Six Original Patterns')

Ch 74 'Zhi Zhen Yao Da Lun' ('Most True Essentials')

Liu Wan-shu (not to be confused with Liu Wan-su, 1120–1200, discussed earlier) pioneered the medical applications of *wuyun liuqi* in the Song dynasty and published his *Suwen Rushi Yunqi Lun Ao* (Penetrating the *Suwen*'s Mysterious *Yunqi* Patterns) in 1099. Here Liu claimed that '*yunqi* is the most crucial factor in supplementation and draining', and wrote that his work 'summarises the secrets that I obtained from an ancient cosmology text and collects together elegant discussions on *yin* and *yang*. When these principles are understood the beads can be strung together and the subject entirely clarified.' Using his secret texts and the relevant *Suwen* chapters, Liu Wan-shu elaborated on 31 *yunqi* topics and created explanatory diagrams, and so wrote the seminal text on *yunqi* doctrine.

A few decades later, the Jin-Yuan master Liu Wan-su was an even more enthusiastic *wuyun liuqi* advocate and provided influential support to this branch of theory. He contended that chronobiology was equal in importance to *ba gua*, *san cai* or *wu chang* – respectively, the eight trigrams of the *Yijing*, three powers heaven-earth-man, and five norms of Confucianism. He wrote that 'when making a diagnosis the most important thing is our ability to identify *yin-yang*, deficiency and excess…[but] the route to understanding illness is by categorising its *bing qi* (disease *qi*) according to the changes and transformations of *wuyun liuqi*'.

With this in mind, Liu Wan-shu integrated the 19 categories of pathogenesis found in the *Suwen* with *wuyun liuqi* theory, matching the illnesses of the five *zang* organs with the five movements (*wuyun*), and associated the *xu* and *shi* of the organs with the cycles of the six environmental *qi*: cold, summer-heat, dryness, dampness, wind and fire. He introduced various other technical changes in chronobiology – for instance, he founded the doctrine of *zangfu liuqi* pathogenesis which he stated as 'when the *zangfu* and *jing-luo* develop an illness their original *qi* is not necessarily *shi* or *xu*, [and] it may be that the illness is caused by a contention between the six *qi*'; this was a new idea in

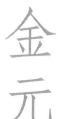

yunqi doctrine. Liu also revised part of *yunqi* theory that is summarised in the epithet *kang ze hai – cheng ze zhi* (in order to avoid harm restrain excess).

The chronobiology scheme can be criticised for its inherent tendency to assess patients on the basis of cosmological and meteorological speculation, a method in which it is easy for the theory to take precedence over the patient's actual body state. Liu Wan-shu's interpretation of the chronobiology style of practice was progressive because it aimed to sidestep such mechanical application of the theory. He disputed its concept of a pre-ordained format of energetic states in heaven and earth and with each year in the 60-year cycle governing a certain *qi* and specific illness patterns. Liu also disagreed with the view of rigid advocates of the system that illnesses were completely governed by *wuyun liuqi,* and wrote that 'people themselves govern their lives… Practising Buddhism or Daoism is a choice, so too is whether to live a short life and die young. People do things to themselves.' Whilst there is undoubted truth in the observation that different disease conditions arise at different times of the year, and that epidemics can be cyclical, it is a mistake to extend this understanding beyond sensible boundaries or to have theories that are disconnected from facts. Liu's introduction of a more flexible approach clearly makes more real-world sense than a blind adherence to the rigid belief that different moments in time generate environmental conditions that result in specific disease states.

Zhang Yuan-su, who we have already discussed as having had a significant influence on much of Jin-Yuan dynasty medicine, also took an interest in *wuyun liuqi* doctrine and incorporated it into his own theories and prescribing style. He used the *wuyun* (five movements of the cosmos) as a method of categorising herbs and the *liuqi* (six earthly climatic influences) as a tool to distinguish formula types. This was a unique innovation that later influenced Li Dong-yuan and the physicians who then inherited his lineage through the Ming.

The Song dynasty Imperial Medical Bureau also lent official support to *yunqi* doctrine. The government-sponsored formulary, *Sheng Ji Zong Lu* (General Collection for Holy Relief), included the sexagenary yunqi chart in a prime position right at the beginning of the text. It included discussions of various aspects of *yunqi* theory including the cyclic patterns of guest and host movements (*zhu yun* and *ke yun*), and the ideas of *si tian* (rule of heaven), *zai quan* (springtime dwelling of the dead) and *ke zhu jia lin* (guest *qi* joining into host *qi*). Additional official support for *yunqi* theories is also seen in the fact that the Song–Jin-Yuan medical schools included it as an exam subject, and such validation helped give it more widespread support, leading to a popular medical aphorism of the time, 'There is little value in consulting all the formula books without studying *wuyun liuqi.*'

Yunqi doctrine at this time not only influenced medical practice; it was also widely applied to other areas of the natural sciences. Shen Kuo (aka Meng Xi), the remarkable Song dynasty polymath scholar, said in his *Meng Xi Bi Tan* (Charts from the Pen of Meng Xi), 'The changing climate of heaven and earth; cold, summer, wind, rain and wind in the north; and [plagues of] worms and locusts all obey certain rules.' The belief of silk-clad scholars that the mechanics of the universe could

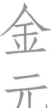

be reliably modelled by the *wuyun liuqi* system, and that it was able to accurately predict climate, epidemics, crops, pests and so on, allowed sceptics to highlight those occasions when it failed and to say that the method was worthless – examples of a beautiful theory struck down by inconvenient truth. To counter such attacks, special get-out clauses were installed into the theory to counter attacks by critics, but eventually, over the following centuries, most physicians arrived at a compromise by recognising *yunqi* theory as a partially successful attempt to reconcile the calendar with climatology, phenomenology, nature, agriculture and medicine, but one that should not be too rigidly applied.

Other notable Jin-Yuan physicians
Yan Yong-he (c. 1206–1268)

A native of Lushan in Jiangxi province, Yan Yong-he was a contemporary and follower of Li Dong-yuan who was also interested in understanding the regulation of the middle *jiao* and of its relationship with the ministerial fire. Like Li Dong-yuan, he favoured the use of the spleen *qi* tonic *bai zhu*, and often paired it with the *qi* regulator *ju pi*. He believed that obstruction of the middle *jiao* by phlegm damp was common, and so also often used *fu ling*, *fa ban xia* and *sheng jiang*. Yan felt that if the middle *jiao* function was weak, it was normally because of weakness in the *ming men huo*, and so he often advocated strengthening the spleen by warming the kidneys; his favoured herbs to do this were *lu jiao*, *rou cong rong*, *tu si zi*, *rou gui* and *wu yao*.

Yan Yong-he wrote the ten-volume (*Yan Shi*) *Ji Sheng Fang* ((Master Yan's) Formulas to Aid the Living) (1253) that discussed the treatment of many conditions and included about 400 formulas. Later Yan published an update, *Ji Sheng Xu Fang* (More Life Preservation Formulas) (1267), with additional formulas and illness discussions. These texts were lost but later reconstructed from quotes in other texts.

FORMULAS FROM YAN YONG-HE'S *JI SHENG FANG*

Formula	Function
Xin yi san	For nasal congestion
Cang er zi san	Wind cold nasal congestion
Di dan tang	Difficult speech due to phlegm
Qi pi yin	Treats oedema
Xiao ji yin zi	For heat haematuria
Gui pi tang	Spleen *qi xu* mental fatigue
Shi pi yin	Spleen *xu* cold oedema
Ju he wan	Cold damp hernia pain
Si mo tang	Lung *qi* stasis breathing difficulty
Tu si zi wan	Kidney *qi xu* exhaustion
Qing pi tang	Spleen heat and damp stasis

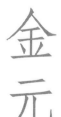

Chen Zi-ming

Coming from an esteemed medical family, Chen Zi-ming became one of the greatest gynaecologists in Chinese medicine history. Drawing on many gynaecology texts, his clinical experience and the knowledge gleaned from his family medical heritage, he published his *Furen Daquan Liangfang* (Compendium of Good Prescriptions for Women) in 1273. Especially strong on understanding and regulating the menstrual cycle, Chen added significantly to the sophistication of gynaecology. He was the first to record the formulas *suo chuan wan* and *si sheng wan* that form part of modern practice.

Jin-Yuan developments in pulse diagnostics

As we have seen, the use of pulse diagnosis can be traced right back to the case histories of Chunyu Yi practising at the start of the Western Han dynasty at the dawn of classical medicine. During the Song, Jin and Yuan dynasties the most popular pulse diagnosis study text was the *Mai Jue* (Knack of the Pulse) that was completed by the famous pulse diagnostician Cui Jia-yan in 1189. In Cui's view, pulse diagnosis teaching was hindered by lack of clarity in the written descriptions of the pulse qualities that were available at the time and this, he said, made them difficult for students to memorise. His solution was to compose four character rhymes in plain language to make learning easier. This single-volume text was published under various titles such as *Cui Shi Mai Jue*, *Cui Zhen Ren Mai Jue* and *Zi Xu Mai Jue*, but was popularly known as *Mai Jue*.

Cui based his work on the *Nanjing*, *Mai Jing* (Pulse Classic) and another *Mai Jue* written by Gao Yang-sheng. He focused on depth and rate as the key qualities and wind, *qi*, cold and heat as the main aspects discernible on the pulse, and subcategorised and described the 24 pulses discussed in *Mai Jing* as well as the long and short pulses in *Mai Jue*. Its lucid and practical style meant that *Mai Jue* became the prime pulse text for the following centuries, and it was reworked a number of times: in the Ming dynasty by Li Yan-wen who renamed it *Si Yan Jue Yao* (Four Character Essentials), and then towards the end of the Ming by Li Shi-zhen who used it as a basis for his *Bin Hu Mai Xue* (Lakeside Pulse Study).

Various other *Mai Jue* books appeared in the Yuan dynasty; one by Liu Kai (1241) also used floating-sinking, slow-rapid for primary orientation, and discussed the different diseases indicated by changes in the three pulse positions (*cun, guan, chi*) on the radial artery. Dai Qi-zong also amended Gao Yang-sheng's *Mai Jue* by publishing his *Mai Jue Kan Wu* (*Mai Jue* Errors Corrected) which was an innovative and meticulous discussion of the individual pulse qualities based on his distillation of the classical sources.

In 1359, the renowned physician Hua Shou contributed his extensive clinical experience to the diagnostic literature by writing *Zhen Jia Shu Yao* (Key Pointers for Diagnosticians). Hua Shou presented the principles of pulse images and pulse identification, and he elaborated and analysed all 29 pulse images and the diseases that they indicated. He also discussed the specific characteristics of pulse diagnosis in women and children.

Where previously textbooks on pulse diagnostics had used words alone to describe pulse qualities, the Yuan dynasty saw the innovative use of diagrams to represent the qualities graphically. Earlier, the Song physician Wang Shu-he is credited with compiling a pulse diagram collection (*Zhangjing Sanshi Liu Maifa Tu*, Zhang Jing's Thirty Six Pulse Diagrams), but unfortunately the original version has been lost. The earliest-surviving illustrated pulse text is *Cha Bing Zhi Nan* (Guide for Checking Disease) by Shi Fa (1241); this is a very practical and clear general diagnosis text that includes significant coverage of pulse diagnostics. Much of its three volumes are devoted to pulse diagnosis, and it describes a system called 'the seven exterior, eight interior and nine pathways, twenty-four pulse sorting method'. It also provided methods for distinguishing life-or-death prognosis in various diseases. In addition, this was the first book to delineate the idea of the four diagnostics (*siwen*) routines of looking, asking, listening-smelling and palpation.

Tongue diagnosis in the Jin-Yuan dynasty

Tongue diagnosis also underwent significant development in the Song–Jin-Yuan period, and many new refinements of this method appeared. For example, Zhu Hong's *Shang Han Lei Zheng Huo Ren Shu* (On *Shang Han*-Like Patterns in People) discussed the differentiation of patterns of *yin-yang* and *xu-shi* according to the presence or absence of a dry mouth and tongue. Discussions of the interpretation of tongue motility abnormalities such as 'stretching tongue' and 'playing tongue' appear in the *Xiaoer Yaozheng Zhi Jue* (The Knack of Paediatric Medical Syndromes) by the great paediatrician Qian Yi. Also, in relation to the significance of altered taste sensations in the mouth, Chen Yan, in his *San Yin Fang*, summarised previous knowledge on changes such as bitterness, salty, sour, astringent, sweet and bland tastes in the mouth.

Li Dong-yuan's *Pi Wei Lun* (1249) analysed the various situations when a dry tongue was present. He said that a dry tongue along with a dry throat was mainly a consequence of improper diet or of exhaustion from labouring and working; a dry tongue with pain in the chest and flanks was mainly due to liver wood travelling recklessly; a dry tongue with bitter mouth or no taste was mainly due to *yang qi* failing to properly extend upwards.

The Yuan dynasty physician Ao Shi distilled the writings of many authors on tongue diagnosis in order to compile his *Jin Jing Lun* (Golden Mirror Treatise). This recorded 12 methods of interpreting the tongues in patients suffering from *shang han* disorders and, to aid clarity, 12 tongue diagrams were attached. Unfortunately this text is now lost, but at the time, *Jin Jing Lun* was the standard work on tongue examination. In 1341, Du Ben re-published a version of *Jin Jing Lun* that added a further 24 illustrations showing coatings and tongue body appearances that were

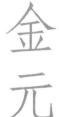

matched together with appropriate formulas for each. This version, *Ao Shi Shang Han Jin Jing Lun*, has survived to modern times, and is Chinese medicine's earliest extant text specifically on tongue diagnosis. Tongue colours such as pink, crimson and purple were painted in and described as well as the coating colours such as white, yellow, grey and black. Descriptions of tongue textures included in the discussions were red prickles, cracks, dryness, slipperiness, astringent and prickly. The text covered most of the main pathological phenomena understood at the time. Accompanying each picture were the associated pulse qualities enabling the differentiation of cold and heat, deficiency and excess, and internal or external injury contracted, along with discussions on suitable treatment methods, on appropriate prescriptions and on the associated severity, urgency or malignancy of the condition. It was considered an important text through the subsequent dynasties, and the information in Du Ben's book is viewed as generally valid today.

Development of forensic medicine

Published in about 1247, *Xi Yuan Zhi Lu* (On Cleaning Up Wrongdoing) by Song Ci (style name Hui Fu) is considered to be the world's earliest-surviving specialist manual on forensic investigation, although, as we saw in an earlier chapter, the first known writings stipulating the conduct of investigations into suspicious deaths and serious assaults date back to Han dynasty bamboo strips. After the Han it is possible to trace the threads of a long-standing forensic medicine tradition, including a 6th-century text, *Ming Yuan Shi Lun* by Xu Zhi-cai, and later other specialist texts such as *Yi Yu Zhi* by He Ning just before the beginning of the Song, and *Zhe Yu Gui Jian* published by Cheng Ke in 1133. So, in writing his manual, Song Ci was able to draw on a long tradition of forensic investigation that generally displays a rational and investigative outlook. In his textbook Song Ci discusses how official investigators should proceed in determining whether a death was an accident, suicide or homicide and, if necessary, tips on how to identify the culprit were provided.

One case presented in *Yi Yu Zhi* by He Ning cites an investigation from seven centuries previously in which a man's body had been recovered from a house fire. His wife was accused of murder by the husband's family, but she denied the charge and refused to confess. Determined to get to the truth of the matter, the investigating official took two pigs, one killed and the other alive but trussed up, and ordered that they both be burned in a shed similar to the house where the fire had taken place. The animal that had previously been killed had no ash in its mouth and nasal passages or fire damage to the trachea, whereas the live animal had damage that corresponded to that found on autopsy in the dead man. Faced with this evidence the woman confessed to having killed her husband and attempting to hide the crime in the fire.

Song Ci came from a scholarly family from Fukien in south China, and in 1217 graduated from the *jin shi* (doctorate) exams from the imperial university. He was appointed as a registrar in Kangxi where his evident skill in resolving various local difficulties allowed him to rise to become a senior official. One of the tasks of regional government officials was to lead the investigation of suspicious deaths and to conduct inquests. Presumably his desire to carry out this task well inspired him to write and compile his forensic manual by setting down guidelines and official rules based on previous forensic knowledge and his own experience in the field.

Much of the content of *Xi Yuan Zhi Lu* is eminently sensible and organised. Detailed procedures are stipulated for different circumstances including a two-stage inquest system, filing of triplicate-signed reports and formal autopsy procedures involving local people in possession of anatomical skills such as midwives and butchers.

In the less contentious deaths there would be an investigation that included gathering opinions based on interviews with reputable local people and, if there was no reason for suspicion, the case would usually not proceed to inquest. Expert witnesses might be called, for example, to rule out medical malpractice by checking for inappropriate moxibustion treatment or acupuncture needle injuries, or to check that improper medicines had not been administered. Officials whose investigations were found to be negligent, such as by lax investigation or punishing the innocent, faced standardised judicial beatings or even years of penile servitude. False accusers and those who bore false witness also faced severe punishments.

> In one case a man was found murdered by multiple sickle wounds. Given the frenzied style of attack, Song-zi concluded that anger, not robbery, was the likely motive, and that the murderer would most likely be known to the victim. His widow was asked if he had had any enemies; she said no, but that he had recently refused to lend some money to a neighbour. The neighbour denied any involvement. Song-zi immediately impounded all the 80 or so sickles from those in the surrounding area, stipulating that anyone found concealing a sickle would be considered the culprit. The suspect was summoned, and he again denied any involvement. 'Is that your sickle?' Song-zi demanded, pointing to the one sickle that was now covered in flies. Realising his guilt had been cleverly exposed, he made an immediate confession.

Xi Yuan Zhi Lu collects numerous tips on crime scene examination, witness interrogation and examination of corpses. Detailed descriptions of anatomy and anatomical terms are included, together with methods of ascertaining cause of death. Most of the methods appear to be valid, although some others are dubious to modern eyes. An example of the latter is a test that was intended to determine whether those who claimed to be relatives of the deceased were telling the truth. Song Ci suggested that a few drops of blood from a living relative dropped on to dry bones would soak in, whereas if they were unrelated it would not. Other procedures, such as those proscribed to determine if a body with only bones surviving had suffered injury before death, seem to make more sense.

> If bones have already been washed and examined repeatedly they will become white and appear uninjured. How can the truth be then determined? Pour oil on

the bones being examined for possible injuries. Bones have cracks and pores. When these are full and excess oil begins to drip out, have the bones wiped dry. Hold them up towards the light. Where there were injuries the oil will stop and not pass through. Clear areas are those where no injuries occurred. Another method: daub some good thick ink on the bones. After it has dried wash it off. If there are injuries the ink will seep into the bones at those points. Where there are no injuries the ink will not seep in. Another method: take some new cotton and pass it over the bones. Where there has been an injury some of the cotton fibres will always catch and be pulled out. When the bones have been broken always look at the colour of both broken ends. Also, take note of whether the protruding bone fibres point inwards or outwards. Where the break was caused by a blow the splinters will point inwards. Where they point outwards the injury was not caused by a blow. Where the bones of the skull have been struck they will be blue. Where bones have been broken there will be extravasated blood. Carefully examine the surface of the bones for livid or purple-black haloes. If they are elongated they are caused by 'other weapons', if round, by a fist, if larger by butting with the head and if small, by kicking with the point of the foot. When among the bones on the four sides of the skeleton there is a break; whether it was a mortal injury or not, have the coroner's assistant or the attendants indicate it and announce it aloud. (Translated by McKnight 1981)

In addition to sensible forensic logic, we find in Song Ci's writings evidence of a fairly accurate understanding of human anatomy as well as some significant faults and misapprehensions. For example, one section in the text provides a long list of the names of the bones in the human skeleton. The fact that assistants were called on to conduct the examination of bodies suggests that anatomical knowledge was considered less the professional province of a scholar physician and more that of midwives, butchers and traumatology specialists. Whilst it is true that the 16th-century Italian anatomists were more meticulous in their explorations of anatomy, it is fair to claim that the Chinese sources were superior prior to this time.

Xi Yuan Zhi Lu continued to be repeatedly published in numerous editions and revisions in subsequent centuries. Marked similarities have been found between these Jin-Yuan forensic practices and medical jurisprudence in mediaeval Europe, so it has been suggested that Song Ci's forensic methods may have spread first to the Arabic world, through Arab links with Sicily, and on to Britain with the Normans in the 14th century. Speculation aside, Song Ci's text did later achieve such renown that in the 19th century it was translated into various European languages, and it made an undisputed contribution to the development of modern forensic medicine. These are detailed in McKnight's (1981) translation of Song Ci's manual.

In sum, the Jin-Yuan period was a period of innovation and development of Chinese medicine that had not been seen since the Han dynasty. There was imperial support for medical scholarship, and a desire to make professional medicine available to a wider population; the period also saw a significant re-examination of the medical tradition, many new ideas were introduced and specialist areas such

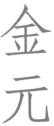

as paediatrics and gynaecology developed. In 1368 the era was brought to an end with the founding of the Ming dynasty after another invasion of northern tribes, during which medical endeavour settled in for centuries of individualism and fragmentation, with numerous styles of practice forming, most of which were based on interpretations and developments of the key schools of thought founded in the Song–Jin-Yuan.

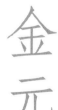

7

MING DYNASTY

The Ming dynasty was founded in 1368 by a peasant called Hong Wu (Zhu Yuan-zhang) who led an uprising that succeeded in defeating the Mongol rulers. Hong Wu instituted reforms that provided a new stable era, and this in turn allowed the second Ming emperor, Yongle (ruled 1403–1424), to inherit a prosperous state and to start spending copiously in an attempt to create an illustrious, powerful and lasting dynasty. He moved the capital from Nanjing to Beijing, and then proceeded to initiate cripplingly expensive projects such as building Beijing's Forbidden City, re-building the Great Wall and creating a large maritime exploration fleet headed by Admiral Zheng He. The teak forests of Vietnam were decimated by the need for hardwood for these ventures, and the country's financial reserves were almost exhausted by his profligacy. Eventually the dynasty succumbed to mounting threats, culminating in its overthrow by the Manchu after roughly two centuries.

Now that printing was commonplace, individual physicians in the Ming dynasty wrote and published many more books than previously and, because of their numbers, a much higher proportion of these writings have survived to the present day. Numerous *bencao* editions appeared, and many specialised medical texts were written that aided the progress of a whole range of medical specialisms; discussions on internal medicine (*nei ke*) were especially prolific. Acumoxa remained popular in the Ming dynasty, and scholar physicians paid more attention to improving this therapy; this interest resulted in the appearance of some major acupuncture texts in the Ming dynasty, some of which are outlined here. In addition, the legacy of the various styles of practice that had been founded in the preceding Jin-Yuan dynasty was carried forward, and this led to diverse schools of thought in medical practice co-existing and contending for popularity. This, too, is a theme for this chapter.

Imperial medical sponsorship of medicine and other areas of academic study continued sporadically through the Ming dynasty, with the general trend being increasingly away from state involvement. One notable official milestone in state publishing was the compilation of *Yongle Dadian* (Yongle Reign Great Compendium) in 1408, a monumental encyclopaedia that incorporated, among its numerous other subjects, history, medicine, mathematics and astronomy. Just a couple of years prior to this another big compilation had been published, *Pu Ji Fang* (Prescriptions for Universal Relief), which brought together over 70,000 medical prescriptions, more than ever before. Compiled by Teng Hong, this ran to 426 volumes and included a significant amount of content on acumoxa.

State medical education in the Ming

Under the Ming regime state control of medical education was allowed to decline sharply, and private medical study became once again the more usual route to professional scholarly practice. Previously the grand Tai Yi Su medical school had provided a well-ordered and high-level training; now it was Tai Yi Yuan imperial hospital that instead took on a training role. Here physicians could specialise in gynaecology, sores and ulcers, acupuncture, ophthalmology, dentistry, orthopaedics, *shang han* diseases, throat diseases, injury, massage and what were termed 'big formula' and 'small formula' departments (*da fang mai* and *xiao fang mai*), referring to paediatric and adult medicine respectively. Necromancy (*zhu you*) was also studied, which involved communicating with the spirits of the ancestors and, at this time, such study was seen as a dignified and serious career for a scholar specialist.

The egalitarian, but in practice unworkable, Song dynasty 'access-for-all' principle was now abandoned, and entrants to education at Tai Yi Yuan in the first part of the Ming dynasty were again drawn mainly from the well-connected sectors of society such as sons of famous physicians. A more easy-going attitude to medical education can be seen from the fact that trainee physicians were allowed to choose their own teachers. Nonetheless, medical students were subject to formal examination of their knowledge and skill, and those who failed were expelled. As the Ming dynasty progressed, additional selection and teaching procedures were established, and by 1527, a set curriculum with quarterly exams was in place. A few years later, regular testing of everybody working in the imperial hospital was introduced, with the results submitted to the regulatory authorities. Those who were deemed to be performing inadequately suffered proscribed penalties such as suspension of their monthly food allowance, and any who attempted to avoid exams were also subject to set punishments. Students who had successfully completed three years of study sat a final examination that was overseen by the medical officers in the imperial hospital, and on the basis of their scores graduates were divided into three grades. Those graduating with the highest grades were assigned to work as physicians in the imperial pharmacy, those with middle grades were awarded 'yellow hat ribbon' (*guan dai*) official status, and low-grade graduates were sent back to the imperial hospital to perform mundane medical duties. Outside of the select confines of the imperial court, though, the Ming government had largely abandoned the ideas of official concern for public health and welfare that had been such an important ideal of the Song. The era of government benevolence was in decline.

Partly because of this hands-off approach and partly because of the wide availability of affordable printed medical texts for self-study, medical scholars in the country at large found local mentors, and many diverse styles of medical practice contended for dominance. Most commonly, these styles were derivations of the schools of practice founded by four famous doctors of the Jin and Yuan dynasties, and in this way literate medical practice began to polarise into a handful of schools of thought. The progress of these currents of medical thought provides the initial theme for this chapter.

Yin nourishing school

Previously we discussed the teachings of Zhu Dan-xi (Zhu Zhen-heng), the last of the four masters of the Jin-Yuan period, who promoted the idea that *yin* was prone to depletion whilst *yang* tended to excess. This general current of medical thought, which came to be known as the *yang yin* (strengthen the *yin*) style, was championed by two of Zhu's most esteemed pupils, Tai Yuan-li and Wang Lu, and was then adopted by many other prominent physicians to become one of the predominant styles of the Ming dynasty.

Tai Yuan-li (1322–1405)

Having gained considerable fame before the onset of the Ming dynasty, Tai Yuan-li (Dai Si-gong) was an official court physician who rose to become president of the imperial medical college. In homage to his teacher, Tai Yuan-li wrote a short work called *Tui Qiu Shi Yi* (A Thorough Examination of the Master's Medical Opinions) that summarised Zhu Dan-xi's teachings in relation to the aetiology and the treatment of 50 illnesses. As well as common adult diseases such as tuberculosis, malaria, diabetes and gynaecological disorders, one section discussed various children's illnesses including threadworm, for which he recommended herbs with ascaricidal properties.

> **OTHER TEXTS BY TAI YUAN-LI**
>
> *Zheng Zhi Yao Jue* (Secret Tips for Diagnosis)
>
> *Zheng Zhi Yao Jue Lei Fang* (Secret Tips with Classified Treatments)
>
> *Zheng Zhi Lei Yuan* (Secret Tips Classifying the Source)
>
> *Lei Zheng Yong Yao* (Categorised Tips on the Use of Medicines)

These writings served to clarify, structure and embellish Zhu dan-xi's doctrine, and so helped consolidate the *yang yin* style's position in Ming dynasty medicine.

Wang Lu (1332–1391)

Wang Lu (Wang An-dao) of Kunshan in Jiangsu province was another prominent advocate of Zhu Dan-xi's legacy. He agreed with the view held by Liu Wan-su and Zhang Yuan-su that most contemporary epidemic febrile diseases could not be effectively treated using the ancient classical prescriptions from the *Shang Han Lun*. Wang Lu came to an important realisation – the problem was not so much that the *Shang Han Lun* was wrong in de-emphasising *warm* disease in favour of cold attack (Zhang Zhong-jing had included some warm diseases in his scheme), but simply that in the Han dynasty these had been much less prevalent. Problematic, too, was the fact that imperial scholars who had promoted *Shang Han Lun* study in the Song dynasty a few centuries earlier had taken the term *shang han* to refer only to exterior cold when in fact it also included the possibility of acute warm diseases. This point was easily overlooked as the *Shang Han Lun* had mentioned such a possibility only in passing. The Song scholars whose task it was to decipher the *Shang Han Lun* had been blinkered by their great respect for this most venerable of classical texts, and had taken insufficient account of the current clinical realities where warm febrile diseases were far more common. The fact was that different illnesses prevail at different times in history and, in addition, disease patterns alter in response to different climatic and lifestyle conditions. So, instead of taking a fresh and objective look at patients' clinical presentations and considering new treatment approaches, physicians had continued to diagnose acute exterior disease as *taiyang*-stage wind-cold leading to knee-jerk treatment with pungent-warm exterior-releasing medicinals. Actually, the Song scholar Pang An-shi had previously highlighted the existence of *wen bing*-type presentations in his discussions on the *Shang Han Lun*, but when he did this, it was more to emphasise their usually fatal outcome than to propose viable treatments. Also, the Jin-Yuan master Liu Wan-su had previously highlighted his concerns about the inappropriate use of warm-pungent exterior-releasing medicinals in epidemic fevers, and had begun to advocate cool-pungent exterior release.

This omission from febrile disease theory was the issue Wang Lu now attempted to tackle by advancing the ideas of earlier thinkers such as Liu Wan-su, clarifying the distinctions between *shang han* and warm epidemic patterns, and proposing that they should demand distinct and different treatment – namely, heat clearage from either the interior or exterior levels of the body. In 1368 Wang published *Yijing Suhui Ji* (Going Against the Stream of the Medical Classics) and then his *Bai Bing Guo Xuan* (Hooking the Profundities of a Hundred Illnesses), but it would take roughly another 400 years before this seed was to geminate into a mature *wen bing* theory.

Warm supplementation school

Taking what appears to be a contrary stance to the *yin* nourishing school, the *wen bu* (warm supplementation) school believed that human vitality was essentially a *yang* function, that *ming men* fire, the 'fire at the gate of destiny', was easily weakened but very difficult to replenish. This school of thought claimed that physiologic warmth was the key difference between life and death; warmth and vitality were clearly *yang* functions, they claimed; therefore the avoidance of death involved treatment aimed at *yang* warming. Furthermore, *wen bu* advocates held that the excessive use of cold-natured heat-clearing medicinals by the styles advocating heat clearance was harmful to the body's *yang qi* and therefore to vitality and longevity. This style also drew on Li Dong-yuan's digestion-strengthening style, and focused on the application of many of his favourite herbs and prescriptions. The most prominent members of this *wen bu* school were Xue Ji, Zhao Xian-ke and, most famously, Zhang Jie-bin. These figures are discussed next.

Xue Ji (1488–1558)

The son of Xue Kai, a famous imperial hospital physician, Xue Ji (Xue Xin-fu) was exposed to medical learning from an early age. Initially a *yangyi* (sores and ulcers) specialist, he progressed into the study of Li Dong-yuan's writings. As well as using variations on Li's flagship formula *bu zhong yi qi tang*, Xue Ji's favoured formulas included *gui pi tang* (which originally came from Yang Yong-he's *Ji Sheng Fang*); he also often used the harmonising formula *xiao chaihu tang* from the *Shang Han Lun* as well as the basic *qi* and blood-restoring formula *ba zhen tang*. In his style he also favoured the use of the Song paediatrician Qian Yi's *liu wei di huang wan*, a prime formula to nourish *yin*, and in doing so Xue Ji further extended the scope of Li Dong-yuan's doctrine by adding an increased element of kidney supplementation. As a result of his developments of the stomach and spleen style, Xue Ji is credited with founding the *wen bu* or warm supplementation school of thinking.

It was Xue Ji who wrote the first ever text that was explicitly devoted to *nei ke* (internal medicine), his *Nei Ke Zhai Yao* (Précis of Internal Medicine) that summarised 200 examples of internal disease. The deficiency illnesses he described included *yuan qi* depletion and various forms of consumptive disorder (*lao*) such as: famine and exhaustion *lao*, spleen-stomach *lao*, spleen-kidney *lao*, spleen-lung *lao*, liver-kidney *lao* and liver-spleen-kidney *lao*. Under these headings he provided discussions on their pathogenesis, treatment and prognosis, and on the outcomes of erroneous treatments. As an exponent of Li Dong-yuan's tonify earth school, Xue Ji's style focused on *xu* conditions of true *yin* and true *yang*.

> Symptoms that ease in the morning but are urgent in the evening reflect *yin xu*, whilst those eased in the evening but urgent in the morning indicate *yang xu*. Urgency during both morning and evening is *xu* of both *yin* and *yang*.
>
> Adapt tonifying methods to the time of day; for *yang xu* use *liu jun zi tang* in the morning and modified *shen qi wan* in the evening; for *yin xu* use *si wu tang* plus *ren shen* and *bai zhu* in the morning and *bu zhong yi qi tang* in the evening. (Xue Ji, *Chuang Yang Ji Yao* – Key Essentials of Sores and Ulcers)

Using warm tonification and *zangfu* regulation to support the *zheng qi* was Xue Ji's basic treatment strategy, an approach he advocated even in cases of sores and ulcers, conditions which are often illnesses with hot and pathogenic qualities rather than being primarily *xu* in nature. This he justified on the basis that this strategy was aimed at strengthening body resources against the pathogen attack. He applied similar principles to all the medical specialities including surgery, gynaecology, paediatrics, ophthalmology and oral medicine. With a

TEXTS BY XUE JI

Zheng Ti Lei Yao (Categorised Essentials of Traumatology) (1529)

Nu Ke Cuo Yao (Women's Diseases – Proven Essentials) (1548)

Li Yang Ji Yao (Leprous Sores – Pivotal Essentials) (1550)

Chuang Yang Ji Yao (Sores and Ulcers – Pivotal Essentials)

Waike Shu Yao (External Illnesses – Pivotal Essentials) (1571)

Neike Zhai Yao (Essentials of Internal Medicine)

wide interest in many areas of medicine, Xue Ji wrote numerous textbooks which were to be merged together by later generations into a single textbook called *Xue Shi Yi An* (Mr Xue's Medical Cases).

ZHANG JIE-BIN (1563–1640)

Later to become one of the most famous Ming physicians, Zhang Jing-yue (Zhang Jie-bin) was 13 when he moved with his father to Beijing where he studied medicine for a while under the physician Jin Ying. In adulthood, though, he settled into a career as a military general, and it was only later in life that he returned to medicine. At first he based his style on Zhu Dan-xi's doctrine *yang usually excessive–yin usually deficient*. Later, though, Zhang said that after reflecting on a *Neijing* passage that states '*jing-shen* remains stable when there is calm *yin* and sound *yang*', he came to disagree with Zhu's view. Presumably as a result of his clinical experience, Zhang reached a different perspective – namely, '*Yang* is not [always] excessive…but true *yin* is [often] insufficient and people generally suffer more *xu* and less *shi*.' From this point on his writings repeatedly stress the importance of sufficient and harmonious primal *yin* and *yang* in the kidneys representing water and fire at the *ming men*; the strength of this root *yin-yang* dynamic Zheng believed to be the source of generative and transforming activities of the whole body when in robust health. In his *Jing Yue Quan Shu* (Complete Book of Jing Yue), Zhang states his core principle: 'Those who are good at tonifying *yin* should seek [to nurture] *yin* from *yang*. Then with [sufficient] *yang*, *yin* can ascend and the source is not exhausted.' In other words, Zhang recognised the interdependence of primal *yin* and *yang* and that *yin* nourishment was rooted in strong *yang*. His formulas generally reflect this idea.

> *Ming men* governs two kidneys and the two kidneys belong to *ming men*. This is the home of water and fire, the dwelling of *yin* and *yang*, the sea of essence *qi*, the whole of death and life. If the *ming men* is consumed, then the five viscera and six organs will lose what they rely on, and there is then nowhere that illnesses of *yin* and *yang* can't reach.

> …these days eight or nine out of ten of the illnesses suffered by people are *yin* deficiency…six or seven out of ten illnesses are caused by *xu*-fire…and *xu*-fire results from the consumption of true *yin*… Support both the true *yin* and *yang*; even when nourishing *yin* include some *yang* strengthening substances and whilst supplementing *yang* add some *yin* nourishing medicinals… This is the wonderful application of [the concept of] the mutual support relationship of *yin* and *yang*. (Zhang Jie-bin, *Lei Jing Fu Yi*)

Zhang Jie-bin's advocacy of the herb *shu di huang* (prepared Rehmannia glutinosa root, a *yin* and blood tonic substance) earned him the nickname of Dr Zhang Shu-di. As his style matured he came to the conclusion that *yang* should really be considered the primal body constituent, and cited the growth and vitality seen in spring and summer as evidence of the primal importance of *yang*. *Yang*, he said, was the origin of life itself and death was characterised by its absence, so his advocacy of the *yin* tonic *shu di huang* may appear paradoxical, until we understand his realisation that the power of *yang* is rooted in *yin* much as the brightness of a lamp depends on a sufficient supply of oil.

Here is Zhang's summary of the rationale for his frequent use of *shu di* (from *Jing Yue Quan Shu: Bencao Zheng*):

- *Shu di* has rich flavour and thin *qi*… There is *yang* within *yin* able to tonify the true *yin* of five *zang*.
- For *yin xu* with scattered spirit, nothing else can confine the insufficiency and gather it.
- For *yin xu* with ascending fire, nothing but *shu di* weighing down the *xu* can direct it downward.
- For *yin xu* with restlessness nothing but *shu di*'s effect of quietening the *xu* can suppress it.
- For *yin xu* with firm urgency nothing but *shu di*'s sweetening of the *xu* can moderate it.
- With *yin xu* and water *xie* overflowing – how can we achieve self-regulation without *shu di*?
- In *yin xu* with true *qi* scattered and lost – how can we restore this without *shu di*?
- In *yin xu* with consumption of both *jing* and blood, wasting and emaciation – how do we thicken the intestines and stomach without *shu di*?

Zhang Jie-bin's early career as a military general meant that his style was characterised by the application of military thinking to medicine, and he likened the treatment of disease to the strategies used in warfare. With this mindset he outlined eight treatment approaches that were designed like pre-set battle plans. His comparison of medicine to warfare was not actually a new one, however, as we saw when discussing the earliest origins of the classical medical tradition; this had always been a commonly used analogy, and many of the concepts of Han dynasty medicine had been borrowed from Zhanguo military terminology.

ZHANG'S EIGHT TREATMENT 'BATTLE PLANS'

Bu zhen – strengthening plan

He zhen – harmonising plan

Gong zhen – attack plan

San zhen – scattering plan

Han zhen – cooling plan

Re zhen – warming plan

Gu zhen – consolidation plan

Yin zhen – reasoning plan

Zhang's scheme seems to have been inspired by the *Bencao Zhi Yao* (Collected Essential *Bencao*) published by Wang Lun in 1496 that introduced a system of broadly grouping the herbs into 12 categories according to their general effect – a method that was itself derived from Tao Hong-jing's 6th-century revision of the *Shennong Bencao* text. The fact that Zhang Jie-bin urged clinicians to keep such a varied range of treatment plans in mind tells us that, although remembered for his kidney-strengthening style, in practice his treatment style was not limited to this. It is often the case that physicians become known for one style with the implication that they advocated this for all their patients when often their approach was much less one-dimensional.

Later, in the subsequent Qing dynasty, Zhang's eight treatment strategies scheme was further refined by Cheng Zhong-ling to create the eight methods of treatment (*ba fa*) that have come down to modern practice, namely sweating, emesis, heat clearage, draining down, harmonisation, warming, tonification and dispersal.

Zhang Jie-bin is most celebrated for writing *Lei Jing* (Categorised *Neijing*, 1624) in which he aimed to 'reveal the hidden and simplify the difficult' by explaining the meaning of the *Neijing* on a range of issues. He is also known for a compilation of his writings published by his grandson, Lin Re-wei. Zhang's systematic approach to practice attracted a large following, and his ideas have continued to exert a significant influence on medical practice right up to the present time. Essentially this style of practice assumes that any age-related, chronic or recurrent illness is likely to require kidney-strengthening treatment to underpin treatment of the branches or symptoms. Also, this style stresses the interdependence of the basal *yin* and *yang*, insisting that one cannot be strengthened without attending to the other.

Another important contribution Zhang made to standard practice in modern Chinese medicine was his delineation of asking diagnosis expressed in his *Rhyme of Ten Questions* in which he proposed a scheme for ensuring that a suitably complete reconnaissance of the bodily terrain be gathered prior to therapeutic engagement. This has been refined in more recent times and has been adopted as the standard questioning scheme to be used alongside looking, palpation and listening-smelling diagnosis.

Zhang Jie-bin's main texts were:

- *Jing Yue Quan Shu* (Jing-yue's Comprehensive Text)

- *Lei Jing* (Categorised Classic)

- *Lei Jing Fu Yi* (Appendix to the Categorised Classic)

- *Lei Jing Tu Yi* (Categorised Classic Illustrated Appendices)

- *Zhi Yi Lu* (Clearing Doubts with Questions).

WANG LUN'S 12 TREATMENTS

Harmonise

Warm

Affect blood

Clear heat

Resolve phlegm

Remove damp

Release wind

Moisten dryness

Remove abscesses

Counteract poisoning

Regulate gynaecology

Treating children

ZHANG JIE-BIN'S *RHYME OF TEN QUESTIONS*

First ask cold or hot

Second ask sweat

Third ask head and body

Fourth ask after bowels and urination

Fifth ask diet

Sixth ask chest

Seventh deafness

Eighth thirst should be identified

Ninth ask causes, pulse and complexion to inspect *yin-yang*

Tenth follow the smell

He introduced many well-known and commonly used kidney-strengthening formulas such as *zuo gui yin*, *zuo gui wan*, *you gui wan* and *da bu yuan jian*. All were inspired by the thinking behind the classic *Shang Han Lun* formula *jingui shenqi wan*, namely the mutual generation of *yin* and *yang*. As well as contributing these important kidney tonic formulas, Zhang's other contributions to the modern formulary include:

- *chai-hu shu gan san*, used to treat pronounced liver *qi* stasis

- *ji chuan jian*, for liver *qi* stasis constipation associated with liver *yin*-blood *xu*

- *tong xie yao fang*, for bowel disturbances due to liver-spleen disharmony

- *yu nu jian*, for bleeding gums due to stomach *yin xu*

- *zan yu dan*, for male infertility or impotence due to ageing

- *zhou che wan*, for purgation.

ZHAO XIAN-KE (C. 1570–1645)

Another doctor working at the end of the Ming dynasty was Zhao Xian-ke (Yang Kui) who, like Zhang Jie-bin, was interested in *ming men* theory as well as Xue Ji's *wen bu* (warm tonification) doctrine. Some sections of the *Suwen* had emphasised the role of the heart *shen* in maintaining *yin-yang* harmony and preventing chaotic *qi* (*qi luan*) in the body, but Zhao took the view that it was in fact the *ming men* that lay at the root of these functions. With this in mind, Zhao's writings addressed the importance of nurturing *ming men huo* (life gate fire) by both treatment and lifestyle advice. He believed that the more powerful the *ming men* was, the greater the person's overall vitality. Like Zhang Jie-bin, his herb formula prescribing also drew on the idea of strengthening *yin* or *yang* or providing simultaneous *yin* and *yang* support. Most often he used *jingui shenqi wan* and other variations on *liuwei dihuang wan*, *ba zhen wan* and other warm tonics, and emphasised warm prescriptions. Zhao's ideas were published in his *Yi Guan* (Medical Connections, 1687), and formed the basis of a vigorous *yang* warming school that was later to gather momentum in the final decades of the Qing dynasty.

Progress of the attack and drain style (gong xie pai)

Some Ming dynasty physicians continued the lineage of the Yuan dynasty founder of the *gong xie pai* (attack and drain school), Zhang Cong-zheng, who held that the roots of most illness could be traced to the presence of *xie qi* that, if not adequately expelled, would linger and prevent proper recovery. The most favoured medicinal for this style was *da huang* (Rheum officinalis root), a herb that possesses numerous therapeutic effects in addition to its purgative effects. Traditionally it is said to drain internal heat, cool blood heat, drain damp-heat, invigorate blood circulation and expel blood stasis, and modern pharmacology studies have also found multiple effects. The existence of the attack and drain school probably contributed to the acceptance of *da huang* as an item traded along the Silk Road in mediaeval times (discussed later in this chapter).

Near the start of the Qing dynasty, an epidemic in 1664 allowed a head-to-head comparison to be made between the efficacy of the warm supplementation style and that of the attack and drain style. In this uncontrolled clinical trial it was adjudged that supplementation styles had lost out to the attack-based approach championed then by Wu You-ke who, by writing his *Wen Yi Lun* (On Warm Diseases), was to help found a new school of warm disease treatment.

Trust the ancients school (xin gu pai)

Proponents of this style believed that the greatest wisdom was to be found in the most ancient classical texts. They believed that Han dynasty medicine was pure and complete in itself and that, as a result of the Song–Jin-Yuan revisions, medicine had lost its way and become corrupted by the neo-Confucianist medical scholars of that era. One key proponent of this idea was Fang You-zhi (1523–1593) who wrote a text called *Shang Han Lun Tiao Pian* (Analysis of the *Shang Han Lun* Sections). This was an attempt to re-construct the *Shang Han Lun* to what he believed to be its original from before its re-edit and division by Wang Shu-hu. Earlier scholars, he wrote, had mistakenly seen the *six jing* as the six channel pairs when they actually referred to the *zangfu*. Fang also wrote a text on herb processing called *Paozhi Da Quan*. Miu Xi-yong (1546–1627) was another Han *xue* (Han study) scholar who advocated a return to old-style practice and wrote *Bencao Jing Su*, an attempt to reconstruct *Shennong Bencao* in a decontaminated form. Styles of practice that emphasised Han dynasty medicine flourished especially in Japan, largely because the most influential period of Chinese medicine's importation to Japan happened in the three centuries before the start of the Song dynasty. In modern China, too, in the last few decades, there had been an increased focus on Han dynasty medical scholarship, with many doctors choosing to specialise in styles derived from the *Shang Han Zhabing Lun*. Their work has led to an increased interest by some medical scholar practitioners in the West on this style of practice.

The moderate sect (zhe zhong pai)

Alongside the advocates of specific styles of practice some believed that best practice meant a non-doctrinaire and flexible application of any of the various styles as appropriate to the individual case. They believed that the various schools that had formed were too limiting and that it was not helpful to have a medicine that too heavily emphasised 'spleen supplementation', 'heat clearage', '*yin* nourishment' or just Han dynasty medicine. Ni Wei-te and Wang Ken-tang were two of the important late Ming dynasty proponents of this current of medical thought.

Ni Wei-te (c. 1320–1390)

Working at the end of the Yuan dynasty and the start of the Ming dynasty, Ni Wei-te was one of the first to object to the division of medicine into different schools. Each, he thought, took too narrow a viewpoint. Ni Wei-te was also concerned about the increasing tendency for physicians to work as specialists in areas such as gynaecology or paediatrics, and so lose track of general practice. As a strong advocate of Song dynasty neo-Confucianism, he felt that a scholar should have as broad as possible understanding of medicine in order to serve his parents and relatives when they became ill, and this meant being prepared for any eventuality. He was author of the *Yuan Qi Zhi Wei* (1370) and is seen as one of the first proponents of the *zhe zhong pai* or moderate sect.

Wang Ken-tang (1549–1613)

Wang Ken-tang had taken a keen interest in medicine throughout his youth, but his father was concerned that it might interfere with his scholarship exams and so discouraged his interest. Wang became a Doctor of Literature in 1589, but later became a prolific medical scholar, publishing his 120-volume text, *Zheng Zhi Jun Sheng* (Essential Tools for Delineating Patterns and Treatments), in 1602. Four years later he produced an expanded edition. Wang Ken-tang's book was successful in bringing together a summary of the ideas of the whole Chinese medicine tradition to date. A prolific writer, he also wrote many other texts on subjects such as surgery, paediatrics, gynaecology and the *Shang Han Lun*.

Wang Ken-tang was notable for his ability to take a balanced and inclusive approach, distilling out the most useful aspects from the whole historical tradition. He was also one of the first Chinese physicians to take an interest in the Western scientific ideas that were being introduced by European missionaries.

The above outlines the main currents of medical thought that contended for a place in Ming dynasty medicine. Elements of all of these schools have survived into modern practice, so in a sense the most successful turned out to be the most flexible, namely the moderate school. Next we move on to discuss some of the other advances from this period.

> **TEXTS BY WANG KEN-TANG**
>
> *Zheng Zhi Zhun Sheng* (Essential Tools for Delineating Patterns and Treatments) (1602)
>
> *Nu Ke Zheng Zhi Zhun Sheng* (Delineating Patterns and Treatments in Gynaecology)
>
> *Wai Ke Zheng Zhi Zhun Sheng* (Delineating Patterns and Treatments in External Illness)

> **IMPORTANT FORMULAS INTRODUCED BY WANG KEN-TANG**
>
> *Jian pi wan*
>
> *Qing gu san*
>
> *Si shen wan*
>
> *Zhu jing wan*

Specialist texts in the Ming
Surgery

Through the Ming dynasty there was increasing interest in pairing internal medicine treatment with external treatments such as surgical techniques and the external application of herbal compresses; these efforts led to improvements in haemostasis, wound care and asepsis. Important advances in surgical techniques were made by Chen Shi-gong (1555–1638) who wrote *Waike Zhen Zong* (Comprehensive External Medicine) to summarise his 40-year experience in surgical practice. Published in 1617, this was the first true surgical manual in Chinese medicine history. Procedures that were described included removal of nasal polyps, excision of cancers of the breast and mouth and lips, and the surgical treatment of injuries.

Ophthalmology

Yinhai Jingwei (Essentials of the Silvery Sea) is an important two-volume text on ophthalmology and is generally agreed to have first appeared in the Ming dynasty, although some place it in the Yuan. Its author is unknown, and in pre-modern times it was incorrectly attributed to Sun Si-miao of the Tang dynasty. The words *yinhai* derive from a poetic Daoist name for the eyes, the silvery sea, and *jingwei* implies this book contains the subtle essence of the theory, treatment methods and prescriptions used in ophthalmology. This book incorporated all the achievements in ophthalmology during and prior to the Ming including great detail on the theory, diagnosis and treatment of many eyes diseases, including the use of surgical techniques.

Yinhai Jingwei discusses 82 eye diseases, including:

- 12 eyelid ailments
- 2 illnesses of the *blood wheel*, the inner and outer *canthi*
- 13 of the white of the eye, the *qi wheel*
- 20 of the *wind wheel*, the iris and cornea
- 13 of the *water wheel* of the eye or pupil
- 7 involving painful eye
- 2 of eye itching
- 3 of eye trauma
- 4 of protrusion of eyeball
- 6 eye diseases linked to systemic disease.

The text provides clear, detailed and generally accurate discussions of many eye diseases, each accompanied by an illustration indicating their location and appearance. Most of the descriptions would be recognisable by a modern ophthalmologist.

Yinhai Jingwei said that 'the eyes are the essence of the five *zang*', an idea that was elaborated using the theory specific to ophthalmology of the 'five wheels and eight ramparts' that claimed a correspondence between parts of the eye and dysfunction in specific organs. Treatment should 'trace the aetiology; if there is wind then dissipate it, if heat then clear and cool it, if there is *qi* stagnation then regulate it.' Topical and internal medicine were often applied together, and for many eye conditions various eye drops were suggested. Surgical procedures such as acupuncture needling, *luo* (ironing) and *lian* (irrigation) were sometimes applied. Useful miscellaneous clinical tips were collated such as the most important medicinals and formulas used in ophthalmology, and these were given in rhyme format for ease of memorisation. Also included were surgical methods that used golden needles to unblock ducts and blood vessels around the eye. Today, numerous editions of *Yinhai Jingwei* survive from the Ming and Qing dynasties.

Because of its very practical style, this book became a very popular handbook for physicians; its formulas were judged to be straightforward and effective, and it gave a very detailed approach to pattern identification. The inclusion of illustrations further added to its usefulness, helping it to become established as the standard pre-modern reference text for Chinese medicine ophthalmology.

Tongue diagnosis

Diagnosis by observation of the tongue is a cornerstone of the 'looking' aspect of modern Chinese medicine practice, but unlike pulse diagnosis, which was in use at the start of the Han dynasty, this method was mainly developed in the Ming dynasty. There are passing references to diagnostic signs in the tongue in the *Neijing* and *Shang Han Lun*, but a detailed exploration of the tongue's value as a diagnostic window did not begin until the Song dynasty. One catalyst for the development of this subject seems to have been the appearance of a text attributed to Ao Ji-weng called *Shang Han Diandian Jin* (Cold Attack – Some Golden Nuggets) that discussed the meaning of 12 basic types of tongue appearance. Circulation of this short essay was restricted to a small circle of scholars, but in 1341 Du Qing-bi, having obtained a copy, used it as the basis for a longer work, the *Ao Shi Shang Han Jin Jing Lu* (Master Ao's *Shang Han* Golden Mirror Records), with more detailed discussion of more tongue types. Circulation of this text also remained restricted until 1529, when an edition was published by Xue Li-zhai, after which it achieved classic status. In the Ming, tongue diagnosis became a cornerstone of pattern differentiation, and after the epidemics of the 1640s it became a key indicator used to monitor the progression of febrile disease as well as the patient's response to treatment.

Li Shi-zhen (1518–1593)

Li Shi-zhen was a native of Qi Zhou in He Bei province; his father and grandfather were both doctors, his grandfather being a well-respected itinerant bell doctor whose success allowed the family to become landowners. This meant that Li's father, Li Yan-wan, could then achieve status as an official scholar and physician employed for a while in the imperial medical service and was able to publish a number of books on medicine. Being a sickly child led Li Shi-zhen to read medical textbooks, and in his youth Li assisted his father in writing out prescriptions on his medical rounds. At his father's insistence Li took and passed the county-level imperial examinations at the age of 14, but he repeatedly failed the higher-level ones, and so was forced to abandon this career route. In his early twenties, with his father's assent, he decided to focus on medicine, and spent a decade in continuous and obsessive study of the classic medical literature. When he was 30, Li had become a very well-respected local physician, and he then further rose to prominence after successfully treating a prince of the Zhu state. He was appointed to a high official medical post in the region, and was eventually awarded the assistant directorship of the imperial medical academy in Beijing, but he resigned this position after one year and returned home. His brief official appointments allowed Li privileged access to the many rare texts that were held in the imperial libraries.

Li was especially interested in understanding the *bencao* medicinals, but felt that the existing texts on this needed revision and a greater level of scholarly attention. Apart from finding many discrepancies between texts, he was concerned that there were also practical problems in the correct identification of the substances that could lead to ineffective medicine or even dangerous mistakes being made. So, starting in his mid-thirties, and continuing throughout his life, Li travelled widely across China, interviewing local experts, recording his data and collecting notes aimed at ironing out the difficulties. His aim was to write the ultimate reference text that was more complete and accurate than ever before and that also allowed improved methods of identification. Li's main textual point of reference was Tang Shen-wei's *Jingshi Zhenglei Beiji Bencao* (*Bencao* Arranged According to Pattern), but the information from this was meticulously cross-checked with that from his personal library of over 800 texts. In 1596, three years after his death, his sons eventually succeeded in getting his 52-volume masterwork, *Bencao Gangmu*, privately published after years of failed efforts to have the work officially published by the state. This masterwork included 1898 medicinal substances, meticulously described and illustrated with the addition of over 11,000 prescriptions. Acumoxa treatment and external herbal treatments were also presented, and his text preserved a substantial amount of old literature that might otherwise have been lost. The 1160 woodblock print illustrations were the work of one of Li's sons and have been criticised for their relatively poor quality compared to the text itself. New and better quality editions appeared over the 50 years after publication, and the importance of Li Shi-zhen's work became widely known.

Interested in classifying and structuring the information in a clear and scholarly manner, Li is sometimes compared with the inventor of species taxonomy in the West, Carl Linnaeus (1707–1778). Li's categorisation of the substances into groups and subgroups were, however, less orientated towards finding relationships between families of things in nature and more about the distinctions that were needed to be able to navigate through a vast reference text. Also, as a physician, his attention was more directed at confirming the therapeutic properties of the substances found in nature as opposed to the minutiae of their taxonomy. Li Shi-zhen's *Bencao Gangmu* project expanded the boundaries of the traditional *bencao* to encompass much more; ultimately what he created was an encyclopaedia covering not only medicine but also, for example, botany, zoology, metallurgy and the study of minerals. His work greatly expanded the nature of China's proto-scientific understanding of nature. His discussions touched on what would now fall into the category of genetics, selective breeding and natural selection. He re-affirmed the toxic nature of substances such as lead, and wrote of the harm caused by following the mineral longevity drugs advocated by the ancient Daoist alchemists. Li also identified the link between tooth decay and excessive consumption of sugary foods, and advocated the steam sterilisation of febrile patients' clothes to prevent transmission to others. Li Shi-zhen was also the first to identify correctly the medical significance of gallstones.

Apart from the poor illustrations, various other problems with Li Shi-zhen's *Bencao Gangmu* became evident. Although he questioned and rectified numerous small details of fact, his reverence for ancient texts meant that some basic historical medical doctrine remained unquestioned. Although scientific in some ways, Li Shi-zhen accepted uncritically the prevalent cultural beliefs in ghosts and malevolent spirits, and included treatments for these in his work. Also, his text was so comprehensive and detailed that it was far too unwieldy to function as a practical clinical manual for working physicians. This was recognised by later *bencao* authors who simplified the text by focusing on the most important medicinals and editing Li's verbose discussions down to more manageable dimensions. The first of these précis texts was *Bencao Beiyao* published by Wang Ang in 1694, discussed in the next chapter.

Li Shi-zhen completed 11 medical texts, only three of which survive today, as well as some works devoted to poetry and literature. His surviving texts on pulse diagnostics (*Maijue Kao Zheng*, On the Pulse and Diagnostic Patterns) and the eight extraordinary channels (*Qijing Bamai Kao*) are discussed below.

Ming dynasty developments in diagnostics

Pulse taking had become very popular in the Ming dynasty as the main method to diagnose, but not all physicians agreed that this was the best approach; indeed, many textbooks stressed the need for a synthesis of the information obtained from all of the four examinations: looking, asking, listening-smelling and palpation. Even the key pulse manual of the time, *Binhu Mai Xue*, pointed out that although 'the world's doctors and patients consider the pulse to be the most important, they are unaware that pulse examination is actually the last of the four examinations. Proficient doctors need to understand the whole picture and so we cannot dispense with any of the four examinations.'

Sun Zhi-hong's *Jian Ming Yi Gou* (Concise Medical Accuracy, 1629), in the chapter entitled 'Essentials when Approaching a Patient', discussed the four examinations in detail and suggested a scheme:

Although pulse taking is important, inspection, listening-smelling and interrogation come first in the list. We should carefully trace the origins of the illness and identify the signs it manifests. Check if the patient's complexion is bright or dull, listen to whether his sounds are forceful or weak, whether the appetite is sufficient, the preference for heat or cold; check for chest and abdomen pain, for bowel and urination function, constipation or diarrhoea; check the eyes, nose, tongue and breath, [whether his posture is] crouched or stretched, flexed or extended. Secondly use pulse diagnosis to clarify the exterior or interior, deficiency or excess, cold or hot, *yin* or *yang*, *shi* or *xu* to see if it matches the symptoms shown on the outside. Consider whether the disease is deep or shallow; distinguish the similarity and difference between diseases, genuine or alike. Look back to how things were the day before the illness happened and forward to predict how it will develop... In severe cases we should take the pulses at the *tai xi* acupoint (Kid 3), at *tai chong* (Liv 3) and *chong yang* (St 41) [and] on both feet as well. Check what medication has been taken already, inspect them carefully and get all the details of the condition and only then start to write the prescription and set up the case record.

Advice was also provided for patients:

...be sure to tell the doctor your daily habits and activities, your personality and how the illness started in detail. If you conceal illness and avoid doctors that may serve to reduce blame on ordinary doctors [when things go wrong] but can constrain the bright doctor's elbow and lead him into error.

This may be a reference to the Chinese patients' common habit of holding back information as a means of testing a physician's diagnostic skills. Given the unregulated nature of medical practice in China, one strategy patients used was to fail to mention a symptom or two in the expectation that a good doctor would be able to divine these from his clinical examination and feed them back to the patient. As well as diagnostic skill and experience, some practitioners might also win over patients by using a process somewhat akin to the stage medium's method of cold reading of his subjects based on subtle diagnostic cues, artfully vague language and guesswork.

In order to stress the importance of diagnosis by interrogation, Li Ting mentioned in *Yi Xue Ru Men* (Medicine for Beginners) that people who train to be doctors should be familiar with lines of questioning, and listed 55 things that needed to be asked. This was essentially an elaboration of Zhang Jie-bin's *Ten Questions* scheme.

Responding to market demand, numerous books on pulse diagnosis appeared in the Ming dynasty. Li Shi-zhen's *Bin Hu Mai Xue* (1564) was an important example; according to the foreword, he compiled it because he felt there were mistakes in Gao Yang-sheng's *Mai Jue* (Pulse Rhyme) from the Song dynasty. Also, he wrote it because he felt that his father's general diagnostic text, *Si Zhen Fa Ming* (Clarifying the Four Examinations), although profound, was not easy to understand. So, based on what was recorded in the ancient *Mai Jing* (Pulse Classic), and measured against his own experience, Li Shi-zhen compiled his pulse text. This was divided into two sections: the first discussed the 27 classic pulse images, the second part (*Si Yan Ju*

Yao – Essentials in Four Characters) reprinted the pulse writings of his father, Li Yan-wen, that in turn were based on Cui Jia-yan's *Mai Jue*.

For each pulse image in *Bin Hu Mai Xue* Li Shi-zhen first summarised the classic historical opinions. Then, under columns headed 'body shape rhyme', 'similarity rhyme', 'illness governing rhyme' or 'body shape similarity rhyme', Li discussed the characteristics, identification and associated illness of each pulse type. By using rhymes to describe the 27 pulse images, Li made it much easier for beginners to study, understand, recite and recall the information. This lucid and user-friendly style meant that it was very widely read.

Acupuncture in the Ming

The popularity of acupuncture continued in the Ming dynasty, and there was some official support of acumoxa practice. In 1443 the Imperial Medical Bureau commissioned some specially appointed specialists to make new castings of one of the provincial bronze acupuncture figures that had survived from the Song dynasty because the 400-year-old original was now worn out. A copy of a Song dynasty stone acupuncture sculpture was also made. Both these figures are now in the San Huang Temple in Beijing.

Many more texts on acumoxa appeared in the Ming dynasty than had been written in all the previous dynasties, although these were mostly either re-compilations of earlier works or previous writings re-worked into songs and rhymes. The best-known Ming texts on acumoxa are discussed next.

Zhenjiu Da Quan (Acumoxa Encyclopaedia, 1439)

The six-volume *Zhenjiu Da Quan* was compiled by Xu Feng (aka Yang Rui) of Jiang Xi province and published in 1439. Volume one presents the basic acupuncture knowledge in songs and rhymes.

As was usual, large sections of the *Encyclopaedia* were pasted in from other texts. The *Liu Zhu Zhi Wei* rhyme section, for example, is the *Liu Zhu Zhi Wei Fu*, a chronobiology text that had been written by He Ru-Yu in the Jin dynasty. *Tong Xuan Zhi Yao Fu* (Essential Points for Penetrating the Mystery) and *Ling Guang Fu* (Sanctification Light) were also borrowed from elsewhere.

> **ZHENJIU DA QUAN**
> **VOLUME 1 CONTENTS**
> Acupoints in rhyme
> Rhyme of the 12 channels
> Rhyme of the 15 collaterals
> Rhyme of the *qi* blood balance in the channels
> Rhyme of acupoints forbidden to needle
> Rhyme of acupoints forbidden to moxa
> Rhyme of acupoints forbidden to bloodletting
> Rhyme of the four seas points
> Rhyme of the 11 *qian jin* acupoints
> Rhyme of the 11 rules of treating disease
> Rhyme of *Liu Zhu Zhi Wei Fu* chronobiology
> *Tong Xuan Zhi Yao Fu*
> *Ling Guang Fu*

- Volume two is an annotated reprint of the whole content of a text called *Biao You Fu.*

- Volume three presents the way of navigating the body using the *cun* measurement.

- Volume four gives indications for the points of the 12 channels and the *qijing ba mai* – eight extraordinary channels.

- Volume five presents the *Jin Zhen Fu* (Ode of the Golden Needle). In this volume, the *ziwu liuzhu* method and the burning mountain fire and cooling heaven needling methods were given.

- Volume six discusses point finding, the use of moxa cones, contraindications and prohibitions, treating moxa sores, dietary prohibitions and health preservation.

Volume six advises:

> …after moxibustion it is always best to avoid exposure to wind and cold, alcohol [and] sexual exhaustion, and the seven emotions of joy, anger, sadness, worry, grief, fear and fright should be eliminated. It is good to choose a quiet and peaceful place to recuperate.

This volume gave new methods of locating the points *gaohuang shu* and *shen shu,* and described the moxibustion method of 'riding the bamboo horse' which was taken from Sun Si-miao's *Qian Jin Fang.* The text is liberally illustrated and is provided with a cross-reference acupoint index for the alternate point names, and also lists point names that are the same for two points. *Zhenjiu Da Quan* became one of acumoxa's main reference texts.

Wang Ji's Zhenjiu Wen Dui

Wang Ji (1463–1539) was motivated to write his *Zhenjiu Wen Dui* (Acumoxa Questions and Answers, 1530) because he felt some acupuncturists were not sufficiently well versed in the Han dynasty classics, so he edited these for contemporary minds, and offered discussions on them using a question-and-answer format. Included in the 80 questions were themes arising from the *Neijing* discussions on acumoxa and other early classical writings to which he added his own annotations and interpretations. Much of the book is devoted to extensive *Neijing* quotes on acupuncture theory, channels and collaterals, acupoints, the nine needles, manipulation methods, treatment for various illnesses, needling methods, cautions and contraindications for acupuncture on people with different constitutions.

Discussing acupuncture's *bu fa* and *xie fa* (tonification and reduction) techniques, Wang Ji expressed his view that 'with acupuncture there is reduction but no supplementation; with moxibustion there is supplementation but no reduction'. He wrote:

> The classics say: for *yang* insufficiency warm with *qi*; for *yin* insufficiency nourish with flavour. Needles are made from *bian* stone [or metal] which possesses neither *qi* nor flavour. Breaking the flesh, damaging the skin and opening holes on the body… how can this conceivably bring about supplementation?

Wang Ji said that the main use of moxibustion was for patterns such as *yang qi* sinking with a deep, slow pulse, and when both pulse and symptoms indicated that coldness was on the inside or with flourishing prosperous *yin* cold in winter and *yang ming* sinking into *yin* water. He thought it was better not to apply moxibustion for a patient with a floating pulse or with *yang qi* dispersed on the muscle exterior, and that moxibustion was also inappropriate in summer. He believed that the chronobiology assertion that we should 'open *yang* points at a *yang* hour on a *yang* date [and] open *yin* points at a *yin* hour on a *yin* date' was of little practical value in clinical practice. Wang Ji criticised the behaviour of some practitioners in peddling nonsense, and especially attacked those who deliberately and wilfully mystified acumoxa practice.

> …these days, when some doctors practise acupuncture they often cover the hands with their sleeves, saying they are doing some secret manipulations and that their technique is mysterious and must not be seen in case it is stolen. These people don't actually know what the [true] methods are!

He also criticised what he saw as irresponsible approaches used by some practitioners:

> …these days, some doctors leave needles in the points without keeping an eye on them, or talk and laugh, or drink alcohol, then after half an hour they twist the needles a little, ask the patient to exhale a couple of times, then go back to the banqueting table to satisfy their cravings before taking the needles out. How can that be the proper way to cure illness?

The *Neijing*, he said, taught the correct attitude when it said that practitioners should concentrate and focus carefully when applying acupuncture 'as if on the edge of an abyss, hands as if grasping a tiger, with a spirit not distracted by other things'.

Wang Ji believed that moxibustion should not be applied on the head or for eye problems because 'the head is the place of the hand and foot three *yang* channels and the meeting with the Du channel'. Moxibustion applied to points on the head, he thought, was akin to taking firewood to rescue a house fire – how could that help?

He also disagreed with the use of repeated sore-inducing moxibustion for health preservation used according to the popular maxim 'to stay healthy and calm don't allow *gaohuang* and *san li* to become dry'. Wang Ji condemned this, saying:

> …frequent moxa done this way causes the local muscle to become hard like the nails in a ship; when the blood and *qi* arrives here it cannot move due to the lack of free flow and stagnation… How can it help to do moxibustion if you are not ill?

Wang's ability to challenge standard opinion and review the tradition for errors and misapprehensions was valuable, although his views sometimes cross the border from pragmatism to prejudice. The view today on health-preservation moxa is that it does provide health benefits, although the value of the sore-inducing forms is generally taken to be restricted to a few specific conditions.

Wang Ji also went on a quest for ways to tackle the spread of syphilis (*yangmei chuang*), an illness that had appeared first in Guangdong province at the beginning of the 16th century, probably having been brought to China by European mariners. *Yangmei chuang*, he believed, must be treated by a combination of internal and external treatments. Externally he advocated the application of ointments based on *jin yin hua* (lonicera flowers) together with garlic-partitioned moxibustion applied to the lesions. This was supported with the *sijun zi tang* (four gentlemen decoction) to strengthen *qi* and remove dampness. Afterwards, to support convalescence, Wang Ji also popularised the now famous *qi* and blood formula *ba zhen tang*. A century later Chen Si-cheng further progressed syphilis treatment using mercury and arsenic compounds externally, publishing his *Meichuang Mu Lu* (Secrets of Foul Ulcers, 1632). His use of mercuric chloride ointment (calomel) became popular with Western sailors, leading to its adoption in the West. The therapy was so successful that Western physicians felt that it would also make a good internal treatment, a mistake which led to numerous deaths by iatrogenic poisoning.

Gao Wu's writings

Zhenjiu Ju Ying (Gatherings of Outstanding Acumoxa Practitioners) and *Zhenjiu Su Nan Jie Yao* (Essentials of the *Suwen* and *Nanjing* Summarised) are two of the most important acupuncture texts written in the Ming dynasty, and are the work of Gao Wu, whose background was in military strategy, riding and shooting. As a young man Gao graduated from the military academy, but in his middle years he progressed on to study medicine. At the start of his medical career he took the view that herbal medicine was the most important clinical modality, but later he saw many patients who had benefited from acupuncture after herb prescriptions had been ineffective, and this led him to focus more on refining his acupuncture expertise. In doing so he came to understand the importance of tracing the root ideas behind acupuncture and its progression through the generations. In the preface to his *Zhenjiu Ju Ying*, he wrote:

> Unless we track down acupuncture's source [ideas] it is hard to understand the skills of its ancient originators; this is why I have compiled my *Jie Yao* text. Also, without tracing its evolutionary current we remain unaware of any mistakes and changes made by later generations; this is why I compiled my *Ju Ying* text.

His *Zhenjiu Su Nan Jie Yao* (*Zhenjiu Jieyao* for short) of 1529 gave beginners a convenient précis of the important discussions on acupuncture from the *Neijing* and *Nanjing*. His *Zhenjiu Ju Ying* (aka *Zhenjiu Ju Ying Fa Hui*) was published in 1529. In this he wrote:

...there are many discrepancies in the *Neijing, Nanjing* and all the other texts. [My aim is] to survey their similarities, and discuss their difference, which is why it is called *Gatherings from Outstanding Acumoxa Practitioners*.

Gao Wu collected and reviewed acumoxa theory and treatment experience from the previous literature and added his own opinions – which included a firm rejection of superstition. Later, *Ju Ying* was taken as one of the models for the compilation of the greatest Ming dynasty acumoxa text, the *Zhenjiu Da Cheng* of 1601.

Gao Wu's *Zhenjiu Ju Ying* consists of four volumes. Volume one aimed at clarifying the use of acupoints. He took a key Song dynasty text on acumoxa (Wang Zhi-zhong's *Zhenjiu Zi Shen Jing*) in which diseases were listed first, followed by the points used to treat them. Seeing this as an impractical learning tool, he re-ordered it to match the channels and points to the illnesses they treat.

Volume two dealt with acumoxa applications including Li Dong-yuan's needling methods, the indications and methods used for individual points, treatment using *ziwu liuzhu* chronobiology methods and the various point selecting methods for general diseases.

Volume three discussed the practicalities of acumoxa including needling equipment, moxa cones, needling techniques, moxibustion sores and how to deal with incidents in the clinic such as needle shock and broken needles.

Volume four consisted of acupuncture rhymes that he said students found useful as *aides memoires*. Gao Wu collected over 60 such songs from various medical books and brought them together into one volume. This volume concluded with 'rhymes of various illnesses' that recorded the symptoms and treatments of about 20 common illnesses. At this time distinctions were made in relation to acupoint location between males, females and children, so Gao Wu designed copper figures of each to set a standard of point location. These, the earliest privately made copper acupuncture models, have unfortunately since been lost.

Li Shi-zhen's *Qijing Ba Mai Kao*

Li Shi-zhen is most famous for his *Bencao Gangmu* masterwork outlined earlier, but he also contributed to acumoxa's channel theories. In 1578 Li published *Qijing Ba Mai Kao* (Verification of the Eight Extraordinary Channels) based on his research into earlier writings on the eight extraordinary channels that appeared in the *Nanjing, Lingshu* and in subsequent texts. He clarified their trajectories and their disease patterns, and added some opinions of his own on their use. The *qi jing ba mai* are: *yinwei mai, yangwei mai, yinqiao mai, yangqiao mai, chong mai, ren mai, du mai* and *dai mai* (*yin* linking vessel, *yang* linking vessel, *yin* heel vessel, *yang* heel vessel, rushing vessel, conception vessel, governing vessel and belt vessel).

Most medical scholars prior to Li Shi-zhen placed Ren and Du vessels as the primary extra channels mainly because these two were said to govern all *yang* and *yin* channels respectively. Li Shi-zhen instead took the *yinwei mai* and *yangwei mai* as the channels that governed the other six *qijing ba mai*. Li wrote:

> …*yangwei* starts at where all *yang mai* meet, from the outside of the ankle going upward at the protective level; the *yinwei* vessel starts at where all *yin mai* meet, from the inside of the ankle moving upward at the nutritive level. That's why they are the outline (*gang*) and links (*wei*) throughout the body.

His idea of using *yinwei* and *yangwei* vessels as the fundamental outline links of the whole body was derived from the 29th difficulty of the *Nanjing*, which says that patients 'suffer from cold and hot when *yangwei* is ill, and suffer from heart or chest pain when *yinwei* is ill'. Li Shi-zhen also consulted Zhang Yuan-su's (1186) discussions on the *yinwei* and *yangwei mai* from the Jin-Yuan dynasties.

Finding some questionable views in the surviving literature, he took a critical stance but, at the same time, Li took the trouble to avoid overstating the value of his own views. When he discussed the classic *qiao mai* statement 'when *yang qi* is abundant, the eyes are open; when *yin qi* is abundant, the eyes are closed', he pointed out that previous sources had offered very diverging interpretations.

The *Lingshu* had offered the explanation that 'when exposed to cold the tendons become tense so the eyes are not closed; with heat the tendons are slack so the eyes are not open'. On the other hand, the classical pulse master Wang Shu-he considered that 'the spleen manifests on the eyelids, so when they are moving well this tells us the spleen can digest; when the spleen is ill the eyelids are sluggish and [the person] sleeps a lot'. The Yuan dynasty attack pathogens master Zhang Cong-zheng (1156–1228) took the view that 'when worry *qi* arrives there is insomnia and somnolence'. After quoting these ideas from the past Li Shi-zhen commented, 'All these opinions talk about the eyes closing or not closing but they fail to mention the two *qiao* vessels. I guess it must be to do with the theory of *yin-yang*, *ying* and *wei qi*, *xu* and *shi*.' So, after presenting the various views, Li Shi-zhen simply asked his readers to reach their own conclusions.

Li's *Qijing Ba Mai Kao* standardised the points associated with the extra channels and in the process he added some new ones along their course. Whilst the Ren and Du channels had their own points, all the points on the other six vessels were shared with the 12 regular channels. An earlier text, Hua Bo-ren's *Jiaozhu Shisi Jing Fa Hui* (Amendments and Comments on the 14 Channels), had recorded 141 points on the extra channels, including 27 points on the *du mai*, 24 on *ren mai* and 90 other points, but there were repeats and inconsistencies. Li's review of the subject added some more, bringing the total to 158 points:

Extra channel	Points added by Li Shi-zhen
Du mai	*Ping yi* (perineum), *zhong shu* (Du 7), *hui yang* (Bl 35)
Ren mai	*Qi chong* (St 30)
Dai mai	*Zhang men* (Liv 13), *wu shu* (GB 37)
Yangqiao mai	*Jing ming* (Bl 1), *feng chi* (GB 20)
Yinqiao mai	*Zhao hai* (Kid 6), *jing ming* (Bl 1)
Yangwei mai	*Bi shu, nao hui* (SJ 13), *mu chong* (GB 16), *cheng ling* (GB 18), *nao shu* (SI 10)

Li Shi-zhen's work helped to systematise *qijing ba mai* practice, but various omissions, inconsistencies and differences from other important sources remained. The *jiao-hui* (crossing and meeting) points of the extra channels on the main *jing-luo* channels that were included in Li's discussion came mostly from the *Neijing*. However, the idea of the eight influential opening points, that is taught today, is more recent. They were not mentioned in the early classical texts; instead the pairs of points on the upper and lower limbs used in this acupuncture system seem to have first appeared in 1241 in the text *Zhen Jing Zhi Nan* by Dou Han-qing. These paired points were not identified as *hui* (confluence points) for the *qijing ba mai* until they were mentioned in Volume four of Xu Feng's *Zhenjiu Da Quan* (Acumoxa Encyclopaedia, 1439) discussed earlier, and this was probably Li Shi-zhen's source for this idea.

Yang Ji-zhou's Great Compendium of Acumoxa

Yang Ji-zhou was born into a family medical lineage, his grandfather having been an imperial physician, so he studied medicine from adolescence. Initially he based his studies on one of the family acupuncture texts, *Wei Sheng Zhenjiu Xuan Ji Mi Yao* (Mysterious Essentials of Acupuncture's Profound Mechanism), and then from over 20 other acupuncture texts that he later acquired. These included *Yijing Xiaoxue* (Primary Study of Medical Classics), *Shenying Jing* (Divine Resonance Classic) and *Yi Xue Rumen* (Medicine for Beginners). His work was a continuation of Gao Wu's quest, in his *Zhenjiu Ju Ying*, for clarity and practicality in acumoxa practice.

Yang Ji-zhou edited and provided a commentary on his source texts and added illustrative cases from his own practice in order to compile his *Zhenjiu Da Cheng* (Great Compendium of Acumoxa). A great publishing success, this textbook has been reprinted many times, and so there are numerous editions; the most popular version is the ten-volume *Wanli Xin Chou* version printed in 1601.

Volume	Contents
1	Yang Ji-zhou's annotation of some classic *Neijing* and *Nanjing* passages
2 and 3	Acupuncture songs selected and annotated from his text collection
4	On point location methods, acupuncture equipment, needling methods
5	Use of the *jing* well points of the 12 channels and *ziwu liuzhu* methods
6 and 7	Describes the main *jing-luo* points on the channels and their indications
8	Acupuncture treatment protocols for various illnesses
9	'Essentials of pattern treatment'; treatment methods from famous doctors, point locating tips, moxibustion methods and cases from Yang's practice
10	Paediatric acumoxa and massage treatment that was taken from *Chen Shi Xiaoer Anmo Jing* (Mr Chen's Paediatric Massage Classic)

Yang Ji-zhou valued acupuncture treatment highly and stressed his view that the best clinical results were obtained by practitioners able to use both acupuncture and herbal medicine. He wrote, 'Illnesses may be due to many different causes, so treatment should vary; as a consequence of this we should neglect neither acumoxa nor herb treatment.' Additionally, he wrote that because the location and specific nature of illness could differ, this meant that treatments should also differ according to circumstance – it was inappropriate to use the one-size-fits-all methods used by 'lazy physicians and folk practitioners':

> …digestive diseases cannot be helped without herbs but vascular diseases cannot be touched without acupuncture; illnesses in the *couli* [surface interstitial tissues] cannot be reached without *roasting* and applying heat, so no doctor can dispense with either acupuncture, moxibustion or herbal medicine.

In some of Yang's cases only acupuncture was used, and in others only herbs; in others the modalities were combined. It was not uncommon, he said, for acupuncture to succeed after herbal prescriptions had failed, and he cited the examples of Lao Li-yi's painful legs, his patient Lao Yu Shao-dong's problem with 'diaphragm *qi*' (chronic hiccups?) and Weng Wang-xi's painful neck lumps.

> …if one wants to treat disease, acupuncture has no equal. [A problem with herbs, he said, was that they]…may have to come from far away, or they can be out of stock, they differ in their freshness or whether they are authentic or fake. How impractical is this for curing chronic diseases? But if we are proficient in acupuncture we can always have needles to hand just in case. (Yang Ji-zhou, 'Tong Xuan Zhi Yao Fu', *Zhenjiu Da Quan*)

> …of all emergency treatments the really wonderful one is acupuncture…Nothing is quicker than acumoxa for rescuing acute disease. Great classics such as the *Suwen* recorded them for the first time and Huang [Fu-mi], He [Yi He], Bian [Que] and Hua [Tuo] are celebrated as miracle doctors because of their use of acumoxa. When a

needle hits the point patients often get up as if they had responded to a magic touch. As the proverb says: *first needle, second moxibustion, third take medicine.* Many know already how wonderful acupuncture is, so when practitioners see it for themselves how can they fail to let everyone know? ('Biao You Fu', *Zhenjiu Da Cheng*)

Yang Ji-zhou made a particular contribution by developing point-joining (*tou xue*) acupuncture in which a single needle is used to reach more than one acupoint. He derived this idea from an existing method that used one needle to stimulate two points to treat migraine that had appeared in Wang Guo-rui's *Bian Que Sheying Zhenjiu Yulong Jing* (Bian Que's Spirit Resonance Jade Dragon Classic) written in the Yuan dynasty, where it said: 'Treating lateral and central head-wind [headaches] is difficult; the golden needle can be applied to *si zhu* (SJ 23) penetrating sub-cutaneously backwards to reach *shuai gu* (GB 8); it is rare in the world to use one needle for two points.' Based on this idea, Yang Ji-zhou invented many other point-joining protocols. He advocated using different methods depending on the presence or absence of phlegm:

> …to treat the phlegm type of this illness needle *feng chi* (GB 20) for one and half *cun* to penetrate through to the point *feng fu* (Du 16). It should penetrate horizontally. To treat the type without phlegm, needle *he gu* (LI 4) to *lao gong* (PC 8).

Much acupuncture in the Ming dynasty focused on the application of formulas for specific symptoms, but this quote from Yang Ji-zhou shows that acupuncturists were using distinct treatment prescriptions based on the classical differentiation model.

Yang introduced some new needling methods and developed existing ones. In the 'San Qu Yang Shi Bu Xie' section of *Zhenjiu Da Cheng*, he elaborated on 12 classic manipulating methods:

Nail pressing	Used to reduce insertion pain and avoid injury to *ying* and *wei*
Holding the needle	Ready for insertion
Warming the needle in the mouth	Not appropriate today
Insertion	
Finger pressing along the channel	To encourage *deqi* arrival
Nail pressing	Up and down the channel to help the *qi* flow when *xie qi* gets stuck
Withdrawing the needle	From deep to shallow position
Rubbing the needle	To reduce *qi*
Twisting the needle	To move *qi*
Needle retention	
Swinging the needle	To open the hole to let *xie qi* out
Needle removal	

He summarised these methods into his easy-to-recite '12 songs', and 11 of these 12 aspects of needle technique are still used clinically today.

His *Zhenjiu Da Cheng* also introduced various novel needle techniques such as:

…burning mountain fire needling, cooling heaven method, green dragon shakes its tail, red phoenix swings its head, dragon and tiger fight, [and] dragon and tiger ascend and descend. These too are sometimes applied today and are considered to have clinical value. Some have been investigated scientifically and are believed to have specific and measurable effects. Yang Ji-zhou also discusses various other reinforcing and reducing methods, such as those applied according to *ziwu liuzhu* cosmology.

Yang urged care in applying moxibustion to the head:

The head is the meeting of all *yang* (channels) and the origin of the hundred channels. Although people suffer many diseases [that affect the head] its nature should be clarified before applying moxa. Fail to trace its mechanism and mistakenly use moxa and it is hard to avoid accidentally causing dizziness and blurred vision. In carelessly selecting locations for moxa it is hard to avoid the fault of causing stagnation and consumption of *qi* and blood on the weak and thin muscle [of the head]. Because the hundred channels meet at the head too much moxa should be avoided and extra caution should be used when selecting points on the head according to the channels.

Historically, it was not uncommon for numerous moxa cones to be applied, for moxa to be given quite strongly and for pustulating sores to be deliberately induced, although some scholars were against this practice. Yang Ji-zhou's writings had a strong influence on his peers in the way that acumoxa was practised, and his admonitions helped reduce scarring to the thin and delicate muscles in the head. His mention of dizziness and blurred vision is a reference to the observation that moxibustion tends to draw *qi* to the area where it is applied, and this can sometimes cause inappropriate surges of *qi* to the head.

He was also opposed to the then common practice of using fixed numbers of moxa cones, and said that the thickness of the local tissues differed from point to point, and so different sizes and numbers of cones were needed as well as different strengths of moxa treatment:

…practitioners who can adapt [treatment] appropriately, not simply sticking to fixed numbers, are sages and deserve our respect.

More specifically, to avoid injury he advised that only light moxibustion should be applied to delicate points such as: *shao shang* (Lu 11), *cheng jiang* (Ren 24), *ji zhong* (Du 6), *shao chong* (H 9) and *yong quan* (K 1). Some points, however, were more effective if a greater amount of moxa was used. These he listed as: *zhang men* (Liv 13), *gao huang* (Bl 43), *qu chi* (LI 11) and *zu san li* (St 36). Such comments suggest the mind of a thoughtful and experienced clinician.

Yang Ji-zhou also included in *Zhenjiu Da Cheng* a text written by a colleague of his, *Chen Shi Xiaoer Anmo Jing* (Mr Chen's Children's Massage), which is the earliest known book on this subject.

Zhenjiu Da Cheng is seen as the essential pre-modern acumoxa textbook. Although some of its advice is, in modern terms, clearly inappropriate, and some of the discussions are over-ornate and the layout untidy, nevertheless, this work succeeded in assembling together much of best practice that had been inherited from previous generations. Yang Ji-zhou therefore provided considerable inspiration for subsequent acupuncturists not only in China but also in Japan. It has also contributed significantly to acumoxa practice in the West as *Zhenjiu Da Cheng* was one of the main source texts that informed the great 20th-century French scholar Soulie de Mourant in his pioneering transmission of acumoxa to the West.

Wu Kun's Zhen Fang Liu Ji

In 1618 Wu Kun (1552–1620) from Anhui published *Zhen Fang Liu Ji* (Six Collected Acupuncture Formulas), a compilation that included both acupuncture and herb formulas and in which the author advocated the use of both modalities. Like Yang Ji-zhou, he said there were numerous patients who had responded well to acupuncture when long courses of herbal medicine had failed, but that acupuncture, on the other hand, had struggled to successfully treat patients with pronounced *xu* deficiency body states. Previously, in 1584, Wu Kun published *Yi Fang Kao* (Examining Herbal Formulas) and introduced one of the prime formulas used today for treating phlegm-heat obstructing the lungs – *qing qi hua tan wan*.

Developments in febrile disease theory

Towards the end of the Ming dynasty renewed waves of epidemics repeatedly devastated the population, and the epidemic of 1641 was especially widespread. These were probably related to the European great plagues of the time. In 1642 the epidemic affected over 80 per cent of households in Zhejiang, often with every person in the family infected. There were too many people to bury, and so victims were left to rot in their deathbeds. Continuing tragic pestilence in 1643 in Henan left the streets deserted, and it is said that the only sound to be heard was the sound of buzzing flies. Once again, the eternal problem of Chinese medicine's failure to find ways to effectively tackle epidemics came into sharp focus and prompted a renewed impetus to develop better treatment.

Wu You-xing (1582–1652) was one of the first in his era to apply himself to analysing this problem by seeking new theories and more effective treatments for these epidemics. His work then inspired others through the subsequent Qing dynasty to further develop this important aspect of Chinese medicine therapeutics. A fuller account of the development of the resulting *wen bing* (warm disease) theory is given in the next chapter.

Overall, the Ming dynasty was a time of considerable plurality in Chinese medicine, characterised by divisions into various competing styles of practice. Most of these were developments of the styles founded in the Song–Jin-Yuan dynasties; one group campaigned against these styles and advocated a return to the purity of the most ancient classics. Still others argued for compromise and a synthesis of styles that could meet the complex requirements of the clinic. Some medical scholars advanced medicine by focusing on particular specialities such as ophthalmology, gynaecology and paediatrics, and some continued to grapple with the problem of febrile disorders. The decline in state interest in supporting professional medical scholarship and public health meant that there was less access to standardised training, but this lack was offset to some extent by easier access to information that came as a result of easier access to dissemination of ideas through printing. This allowed the numbers of educated physicians in the population to grow significantly. Acupuncture, moxibustion and its allied techniques were widely accepted, and many serious medical scholars advocated these physical therapies as an essential part of the practitioner's therapeutic armoury. Because of this interest, the acumoxa literature and the techniques used developed significantly, resulting in some major new *zhenjiu* textbooks. Herbal medicine also gained some important new literature, most notably in the form of Li Shi-zhen's great new *bencao* compilation.

By the early 1600s the Ming dynasty began to lose stability. Apart from the turmoil caused by the disease epidemics, Emperor Wanli squandered vast amounts of money and became completely out of touch with his people. He lost contact with his ministers, and this allowed the court eunuchs to get out of control; heavy taxes and some very oppressive measures were introduced that were backed up by a nationwide spy network. There was a severe famine in 1628 and rebellion grew amongst the Chinese people, bandits ran amok, and by 1638 the threat from the Manchus (*Manzi* in Pinyin) from Manchuria in the north had reached the point where they were threatening Beijing. In 1644 it was the Chinese rebels who succeeded in capturing the capital, the imperial troops fled and Emperor Chong Zhen abandoned his palace and hanged himself on a hill near the Forbidden City. The Chinese rebel leader enlisted the help of the Manchus in controlling Beijing only to see them betray him and seize the throne for themselves. The Manchus declared the foundation Qing (pure) dynasty, expelled the Chinese rebels and took control of China's existing government systems.

8

THE QING DYNASTY AND
THE EARLY 20TH CENTURY

When the Manchu invaders took Beijing to establish the Qing dynasty in 1644, Shunzhi, the first emperor, was a boy of six with little understanding of, or concern for, the business of government. Reluctant government scholar officials and bureaucrats were recruited from the previous Ming regime and were persuaded to cooperate in administering the country that was now under Manchu rule. As part of their persuasion process the Manchus offered placatory gestures that were intended to foster the goodwill of the previous dynasty's Mandarins, and one of these was to establish the performance of official rites to honour the revered physicians of ancient times, ceremonies that were conducted in a palace next to the Imperial College of Physicians in Beijing. This measure was designed to win support by demonstrating to the government Mandarins and to the people that the new rulers continued to reserve a respectful place in their agenda for the past. Including these rites demonstrated respect specifically for the official medical institutions of the past. It was not long, though, before the Manchu court was distracted by more pressing difficulties, and so the initial government support for the regulation of medicine and public health soon faded away.

The decline in official concern for the regulation of medical matters, together with the easy availability of printed medical texts, encouraged increasing numbers of semi-educated practitioners to establish themselves as medical practitioners. In this way modestly skilled doctors proliferated and competed with the scholar physician classes, a situation that led to confusion as the pretenders adopted the style and mannerisms of highly educated doctors. They created clouds of mystique designed to disguise their lowly talents, and the dilettante practitioners founded secret family lineages whose quality was dependent on the scholarly attainment, or lack, of the founder. With poor state regulation a free-for-all was established so that as well as the proliferation of semi-skilled doctors, medicine also increasingly fell into the hands of completely uneducated folk practitioners. The fact that Westerners began to promote their medicine as a superior form added to the confusion.

As competition increased between the different grades of caregiver, effective marketing became crucial to survival. Lowly practitioners usually aggrandised themselves by boasting of secret family methods passed down from ancient times, thereby allowing a fresh input of nonsense to sully China's classical medical tradition. A flavour of the common physician's style can be seen in these instructions on preparing herbal decoctions (from Wong and Wu):

> After taking the medicine the bowl should be upturned. If there is any left it should be poured on a dog's back. The medicine dregs should be thrown into the middle of the road so that passers-by may tread on them and carry away the disease.

So, lax state regulation of medical practice in the Qing dynasty fostered a buyer-beware culture. Patient tactics aimed at dealing with the problem of charlatans and the under-skilled included consulting with many different practitioners so as to choose the one who was most convincing. Another ruse was to deliberately withhold information to test whether the doctor was able to divine them using his diagnostic skills, such as pulse, tongue and facial diagnosis. Genuine diagnostic acumen could be approximated using the artful cold reading skills of the stage mystic. Nevertheless, despite the proliferation of medical pretenders, much genuine scholarship continued, and the Qing dynasty produced many notable figures who made important improvements to the scholarly medical literature.

Following the death of Emperor Shunzhi in 1661 the throne was taken by Kangxi, another young boy, who in his six-decade rule was to have increasing contact with foreigners, especially the European Jesuits. Shrewd and cultured, Emperor Kangxi very much enjoyed his exposure to the new tide of scientific and philosophical ideas coming from the West from newcomers such as the Jesuits. At first he saw these novel teachings as potentially beneficial for his empire, but the romance then declined as clashes with the church authorities in Rome soured relations. Kangxi became increasingly concerned about the flood of missionaries and profiteering foreigners into China, an influx that in the next two centuries was to first erode and then destroy his dynasty. Early on, the prescient Kangxi wrote, 'My fear is that at some time in the future China is going to get into difficulties with these Western countries.' For many centuries before, Arab and European traders had come to China respectfully and in peace, but in the Qing dynasty the European influx now often behaved like piratical adventurers – arrogant in attitude, convinced of their own superiority, ruthlessly seeking their own profit, carrying firearms and even on occasion randomly slaughtering Chinese peasants for sport on their way to an audience at court.

Medical thinking at the onset of the Qing dynasty

Scholarly medical thinkers at the start of the Qing reflected on the way that Ming dynasty medicine had fragmented into numerous competing schools of theory and practice, that any sense of consensus and coherence to the way that medicine should be practised had been lost in the mix of competing styles. Qing physicians had begun to see a need for reconciliation between the various schools and for greater unification of the medical traditions. The numerous styles of the Ming began to condense into two main strands of thought, one that based its teachings on the Han dynasty classics such as the *Neijing, Jiayi Jing* and *Shang Han Lun* to the exclusion of later advances. This style presented itself as scholarly orthodoxy with a pure and ancient lineage rooted in halcyon times. Advocates of Han methods claimed that medicine had lost its way in the Song–Jin-Yuan period when, as they saw it, the classical teachings had become distorted, obfuscated and sullied by innovation. The other main strand of thought considered that Han medicine did not always suit their patients, that times change, and that newer doctrines were needed in response to contemporary medical needs. They thought that there was a need to incorporate the new discoveries and respond to a changing clinical landscape. This school embraced the advances that had been generated by the ever-expanding clinical experience and ever-growing body of medical literature, for example, in areas such as paediatrics and gynaecology. They considered these innovations and advances essential for effective medical practice. To some extent this debate continues today. In between these camps there were moderates who considered that Han dynasty medicine set down the core paradigms on which the authentic later traditions were founded – they saw no need to exclude one or the other, and that an unprejudiced outlook was paramount.

The most important thread to pick up first is one of the great achievements of Qing medical scholars: the development of a detailed understanding of febrile diseases and their treatment. Although *wen bing* (warm disease) theory tends to be thought of as a Qing dynasty innovation, as suggested in earlier chapters, the idea of warm disease pathogens can be traced right back to the founding classical texts, with some refinements appearing through the Song–Jin-Yuan and Ming dynasties. This is now a convenient place to review the development of this current of medical thought.

Wen bing origins and development prior to the Ming

The term *wen bing* was coined mainly with reference to acute contagious epidemic infections, although Qing dynasty *wen bing* theory also encompasses some fevers that are not due to infections. The term first appeared in the *Neijing* chapter 'Liu Yuan Zheng Ji Da Lun', which mentions 'people suffering from warm disease' (*min li wen bing*) and 'outbreaks of warm disease' (*wen bing nai zuo*). Scattered elsewhere in the *Neijing* are some very brief descriptions of the diagnosis, causes, symptoms, pulse and treatment principles of *wen bing* disorders. The *Nanjing* also mentions acute fevers: 'There are five types of *shang han* illness: windstroke (*shang feng*), cold attack (*shang han*), damp-warmth (*shi wen*), heat disease (*re bing*) and warm disease (*wen bing*).' It took over a thousand years for these early warm disease ideas to be more fully described and a few hundred more before they reached maturity in the 17th and 18th centuries.

We tend to think of Zhang Zhong-jing's *Shang Han Zhabing Lun* (+220) in terms of attack by cold, but Zhang also mentions the symptoms of early-stage *wen bing* disease, saying, '*Taiyang bing* has fever, thirst and no aversion to cold; this is *wen bing*.' It is evident, too, that Zhang prescribed heat-clearing formulas such as *zhuye shigao tang* for epidemic illnesses, and indeed many of these formulas were later to be adopted by the Qing dynasty *wen bing* school. Shortly after the *Shang Han Lun* appeared, Wang Shu-he (+265–317, famed for his pulse classic) introduced some new febrile disease categories by expanding on the *Neijing*'s *wen bing* passages. In discussing *wen bing*, Wang Shu-he proposed the existence of various categories of febrile illness, such as: *shu bing* (summer disease), *wen nue* (malarial warmth), *feng wen* (wind warmth), *wen du* (toxic warmth) and *wen yi* (epidemic warmth).

Then, in the Sui dynasty (+581–618), Chao Yuan-fang devoted a chapter of his pathophysiology text, the *Zhubing Yuanhou Lun*, to warm diseases. In Chapter 10, entitled 'Wen Bing Zhu Hou', Chao wrote:

> …people are sometimes struck by an epidemic pathogenic factor…a disease so highly contagious it can kill whole families before spreading elsewhere.

Some recognition of *wen bing* fevers continued through the Tang dynasty (+618–960); for instance, in Sun Si-miao's *Qian Jin Fang* and in Wang Tao's *Waitai Miyao* we find various formulas aimed at treating *wen bing* illness patterns, even though these were not explicitly identified as such. It is fair to say that epidemic warm diseases had been recognised from early times, but its aetiology and treatment had not been analysed systematically or in detail.

With the refreshed approach to medical scholarship and the new governmental concern for public welfare that came into play in the Song–Jin-Yuan dynasties, much official effort was invested in the re-appraisal of medicine. As part of this, and in response to the public health issue of devastating febrile epidemics, *wen bing* study started to move away from its position as an arcane cul-de-sac of *shang han* doctrine and received more scholarly attention. New solutions were needed for the febrile diseases of the time. As detailed in Chapter 6 on Jin-Yuan medicine, Liu Wan-su, the first of the four famous masters, focused on heat-related pathologies. Liu vehemently opposed what he saw as the misuse of pungent warm medicinals at the onset of *wen bing*; instead he advocated the use of pungent cool substances to release the exterior along with substances intended to cool the interior, nourish *yin* and bring down fever. Liu introduced innovative formulas such as *shuang jie san* (which is the prescription *fang feng tong sheng san* minus *da huang*). Indeed, aspects of the work of each of the four Jin-Yuan masters can be viewed as attempts to explain and more effectively treat fevers. Liu Wan-su emphasised the countering of heat-using cold herbs, Zhang Cong-zheng advocated *xie* pathogen expulsion by the three methods at the core of *shang han* theory, Li Dong-yuan claimed that fevers could be treated by the regulation and supplementation of the middle *jiao* and Zhu Dan-xi proposed that *qi* moving and countering *yang* excess by *yin* nourishment was important. Today the view would be that all of these methods might be appropriate in different circumstances to treat patients with feverish symptoms.

Right at the start of the Ming dynasty, the scholar physician Wang Lu (Wang An-dao, 1322–1391), like the first of the four masters, Liu Wan-su, two centuries before, was also dismayed at the continuing misuse by his contemporaries of *shang han* formulas in acute warm illness. He wrote:

> *Wen bing* ideas should not be mixed up with *shang han* theory…and warm epidemic illnesses definitely should not be treated with formulas designed for *shang han* six channel diseases.

It is reasonable to assume that such conclusions were based on the bitter clinical experience of repeated failure to effectively save lives with the Han dynasty *shang han* formulas. Wang Lu's view was that *wen bing* fevers happened because of pre-existing heat hidden internally in the body that was aroused and re-kindled by an exterior attack, and that febrile symptoms were due to this interior heat emerging to the exterior. With this concept in mind, like Liu Wan-su, he believed that treatment of fevers should mainly focus on clearing internal heat, not on releasing and untying exterior wind and cold.

So, as a result of Song–Jin-Yuan scholarship, *wen bing* theory had started to become increasingly distinct from the *shang han* style, thereby setting more theoretical and experiential precedents for the formation of an independent *wen bing* doctrine later on. At the end of the Ming and the start of the Qing, *wen bing* theory was beginning to blossom, both in terms of the refinement of its theories and in its clinical application. The first notable innovator in this new current of thought was Wu You-ke.

Wu You-ke and li qi theory

A native of Jiangsu province, Wu You-ke (Wu You-xing, 1582–1652) lived at a time when both poverty and epidemic disease were rife. He was considered to be a follower of the Jin-Yuan master Zhang Cong-zheng, founder of the attack and drain style (*gong xie pai*), because his primary clinical orientation was the expulsion of *xie qi* from the body. Between 1408 and 1643 there had been repeated epidemics and that of 1641 had spread particularly widely across the country. According to Unschuld, these epidemics typically involved pains in the head, back, eyes and hips, deafness, vomiting, alternating hot and cold fits, urinary retention, constipation, abdominal pain and unpleasant sensations of fullness. Witnessing these warm febrile epidemics and their very high mortality rate, Wu You-ke wrote:

> …since ancient times there have been few discussions devoted to *wen yi* [warmth epidemics]; practitioners simply read and regurgitate the *Shang Han Lun*. However, in our clinical practice what we see most often is *wen yi*; only 1 or 2 per cent are actually *shang han* cases… The difference between *wen yi* and *shang han* [cold attack], though, is like the difference between the sky and soil.

Dismayed by their failings, Wu wrote that many doctors:

> mistakenly apply *shang han* methods and as a result they never actually see any patients cured. Patients are told their illness will clear by itself in a week or two and so delay treatment, but they have often already died before this time. Some die from being given drastic remedies or from the inappropriate coordination of attack and support. In some cases [the problem is that] the doctor's knowledge is insufficient, so being unsure and overcautious he uses mild slow-acting medicines for acute disease. Although these are not themselves harmful, the problem lingers on, leading to eventual death. Such cases are all too common.

Wu is famous for his view that 'today's diseases are not treatable by the ancient methods', and with this thought in mind he sought new treatments for the new epidemics. An epidemic of 1644 provided a pivotal opportunity to compare the clinical outcomes from *shang han* advocates, from Wu You-ke's methods and from those of Li Dong-yuan's warm supplementation style. The superiority of Wu's approach became very evident; patients treated by pathogen elimination methods were seen to fare much better, and the outcomes for those receiving supplementation or cold attack treatment generally proved unsatisfactory.

Having an understanding of the contagious nature of the pathogens as well as a highly pragmatic outlook, Wu advised physicians facing epidemic *wen yi* disorders to think first of all about prevention of spread:

> [We should] spend less time on theory; instead we should interrupt the transmission of pathogenic *qi* by taking account of the way it enters the body, the parts of the body it attacks and the way it progresses. In this way we can offer effective practical help based on everyday experience.

In 1642, having woven together the traces of *wen bing* theory that he had gleaned from the historical tradition with his own clinical observations and study, Wu published his *Wen Yi Lun* (Warm Epidemic Essays) in which he set down his ideas on *li qi* (pestilential *qi*). This work initiated more systematic study of what was to become known as *wen bing* theory.

Wu's foreword to his *Wen Yi Lun* opens with:

> …it is not wind, not coldness, not summer [heat], not dampness that causes *wen yi* disease, it is caused by *li qi*[, a strange pathogenic *qi* that exists] between the sky and ground.

As well as exploring the idea of warm disease and *yi qi*, Wu introduced the terms *za qi* (miscellaneous *qi*) and *li qi* (pestilential *qi*). In the chapter 'Truth and Falsehood in *Shang Han* Cases' he says:

> What is *yi*? It is contracted from *li qi* in the environment. What is *li qi*? It is not coldness, not summer-heat, not warmness, not coldness, not the *qi* of the four seasons or a mix of these either. It is a special type of *li qi* that is found in nature.

Approximately five centuries previously, the Jin-Yuan master Liu Wan-su had confidently insisted that 'no externally contracted disease agent exists apart from the six *qi*: wind, cold, summer-heat, damp, dryness and fire'. Wu now directly challenged this assertion, saying that Liu was:

> unaware that diseases caused by *za qi* are [now] much more common than the ones caused by six *qi*. The six *qi* are tangible and finite in number whereas the forms of *za qi* are intangible and are infinite in number. If we only recognise the six *qi* whilst omitting *za qi*, how can all the diseases in the world be encompassed?

What was revolutionary about Wu's introduction of *za qi* and *li qi* was that now, as well as the previously recognised exterior pathological agents (the six *qi* in seasonal *qi* theory plus *fu qi* – hidden *xie qi* – and *zhang qi* – miasmic *qi*), there was actually a multitude of individual pathogens, each with its individual characteristics and each manifesting its own species of illness. This was a revolutionary idea for Chinese medicine, a notion of transmissible fever-inducing pathogens that was akin to the germ theory of diseases.

Wu said that although it was 'imperceptible, invisible, silent and odourless', *li qi* had an objective material existence. He said that, by invading through the nose or mouth, it first gained access to the lungs or stomach. It was transmitted by person-to-person contact with infected people and it might be contracted by anyone regardless of their internal energetic state. Illness due to *li qi* manifested in essentially the same way in everyone, and it was this specific clinical picture that was the characteristic hallmark of this particular type of *li qi*.

Through his careful study of epidemic diseases, and without the benefit of a microscope, Wu reached some accurate conclusions about transmissible disease. He noted that when *li qi* infected people, whether it caused disease or not depended on various factors such as the amount of *li qi* exposure, its virulence and the strength of the body's defences. *Li qi* epidemics, he said, may either be widely prevalent or sporadic and scattered, and in the course of *li qi* outbreaks there were differences that related to the areas affected and to temporal factors. Wu noticed, for example, that epidemics spread more easily in towns and cities than in the countryside.

Different types of *li qi* were said to cause different forms of illness and to affect different body organs and systems; hence Wu said that 'different illness manifestations indicate different *qi* causes'. As well as their involvement in human disease, Wu said, similar epidemics could be seen in animals that could also become ill on exposure to different forms of *li qi*:

> In the animal world…we see examples of cow plague, sheep plague, chicken plague [and] duck plague. How can we consider these the same as human epidemics? Especially when we can see that sheep are well whilst cows are ill, ducks are fine when chickens are ill and people are ill but animals are not. It can only be because they have been attacked by different types of *qi*.

Taking the idea still further, Wu said that the various suppurative skin lesions such as smallpox, furuncles and erysipelas were also caused by specific forms of *li qi*. In the past many of these illnesses had been simply subsumed under the generic heading 'fire', but Wu felt this was an inadequate basis on which to understand and treat such conditions, that specific varieties of pathogen required specific treatments.

Wu You-ke's *Wen Bing Lun* text defined some first principles for *yi bing* (epidemic disease) treatment. Agreeing with Zhang Cong-zheng of the Yuan dynasty, he said that *ke xie* (guest pathogens) needed to be expelled as early as possible before too much injury had been caused. For the initial stages of attack by epidemic *xie* he advocated attack and drain (*gong xia*) methods to expel the pathogen as opposed to strengthening treatments. At the same time, Wu said that doctors must remain mindful of the patient's *xu-shi* state, whether the *xie qi* was mild or severe and whether the disease was acute or chronic, and to tailor their treatment accordingly.

Another characteristic of Wu You-ke's theories was his special interest in the concept of the *mo yuan* (membrane source), a putative vital centre in the body where *xie qi* can linger, causing chronic ill health. He believed in assessing how far the *xie qi* is from *mo yuan* before applying medicine so as to avoid the problem of inappropriate treatment vigour.

MO YUAN

Although the *mo yuan* concept, an anatomical-energetic location where warm and turbid *xie qi* may become lodged, was introduced by Wu You-ke, the idea may have been inspired by the very early (Warring States period) theory of illness penetrating to the *gao huang* vital centre said to be located between the heart and the diaphragm. The *mo yuan* described a niche said to be located anatomically between the lungs and the diaphragm and energetically at the half-interior and half-exterior level. It was said to be connected exteriorly with the muscles and interiorly with the stomach – itself the gateway to the *sanjiao*. The *mo yuan* became a reference point for Wu's approach to theory and treatment. This notion of *xie qi* hiding in the *mo yuan* was to strongly influence subsequent Qing dynasty *wen bing* specialists. His *da yuan yin* formula became the reference prescription for opening the *mo yuan*, expelling foulness and dissolving turbidity. Also, his method of giving pear juice, lotus root juice, sugarcane syrup and watermelon to clear heat and nourish *yin* in *wen bing* patients with internal heat was found to be very effective and became the model for Wu Tang later to create a snow pear syrup formula and five juice formula. The very aromatic herb *cao guo* was one of the medicinals specifically employed to transform damp turbidity obstructing the *mo yuan*.

The importance and influence of li qi doctrine

So, even at its founding at the end of the Ming dynasty, the *wen bing* school had accurately identified many of the characteristics of epidemic diseases. Two centuries prior to germ theories of disease in Western medicine, Wu You-ke had recognised that specific individual vectors were responsible for individual illnesses, and that these agents were transmitted from person to person. It was also an advance to move beyond the notion of fire as the cause of all skin infection and inflammation to the idea of specific types of *li qi*, each with their own characteristics – this was getting close to germ theory without the benefit of microscopes.

Comparing *shang han* and *wen bing* theory, Wu investigated the causes, route of entry, symptoms, progression and treatment of the two groups of disease. In setting out his understanding based on his experience of diagnosis and treatment, he provided a foundation for the development of *wen bing* theory by other scholars. All the subsequent Qing dynasty *wen bing* specialists were inspired by Wu You-ke's work, including those whose own models of febrile disease diverged from those in the *Wen Yi Lun*. Wu Tang (aka Wu Ru-tang, 1758–1836), for example, was one of those who espoused views that differed from Wu but, nonetheless, in the foreword to his *Wenbing Tiao Bian* (Systematic Differentiation of Warm Disease, 1798) he acknowledged its importance: 'We should study Wu You-ke's *Wen Yi Lun* long and hard; it is a grand and wide-ranging discussion on issues that had gone unnoticed by previous physicians.'

Wu taught that once a *li qi* or warm disease attack had been cleared, instead of using *qi* tonics for convalescence, it was usually better to give *yin*-nourishing medicinals. This was partly to restore the injury to *yin* implicit in the aftermath of a warmth invasion, and also because some residual *wen xie* often remained during recuperation that could perhaps be re-kindled by the warmth inherent in the *qi* tonification method, leading to congestion, stagnation and binding of the warm *xie* to the *zheng qi*. Any lingering *xie*, although subdued, might develop into a different syndrome later on. This idea of the possibility of residual warmth pathogens became a key part of *wen bing* doctrine, and later the physician Ye Tian-shi was to re-iterate the idea, saying:

> …although the smoke from the stove has died, we should be mindful of fire in the ash… Use blood-nourishing herbs, but use them cautiously in case their richness and heaviness cause stagnation.

Progression of wen bing theory

In the 17th and 18th centuries the *wen bing* disease epidemics became even more numerous and more virulent than they had been in the Ming dynasty. Eighty or more epidemics had occurred in the early Qing dynasty, variously identified at the time as *shang han*, cholera, dysentery, malaria, variola, scarlet fever, measles, diphtheria and the bubonic plague. In the area south of the Yangzi River, with its dense population, warm-damp climate and greater population mobility, *wen bing* diseases were frequent and rife. Amongst physicians practising in south China, working out how to control and treat these epidemics became a crucial life-and-death medical imperative. A physician's reputation to a significant extent rested on his ability to successfully treat fevers.

Wu You-ke's *Wen Yi Lun* founded the new systematic study of epidemic warm diseases, and as *wen bing* theory developed through the Qing dynasty, new styles appeared such as *wen re* (warm-febrile) doctrine espoused by Ye Tian-shi (Ye Gui), Xue Xue (Xue Sheng-bai), Wu Tang and Wang Shi-xiong. It was these new medical thinkers who proposed the idea of a pathogen group they called *wen* (warmth) that differed from Wu You-ke's *li qi* idea. *Wen*, they said, first entered the lungs before spreading, through the reverse *ke* cycle of *wu xing* theory, to the pericardium, causing symptoms such as clouding of consciousness and convulsions. Xue Xue then characterised this *xie qi* as 'a mixture of *wen* and *re*' (warmth and heat).

Ye Gui (1667–1746)

Ye Gui (styled Ye Tian-shi) was born into a medical family lineage based in Wu Xian in Jiangsu province. His father, Ye Yang-sheng, was a noted paediatrician, and his grandfather, Ye Shi, was also a well-regarded physician. Ye Gui is said to have been an especially bright child and a natural scholar; during the day he studied literature with a personal tutor and at home he apprenticed as an assistant to his father. Sadly his father died when he was 14. Although life in his family then became much more difficult, he was determined to devote himself to medicine and was fortunate enough to be able to continue his medical studies under a past student of his father, Master Zhu. When still in his teens, Ye Gui had exceeded Zhu's expertise and had already begun to achieve fame as a physician in his own right. He carried on developing his medical skills by seeking out skilled mentors. Over a ten-year period Ye Gui studied under 17 different teachers, including some of the most famous physicians working at that time in Suzhou, such as Zhou Yang-jun, Ma Yuan-yi and Qi Zheng-ming. In this way he attained a deep level of understanding of the entire classical tradition quite early in his career, and was able to use his eclectic style to rise above blind acceptance of doctrine. Rejecting the idea of adherence to restricted schools of practice, he became one of the most renowned Qing dynasty doctors, and is seen as a key figure in *wen bing* study.

Ye Gui's main contribution was as one of the most medically articulate founders of *wen bing* theory, although his style is known more through his case histories than through theoretical discussions explaining his ideas. Some now consider the formulas appearing in these case histories to be amongst the most elegant in the entire history of Chinese medicine. Whilst various ancient physicians such as Liu Wan-su and Wang An-dao had previously realised that *wen bing* diseases were different from *shang han* illnesses, and had experimented with new treatments, they were reluctant to abandon the classical six channel differentiations of the *Shang Han Lun*. Ye Gui and the new *wen bing* scholars felt no such constraints and felt free to devise new theoretical models, treatment methods and formulas.

Ye Gui's inspired inventiveness led to his formulation of a new diagnostic scheme, the four *qi* (*si qi*: *wei, qi, ying* and *xue*, sometimes rendered in English as 'four levels'), as the theoretical framework for *wen bing* pattern identification. His meticulous approach to diagnosis and prescription design was a significant addition to the range of pattern identification tools available to clinicians. Ye Gui remained respectful of Zhang Zhong-jing's prescriptions, and wrote *Linzheng Zhinan Shang Han Men Fang* (Clinical Guide to *Shang Han* Formulas), a text that was itself an inspiration to subsequent medical thinkers who admired his luminescent prescription writing skills. Apart from this and his work on fevers, Ye Gui was very able and creative, and according to some contemporaries was a divinely inspired, general medicine physician. One of his innovations, for example, was to add the idea of nourishing stomach *yin* to Li Dong-yuan's stomach-spleen theory founded in the Jin-Yuan dynasty.

As a busy clinician Ye Gui had little time to devote to writing. His best-known texts such as the ten-volume *Wen Zheng Lunzhi* (Differentiating Warm Patterns) and *Lin Zheng Zhi Nan Yi An* (Clinical Case History Guides) were actually compiled by his students. The first is said to have been based on the lecture notes taken by his student Gu Jing, and the latter was compiled by Hua You-yun based on the journals of case histories taken down by students in his later years.

Although Ye Gui borrowed from Zhu Dan-xi's *yin*-nourishing style, his broader outlook, including a deep sense of the meaning of the Han classical teachings, allowed him to adopt a much more eclectic approach, one that extended beyond previous doctrine. His approach was akin to some of the earlier 'greats' in that it was firmly rooted both in a deep understanding of the medical tradition and in astute clinical practice. So influential were his published case histories that he is sometimes credited with founding his own current of practice, the *ye pai*, based on his prescription writing style. In general Ye Gui's style involved using mild doses and a light touch that avoided strong-tasting or aggressive herbs. Most often his intent was to open up and unblock the *qi* mechanism (*qi ji*) to allow *zheng qi* to flourish.

Published in 1746, Ye Gui's *Wen Re Lun* clarified the clinical patterns and progression of *wen bing* illnesses and introduced his differentiation system based on the four *qi*. Various clinical *wen bing* patterns and their treatment were described and Ye Gui's scheme soon became the core of *wen bing* theory.

Shortly afterwards, the *wen bing* theory corpus was supplemented by Xue Xue's *Shi Re Tiao Bian* (Systematic Differentiation of Damp Heat) and Wu Tang's *Wenbing Tiao Bian*. These texts introduced an alternative differentiation system based on *xie qi* invasion through the *sanjiao* (discussed in the next section). This *sanjiao* scheme augmented Ye Gui's theory and is now generally seen as especially applicable to the analysis of damp heat diseases. In this way the development of *wen bing* theories had reached maturity by the beginning of the 19th century. Today, there is some divergence of *wen bing* styles, with different physicians preferring one approach or another, and even some who use the six-stage patterns of *shang han* theory as an analytical scheme but who often use *wen bing* formulas for actual treatment.

There is no doubt Ye Gui deserves his status as one of the great physicians of Chinese medical history but, according to Wong and Wu, he was not averse to a little self-promotion. They write that an important Buddhist abbot once came to Ye Gui's home town by the river to attend a big religious festival, and developed a fever shortly after arriving. The young physician Ye Gui was apparently summoned to attend and treated the abbot so that he could complete his duties. He refused payment; instead he told the abbot that he would be across the river when the crowds would be thronging at his departure. Ye is said to have asked the abbot if he would be kind enough to provide some publicity for him by waving and proclaiming, 'Ah, there is the great Dr Ye who so miraculously cured my illness!'

Wu Tang (1758–1836)

Wu Tang (styled Ju Tong) was born in Jiangsu. His father became ill and died when he was 19, a loss that prompted him to study medical texts. Shortly after this a *wen bing* epidemic struck the population, and his observations of the efforts of physicians to treat those afflicted led Wu Tang to conclude that such illnesses were still being inadequately treated by most practitioners. Later on, when he was employed in Beijing to help check and revise a massive state encyclopaedia, the *Si Ku Quan Shu* (Compendium of the Four Libraries), he came across Wu You-ke's *Wen Yi Lun* (Warm Epidemic Fevers) written at the end of the Ming dynasty. He realised that this contained novel insights into epidemics that had not yet been fully recognised, but in his view, Wu You-ke's work needed refinement. Several further significant *wen bing* epidemics then led him to see that Ye Gui's system of pattern identification made sense as a guide to the clinical realities in epidemic fevers. Although he admired Ye Gui's treatment methods, Wu felt that the theoretical discussions needed revision and updating, and he saw scope for increased clarity and systematisation. Wu Tang re-examined the historical literature to extract what he saw as most essential and what matched most closely with his own experience in order to compile his *Wenbing Tiao Bian* in six volumes. His unique contribution was to build on Ye Gui's stated opinion that further development of *wen bing* theory would involve deeper study of the *sanjiao*. Wu Tang did this by devising a new pattern differentiation based on the progress of fevers from the upper *jiao*, through the middle *jiao*, to the lower *jiao*. It is believed that Wu Tang felt this scheme was appropriate because his patient population often seemed to suffer damp-heat febrile disease that progressed in this manner.

Wu Tang's scheme divided *wen bing* into nine categories, and for each he described the causes, pathogenesis, symptoms, treatment method and prescriptions and prescription rationale. His writing style was lucid, systematic and detailed, and he introduced a whole new set of formulas to treat *wen bing* patterns, including *sang ju yin, yin qiao san, qing ying tang, san ren tang, sang xing tang* and *xiao ding feng zhu*. These now-famous and effective formulas are themselves a testament to Wu Tang's great skill.

WU TANG'S NINE *WEN BING* CATEGORIES
Feng wen – wind warmth
Wen re – warmth and heat
Wen yi – *wen* epidemic
Wen du – *wen* poison
Shu wen – summer heat warmth
Shi wen – damp warmth
Qiu zao – autumn dryness
Dong qen – winter warmth
Wen nue – warmth malaria

Agreeing with Ye Gui's view that *wen bing* illnesses tended to consume *yin* fluids, Wu Tang incorporated *yin* and fluid nourishment into his protocols for the later stages of *wen bing* diseases. He also borrowed from Wu You-ke's use of pear and cane juice to treat the thirst and restlessness seen in these conditions. This is seen in his formulas – *xue li jiang* (pear juice), *wu zhi yin* (five juice decoction), *zeng ye tang* (increase fluid decoction), *yi jia*, *er jia* and *san jia fu mai tang* (three shells to restore pulse decoction) – that have all entered standard modern practice for the treatment of febrile diseases. In addition to his innovative and well-crafted prescription writing, Wu Tang further discussed the function and application of *an gong niu huang wan*, *zi xue dan* and *zhi bao dan*. Since its publication in 1798, *Wenbing Tiao Bian* has been seen as a crucial text for *wen bing* study as it provides a lucid, systematic and complete account of the subject.

> **IMPORTANT WU TANG FORMULAS**
>
> *An gong niu huang wan*
>
> *Da ding feng zhu*
>
> *Hua ban tang*
>
> *Qing-hao bie-jia tang*
>
> *San jia fu mai tang, yin xu* and liver *yang*
>
> *San ren tang*
>
> *Sang xing tang*
>
> *Sha shen mai dong tang*
>
> *Xiang fu xuan fu hua tang*
>
> *Xin jia xiang-ru yin*
>
> *Xing su san*
>
> *Xuan bi tang*
>
> *Yin qiao tang*
>
> *Zeng ye tang*

Wu Tang could appreciate the elegance of Ye Gui's ideas, and considered that his principles and the methods were accurate and effective, but he felt they had not been presented to best effect by his followers. For this reason he extracted the treatment methods that were scattered through Ye Gui's cases and gave them new names. In doing so he made the pattern identification and treatment of *wen bing* doctrine more ordered and detailed. This clarification was one of Wu Tang's significant contributions, but he was also a very skilled and innovative general medical scholar who introduced many formulae considered important in modern practice.

Xue Xue (1681–1770)

Xue Xue (style name Xue Sheng-bai) was born in the southern city of Suzhou, and was roughly contemporary with Ye Gui whose mastery he came close to equalling. Xue Xue was a cultured gentleman polymath (*feng ya*); he was an accomplished poet and painter, a martial artist and was skilled at shooting and riding. Later on he moved into a medical career and derived his own style after study of the Han dynasty classics, the Jin-Yuan schools and the styles of modern doctors such as Wu You-ke. Xue Xue gained a reputation for regularly achieving near-miraculous results in internal medicine, gynaecology and paediatrics, and treated many patients with damp-heat epidemic diseases successfully. His representative book, *Shi Re Tiao Bian* (Systematic Identification of Damp Heat), details the differentiation of damp-heat patterns, and his innovative approach helped further develop and refine *wen bing*

doctrine. No original versions of this book survive, but the content was preserved in *Nan Bing Bie Jian* (Identification of Southern Diseases) by Song You-pu, and in *Yi Shi Mi Ji* (Secret Medical Records) by Shu Song.

Later in life Xue Xue wrote *Yi Jing Yuan Zhi* (On Original Yi Jing Knowledge) and he also published some medical cases and lecture notes on various subjects.

Further progress of wen bing theory

Other medical scholars working in south China continued to develop *wen bing* theory in the last century of the Qing dynasty. Liu Bao-yi (1842–1901) from Jiangsu province, although coming top in the state scholarship exams, abandoned his official career in favour of medicine. In his *Wen Re Feng Yuan* (Encountering the Source of Warm Heat) Liu suggested that *wen bing* scholars such as Ye Gui had neglected to fully address the issue of *fu xie* hidden pathogens which he said had been a part of Chinese medicine theory since classical times. He emphasised the distinction between newly acquired acute warm illness and patterns that were due instead to *xie qi* lingering on the interior that could also appear as acute illnesses with some signs of apparent exterior attack. Ye Gui had tended to emphasise the use of light fragrant herbs that affected the exterior, but to treat the deep-lying heat *xie* that Liu felt explained the pathology in some cases, he felt that substances that were able to clear heat pathogens from the interior energetic layers were sometimes more suitable. One example of his approach is seen in his pairing of *dan dou chi* and *xuan shen* to vent deep-seated *xie* heat at the *shaoyin* stage. A distinctive feature of Liu's style is that he generally preferred to use the *Shang Han Lun Liu Jing* framework to analyse the nature and location of *fu xie* in the body. Liu Bao-yi was famed for his unsurpassed rate of success in treating *wen bing* illnesses, and, as often happened through history, his fame developed after he successfully treated an important government official. He retired to his home town of Zhuo Zhuang, where he taught medicine and wrote *Liu Xuan Si Jia Yi An* (Liu's Selected Cases from Four Physicians).

Wen bing doctrine opposed

The *wen bing* style became well established amongst a particular clique of practitioners in and around Jiangsu province in southern China. Although it had been developed to meet a real need by genuine scholar physicians, the style they developed was not universally admired. Doctors in the north remained unconvinced that *wen bing* theory was a worthwhile contribution to the tradition, and opposition to its acceptance continued right through to the mid-20th century. A turning point that marked the final acceptance of this style is said to have occurred in the 1950s when Chairman Mao was successfully treated by a physician using the *wen bing* formula *yin qiao san*.

Also working against the acceptance of the *wen bing* style was the rise of the 'Back to the Han' movement that questioned the value of the neo-Confucianist influence on medicine that happened in the Song–Jin–Yuan dynasties. The four famed masters

清

of this period came under increasing criticism, and many scholars renewed their interest in the *Shang Han Lun*. One of the first to take this view was Fang You-zhi (1522–1590s) who wrote *Shang Han Lun Tiao Pien* (Interpreting the *Shang Han Lun* Chapters). This movement gathered pace and fostered a rejection of Zhang Yuan-su's famous view that the medicine of ancient times did not suit modern patients, a view that was largely based on its failure to live up to expectations in tackling the epidemics of the Song era. The leading thinker Xu Da-chun, discussed later, was especially scathing of neo-Confucianist medicine and the limited therapeutic horizons of most of its famed advocates. This outlook is also understandable given the tendency for some to always prescribe tonics and others to over-emphasise heat clearage or *yin* nourishment.

Other notable Qing physicians
Wang Ang (c. 1615–1700)

Wang Ang (style name Ren An) was born in An Hui at the end of the Ming. A literature scholar in his early years, he published an anthology of poems but, like many others, he did not wish to cooperate with the newly established Qing government of the Manchus, and so abandoned his civil service scholar career to study medicine. Over the next four decades he studied the classical medical texts and gained a good understanding of the *bencao* and *fangji* literature. Wang Ang then concluded that much of the written tradition was unwieldy in its size and its literature rambling and near incomprehensible, so he set himself the task of distilling out the essentials and re-presenting traditional doctrine in more accessible language.

> **TEXTS BY WANG ANG**
>
> *Bencao Bei Yao* (Handbook of *Bencao* Essentials) (1694)
>
> *Yifang Ji Jie* (Collected Explanations of Medical Formulas) (1682)
>
> *Tangtou Ge Jue* (Formulas in Verse)
>
> *Suling Lei Zuan Yue Zhu* (*Suwen* and *Lingshu* Compiled, Categorised and Annotated) (1688)

Together Wang Ang's very popular and highly regarded writings became known as *Wang Shi Si Shu* (Master Wang's Four Books); widely read, they have remained standard texts to the present day.

One of Wang Ang's strengths was his openness to the new influx of Western medical and scientific ideas that were beginning to reach China at this time. He was quick to accept that many aspects of Western medical knowledge were superior to those of the Chinese tradition, but he claimed that some important aspects were missing from the Western style. Anatomy was plainly much more detailed in its descriptions of form and shape, but he pointed out that Western medicine had no understanding of the functions of *qi hua* (*qi* transformation). In his *Bencao Beiyao* (Handbook of *Bencao* Essentials, discussed in more detail later), he included the Western notion that 'the brain is the home of consciousness…inspiration and memory occur in the brain', so in a sense he was one of the first to try to arrange a marriage of the two medical systems.

Having practised meditation from childhood, Wang also had a deep understanding of the use of meditation to preserve health, and he himself continued to thrive in his eighties. He summarised his lifelong experience of meditation in a section appended to his *Yi Fang Ji Jie* text called 'Wu Yao Yuan Quan' ('Original Reasons for No Medicine'). Here he gives advice on meditation and exercise to maintain health.

Cheng Guo-peng (1680–1733)

Born in Anhui, Cheng Guo-peng (style name Zhong Ling) suffered a childhood illness that prompted his wide reading of medical texts from many styles of practice. He was ordained as a monk in the Tiandu Putuo temple, and in 1732 he published what was to become a very popular and important introduction to Chinese medicine, *Yi Xue Xin Wu* (Enlightenment from Medical Study). Although primarily an advocate of the post-classical doctrines such as the Song–Jin-Yuan styles, he also revered Zhang Zhong-jing as the quintessential model of good prescription composition. Cheng's book is constructed on the framework of the eight methods of treatment that is central modern practice. In addition to this introductory text Cheng also wrote *Waike Shi Fa* (Ten Methods in Surgery). Cheng was known for his strict approach with students and he taught a great many leading physicians using a style that combined study, discussion and clinical observation.

> **CHENG GUO-PENG FORMULAS**
>
> *Banxia tianma bai-zhu tang*
>
> *Bei-mu gua-lou san*
>
> *Ding xian wan*
>
> *Jia wei xiang su san*
>
> *Juan bi tang*
>
> *Sheng tie luo yin*
>
> *Xiao luo wan*
>
> *Yi wu chai ge jie ji tang*
>
> *Zhi sou san*

Xu Da-chun (1693–1771)

Xu Da-chun (style name Xu Ling-tai) was born into a venerable and cultured family able to trace its ancestry back to the Song dynasty. Although his family was relatively poor, he managed to acquire a good education and, despite the fact that he did not take the imperial exams, he gained fame as a multi-skilled scholar. Those who knew him said that he possessed extraordinary strength of both body and mind. With a commanding presence and resounding voice he was skilled in many subjects besides medicine, including literature, poetry, geography, music and martial arts, and was also expert at the management of the county's watercourses. Xu Da-chun's skills in medicine were said to be prodigious and his prescription writing was seen as miraculously effective. His renown as a physician meant that he was summoned to the imperial court on a couple of occasions, the last being when he was 78 years old and coincided with his death in the capital. In the years before his death he became known as Huixi Laoren (Old Man of Hui Brook).

Most of his books were studies and clarifications of the ancient classics, such as the *Nanjing, Shang Han Lun* and *Shennong Bencao*, but most interesting is perhaps his *Yixue Yuanliu Lun* (Essays on the Original Medical Currents, 1757), which has been translated into English by Unschuld. In this book Xu is outspoken about the lamentable state of medicine practised by many of his contemporary physicians, and advocates the back-to-the-classics style view that admonishes the Song–Jin–Yuan masters for diverting medicine away from the pure path of the ancients. Only Zhang Cong-zheng, the attack and drain school master, escapes his vitriolic brush-pen. Like Zhang he believed that direct clearance of pathogenic *qi* was the correct treatment.

> Some say, when pathogens accumulate, there must be a depletion of *zheng qi* and so they supplement the *zheng* to expel the *xie qi*. That, however, is a great mistake! When the *zheng qi* is depleted and pathogens accumulate, one must first expel the *xie qi* as fast as possible to protect the remaining *zheng qi*. If, however, pathogenic *qi* is strengthened even further, the *zheng qi* will be even less able to prevail. When the *zheng qi* is entirely depleted it will be impossible to push the pathogens out… One may compare this with a situation where thieves enter a house. One must, of course, expel the robber first, and strengthen the walls only afterwards. It is just impossible to strengthen the walls before the robber has left!… Some might respond to this saying that to push out *xie qi* by strengthening is the same as to increase one's servants to drive off the robbers. This, again, is not the case because if one consumes only tonics we by no means supplement only the *zheng qi* without strengthening the *xie qi*…one not only fails to expel the robbers, the robbers are even supported!… If one fails to investigate, though, whether pathogens are present or not, and whether the person is *shi* or *xu*; and if one adds warm or hot substances of a purely tonifying nature, then one will merely supplement the pathogens and help them settle down. In minor cases, the pathogens will never leave the patient's body again. In serious cases, death is inevitable. (Adapted from Unschuld, *Forgotten Traditions*)

On the whole Xu Da-chun's comments are clear-minded and sensible, advocating a pragmatic and patient-orientated style of medicine, and remain applicable for practitioners today.

The Qing regime's regulation of medicine

The Manchu regime's regulation of medicine broadly initially continued that of the preceding Ming, but became increasingly half-hearted as other state concerns began to take precedence. The state-regulated imperial pharmacy limped on, but in a ramshackle state. Doctors were officially required to hold a government licence, practitioners faced heavy fines for unlicensed practice, and doctors found to be negligent in their treatment of patients could suffer corporal punishment. Alleged iatrogenic fatalities were subject to official investigation with the aim of identifying the prescription or the acupoints applied and to check for any malpractice. If all was found to be in order, the incident would be treated as accidental death, although in some cases the doctor was still liable to be suspended from practice. The law treated those who gave fake medicines or exploited patients for personal gain as common thieves, and those who caused death through negligence or used medicine to deliberately kill could face execution. Apart from the possibility of such criminal investigations, medical regulation was, in reality, lax and un-policed, with innumerable quack-style medical itinerants competing with skilled and semi-skilled physicians in a buyer-beware environment.

Medical education

Apart from a privileged elite, the majority of those who undertook professional medical education in the Qing acquired their skills through family lineages and apprenticeship. The plethora of competing and disparate styles of practice inherited from Ming medical practice continued such that medicine became a confusing lottery. For the educated strata, there was a movement to distinguish skilled professional medical practice from charlatanism. Educated physicians mostly abandoned acupuncture and moxibustion, and began to associate these as relatively lowly manual skills, preferring instead the more intellectually refined practices of herbal medicine. Acumoxa was still practised, but now, being increasingly a cheap medicine of the lower social orders, this perception contributed to a decline in standards.

In 1822 acupuncture practice was banned by imperial edict from the court and removed entirely from the imperial medical college curriculum. Usually this is presented as evidence of official disapproval of acupuncture, although it may equally be taken to highlight concerns about its potential for deliberate harm to members of the court. The edict related to acupuncture practice in court and did not prohibit acupuncture elsewhere, although such a ban would have a negative impact on acupuncture's esteem in high society. There may well also have been specific incidences of accidental infection or injury to members of the imperial court that lay behind the edict. Whatever the reasons, towards the end of the Qing dynasty, the status of acupuncture and moxibustion had declined significantly, and most acumoxa treatment was now delivered by illiterate and poorly qualified mendicants working in the streets or in poverty-stricken rural areas delivering care to the poor.

Elite medical education

Naturally, for those moving in imperial circles, good medical education was available. The government in the early part of the Qing dynasty supported two types of teaching institution (*jiao xi suo*) that provided medical training leading to official recognition as a doctor. The 'internal' medical college existed mainly to teach medicine to the court eunuchs, and here teaching was given by selected physicians from the imperial hospital at the East Pharmacy. Those tutored in the 'external' medical college were students who had been recommended by medical officials, and were either children of these officials or well-connected ordinary people. Set texts for the three-year training included the main ancient medical classics as well as more recent works such as Li Shi-zhen's *Bencao Gangmu* medical encyclopaedia and *Yi Zong Jin Jian* (Golden Mirror of the Medical Clans) written by Wu Qian and commissioned by Emperor Qian Long. As in much of Chinese history, state medical colleges existed primarily to supply medical professionals to the court; in contrast to the ethic of the Song dynasty there was little desire to make the benefits of high-level medicine available to the wider populace. As the Qing dynasty progressed, the size of the imperial medical college dwindled, so that by 1866 there were only five of the original 11 departments left.

Rise of Western medical influence

As the Qing dynasty declined, Emperor Kanxi's foreboding premonitions of almost two centuries before proved well founded. A rapidly rising tide of Western influence occurred after the opium wars (1839–1860), during which the British used their military might to give the Chinese a bloody nose for having the effrontery to resist their disgraceful drug peddling scam – a scam that had made addicts of millions and impoverished the whole country by siphoning off much of its wealth. Many more Westerners now flooded into China, and medical education began to change. Brought down from their grandeur, officials and educated Chinese had now been persuaded to have a sense of inferiority as superior firepower was equated with superior technology, and somehow this was taken to imply superior medicine too. For millennia China had received continual tributes as a world-leading civilisation and as a technological superpower; now there was widespread humiliation as this crown was handed to uncouth and militaristic Western foreign barbarians.

As mentioned, traditional medical education at the imperial hospital and elsewhere had already been in neglectful decline and, for most people, seeking medical treatment meant risking the care of incompetents, or at least getting by with simple folk medicine. This was just at the time when new Western-run mission hospitals and medical schools were becoming an accepted feature of the landscape, especially valued for the care they provided for the poor and needy. These were administered by church-inspired philanthropic Western missionaries keen to use this as a vehicle to gain the respect of the populace, and these bright modern hospitals succeeded in this, quickly gaining a good reputation. It is worth noting, however, that these Western clinics employed many traditional Chinese physicians to work alongside the Western physicians, so in the early days, their success was not specifically attributable to Western medical treatment.

Founding of Western medical schools

At government level, now persuaded of Western superiority, the crestfallen late Qing government decided that the time was right to adopt the foreign medical education model, and so Western-style medical schools began to open. One of the first was founded in 1865 as part of the Science Department of Beijing Academy. The government invited Englishman John Dudgeon to act as Dean of Medical Studies, but this course disintegrated before any students had graduated. China's first successful government-sponsored Western-style medical school was set up in the city of Tianjin in 1881 and graduated its first cohort in 1885. Twelve years later it was renamed the Bei Yang (North Western) Medical School before becoming the Chinese Navy Medical School (the fashion then being to associate medical training with military sponsorship). This survived until 1930.

In 1898 Jing Shi Daxue Tang (later to become Beijing University) was founded, and this included Chinese medicine as one of its eight departments. Five years later a dedicated medical institute was added, teaching both Chinese and Western medicine and also foreign languages. This is the origin of today's Beijing Medical School.

At the end of the Qing dynasty various other Western medical schools were set up, one after another, in provinces across China, including the Hu Bei Medical School and the Guan Dong Army and Navy Medical School. In 1905 Yuan Shi-kai founded a medical school that was staffed by Japanese tutors. Some Chinese medicine schools were also established, such as Li Ji Yi Xue Tang in Zhejiang province, which was established in 1885. Well structured, this had its own textbooks that had been especially written for the course, and its own Chinese medicine journal. This school trained many very skilled *zhongyi* (traditional Chinese) doctors who were able to bring the scholarly tradition into the 20th century, one prominent example being Chen Bao-shan.

Notable pre-modern medical figures
Fei Bo-xiong (1800–1879)

Fei Bo-xiong (style name Jin Qing) was born in Meng He in Wu Jin county in Jiangsu province. As the sixth generation of the local Fei family medical lineage, he embodied the Fei family academic style. In his youth he studied to be a scholar and was noted for his abilities in poetry, literature, music and chess. When he turned his attention to medicine, he very quickly became famous in the region for his skilful practice.

Fei Bo-xiong's view, like so many others before him, was that medical practice had become confused and overcomplicated, so he advocated a re-examination of the tradition with the aim of returning to a pure and moderate (*chun zheng*) medicine. He also believed in using a straightforward practical approach to common illnesses without being beguiled by the various rare, complex and exotic treatment styles to be found in the medical tradition. With this pragmatic outlook, Fei spent his life in pursuit of this pure medicine and completed a 24-volume draft of his *Yi Chun* (Pure Medicine), which he submitted for publication. Unfortunately, before publication, his manuscript was destroyed in military action taking place at the time. Attempting to recall the content of the lost text, Fei wrote his four-volume text *Yi Chun Sheng Yi* (Pure Medicine Remainders). In addition to this he rewrote a popular formula text, *Yi Fang Ji Jie* (Collected Explanations of Medical Prescriptions), improving the explanations and editing out the less practical content to create his four-volume *Yi Fang Lun* (Discourse on Medical Prescriptions). Fei also advocated dietary therapy and published his experiences on this subject in *Shi Liao Bencao* (Diet Therapy *Bencao*).

Fei's prescriptions were generally clearing, moistening and moderate, with a strong orientation towards the main clinical objective. His contemporaries said that his sometimes miraculous results came from his skilled use of the ordinary, referring to his ability to apply commonplace herbs and prescriptions in an extraordinarily skilled way. Fei's reputation was built on his experience in treating chronic diseases, especially *xu lao* (vacuity consumption). He was twice called to the imperial palace where he successfully treated the emperor's mother for *fei yong* (lung boil, pulmonary abscess) and Emperor Dao Guang himself for loss of voice. Fei was awarded with the customary testimonial plaque from the imperial court that read *Shi Huo Guo Shou* ('The hands that saved the country') for display in his clinic.

Fei's fame peaked in the decade from 1851. His clinic backed on to the river in Meng He, a town to the southeast of Nanjing, and it is said that the area around Fei's house was filled with the boats of his wealthy clients queuing for his attention. Fei's activities were so significant that they contributed to the local economy and, as a spin-off, helped to bolster the renown of many of the other physicians in the region. His skill and good fortune was later compromised by the chaos of the Tai Ping rebellion conflicts and, eventually suffering from crippling problems with his feet, he was confined to his bed.

The official Qing dynasty historical annals (*Qing Shi Gao*) declare that 'Bo Xiong was the most outstanding of the famous doctors in the late Qing in the Jiang Nan region'. His grandsons Fei Sheng-pu and Fei Zan-chen also became famous as medical practitioners. According to Volker Scheid's meticulous studies of Qing dynasty medicine, Fei's style went on to exert a strong influence on the style of Chinese medicine in the 20th century by creating a lineage that was to significantly influence the traditional medicine colleges in Shanghai and Hangzhou.

Zheng Qin-an (1824–1919)

Zheng Qin-an was interested in the kidney tonification *yin-yang* balance school that had been championed roughly two centuries earlier by Zhang Jie-bin. He also incorporated Li Dong-yuan's *yin* fire idea that explained heat signs in the upper *jiao* as being due to a weakened middle *jiao qi* mechanism leading to weakened *ming men huo* (life gate fire). Zheng thus originated the *huo shen pai* (fire spirit school), a style that arose in Yunnan province where the highest quality medical aconite species (*fuzi* and *wu tou*) are grown, and where aconite tubers are sometimes even used in cooking.

Zheng wondered why the *fuzi*-containing *Shang Han Lun* formula *si ni tang* (four rebellions decoction, used in post-febrile patients with icy-cold limbs) was not applied until the patient had actually collapsed. Zheng concluded that *fuzi* was better to warm the fire of *ming men* than any other *yang*-warming herbs, even though it was generally considered by others to be less a substance to supplement *yang* and more a herb to warm coldness and dispel damp. In Zheng's view, *fuzi* was a crucial herb not only because it was hot and had a tonic quality but because, like *gan cao* (liquorice), it entered all 12 channels and so had a universal quality, able to warm and tonify as well as attacking cold and damp. He quoted Zhang Cong-zheng's maxim that 'when the *xie* is expelled the *zheng* recovers', and so supported the attack and drain school (*gong xie pai*) idea that tonification could be indirectly and elegantly achieved by pathogen removal.

Despite its deepest theoretical basis in the *Yijing* and in early classical ideas from the *Neijing*, the *huo shen* style has remained fairly marginal in the 20th century. It was seen as feudalistic, going against the communist *zeitgeist*, and also possibly dangerous with its use of high doses of hot medicinals such as *fuzi*, *ruo gui* and *gan jiang*. The doses of *fuzi* that are often advocated by this school tend to be well in excess of standard practice. For safety, the proponents of *huo shen pai* advocated long cooking times of *fuzi* and pre-testing before ingestion to ensure that there was no mouth-numbing effect from the decoction. Mouth numbing indicates that the toxic alkaloids have not yet been broken down into the desired safe active constituents. In addition, *huo shen* advocates also claim that the fine-quality *fuzi* grown and expertly processed in Sichuan is much safer and more therapeutically effective than current standard commercial grades in common use.

The *huo shen pai* style has been continued in the 20th century by a handful of advocates including Wu Pei-heng (Wu Fuzi, 1886–1971) who was also known as an expert at treating *fuzi* poisoning based on his experience of incidents related to the inexpert food use of *wu tou* aconite in Sichuan province. Other members of this school were Lu Tao-zhi (1876–1963), Fan Zhong-lin (1895–1989) and Zhu Wei-ju (1884–1954).

Advocates suggest this style is most appropriate for complex disorders, especially those with *yin* fire signs such as heat above and cold below where weakened middle *jiao* function has drained kidney *yang*, allowing fire to rebel upwards leading to symptoms such as mouth ulcers. Some Western scholar practitioners such as Heiner Fruehauf have been exploring this style in recent years.

Yun Tie-qiao (1878–1935)

Yun Tie-qiao came from the Meng River area in Wujin County in Jiangsu province. Yun's father died when he was five and his mother died when he was 11. In his teenage years Yun was very studious, and aged 15 he was admitted to Nanyang

University to study foreign languages and literature. Later, when he was working as the editor of a literature journal, his eldest son died and this prompted him to turn his attention to medicine. In 1920 he began a practice specialising in paediatrics.

He authored a great many medical texts on a wide range of subjects and, in addition, many of his lectures were taken down and published. In 1932 he became ill; exhausted from overwork he moved to Suzhou to recuperate. Unfortunately his health remained poor, so he dictated a final book from his sickbed and died in 1935.

Yun was interested in the connection between medical theory and practice, especially the way that study of Western medicine might offer a means to advance Chinese medicine. He believed that each system had its strengths and weaknesses. The first contributing its superior understanding of anatomy, physiology, pathology and localised lesions, Chinese medicine by the holistic perspectives it offered on the links between the body and the environment and the changes that could be modelled using *yin-yang* theory.

Yun Tie-qiao was one of the first to defend the Chinese medical tradition against the political forces working to replace it with biomedicine, forces that were led by Yu Yun-xiu who claimed that Chinese medicine was unscientific and should be completely abandoned. Other notable figures who fought to protect the tradition included Yang Ze-min, Yu Yuan-lei, Wu Han-sen and Lu Shi. This subject is discussed later. First, though, we step back again to the start of the Qing dynasty to review developments in *bencao* and *fangji* literature.

Qing improvements in herb and formula studies

The publication of Li Shi-zhen's monumental *Bencao Gangmu* in the Ming dynasty inspired many physicians in the Qing dynasty to study the *bencao* in more detail. Taxonomy was improved by the publication of Wu Qi-jun's *Zhi Wu Ming Shi Tu Kao* (Illustrated Reference of Botanical Nomenclature). Outlined next are some contributions to the *bencao* literature made in the Qing dynasty.

Bencao Bei Yao (1694)

Wang Ang, whose biography was given earlier, greatly admired the encyclopaedic nature of Li Shi-zhen's *Bencao Gangmu* but felt that it was far too unwieldy to be useful as a practical clinical manual for physicians. On the other hand, he felt that more concise texts, such as *Zhu Zhi Zhi Zhang* (Bible of Herb Indications) and *Yao Xing Ge Fu* (Songs and Rhymes of Medicinal Properties), had sacrificed a lot of important detail to achieve brevity. With these factors in mind Wang Ang compiled *Bencao Bei Yao* (Handbook of *Bencao* Essentials) by re-editing *Bencao Gangmu*, deleting excessive detail and simplifying the text. Now the core *bencao* information was made available in a way that was clear, detailed and precise, and with a practical focus on the more commonly used herbs. In a well-illustrated text, Wang Ang discussed the herbs in the classic style in a succinct paragraph or two, but also added some refinements that took the study of medicinals to a new level of pragmatism. Rather than simply listing the actions and indications of each substance, Wang Ang's discussions make much more explicit connections between the herb functions and the traditional principles of physiology, pathology, diagnosis and treatment. The ideal of pattern identification, rather than a simple focus on indications, was a touchstone throughout the text so that readers could more easily integrate theory with practice. This gives the work a very practical value – a focus that made *Bencao Bei Yao* one of the most popular *bencao* texts in history. His pragmatism shows too in the fact that whilst he listed the archaic *18 Incompatibles* and *19 Antagonisms* from the *Shennong Bencao*, he pointed out that the contemporary consensus opinion, based on clinical practice, was that these rules were outmoded.

Bencao Gangmu Shi Yi (Omissions from the Grand Bencao)

This work by Zhao Xue-min (1719–1805) was another text that was specifically intended as a refinement to Li Shi-zhen's *Bencao Gangmu* masterwork. He altered some of the chapter classifications, adding categories for *teng* (vines) and *hua* (flowers) and deleting the *ren* (human-derived) medicines section. Zhao's version, published in 1765, added over 700 new medicinals that had not been detailed in the *Bencao Gangmu* including many herbs that had been drawn from the folk traditions such as *ji xue teng*. He also showed his eclectic outlook by recording many exotic new medicinals such as *pang da hai* and *jin ji le*, the plant from which quinine was derived and that had been introduced into China by Western physicians. Zhao's text also described another import from foreign physicians – the Western method of making herb tinctures.

Apart from refreshing the *bencao* with many novelties, Zhao's particular concern was on the problem of the great variability that is to be found in the literature of herb qualities in different eras and in different regions. He wrote, for example, that 'various products are different nowadays; the *shi hu* that comes from Huo Shan is smaller and sweeter [than other varieties]; the *bai zhu* from Yu Qian has spots on the root and is more potent'. His commentaries reveal that he had some insight into the way that species can evolve and adapt to different environments; because of this, Zhao's ideas have sometimes (weakly perhaps) been compared to those of Charles Darwin.

Zhao Xue-min's *Bencao Gangmu Shi Yi* further developed Li Shi-zhen's masterwork by adding in many of the developments in *bencao* knowledge gathered over the previous two centuries. In addition to his *bencao* work, he also is credited with compiling two case history collections.

De Pei Bencao (Materia Medica of Combinations)

This is a ground-breaking and innovative collaboration of three scholar physicians that was compiled jointly by Yan Xi-ting, Shi Zhan-ning and Hong Ji-an and published in 1761. Their ten-volume *bencao* selected 647 herbs from the *Bencao*

Gangmu and discussed their properties, actions and indications in the light of their own experiments and clinical experiences. It differed from other *bencao* texts in its special focus on clarifying the way medicinals function together and interact with each other. The authors used the classical *qi xiang* (seven relations) idea as a basis, and added in various other ways of representing the synergy of herbs and their pairing dynamics. Also included were discussions on contraindication and the various processing methods used to alter the qualities of the substances, as well as a chapter on the affinities of some of the medicinals to the extraordinary channels (*qijing ba mai*).

Especially innovative was the authors' use of a collaborative investigation approach that included what we would describe today as a peer review process. Whenever they encountered difficult or complex cases in their own practices, they debated their observations of patient responses together, and also experimented to improve their understanding. Their conclusions of this work were compiled into their book. In this way *De Pei Bencao* added to the practical value of the whole tradition by testing and strengthening the connection between received doctrine and clinical practice. Space was left in the publication for practitioners to add their own notes with the intention of encouraging others to carry on the work of checking theory against reality. This work represents quite an enlightened and forward-looking innovation; apart from the clinically based collaborative aspect it also implied that they saw their studies as a process rather than simply a product. Its clarity and practical focus made *De Pei Bencao* very popular amongst later physicians, and it remains an important text today.

Chinese medicine and smallpox inoculation

Modern biomedicine usually attributes the introduction of smallpox inoculation to the English physician Edward Jenner, who published his method in 1798 apparently after observing how children exposed to cowpox had developed resistance to smallpox. However, a technique akin to Jenner's vaccination had been practised in Britain decades before the publication of Jenner's work, and almost certainly in China centuries before that.

The earliest known description of smallpox in Chinese medical history appears in Ge Hong's *Zhouhou Beiji Fang* in +326 where it was described as having a peak incidence at around the start of the Chinese New Year with pustules appearing first on the face and then spreading rapidly all over the body. Ge Hong said the lesions looked like burns covered with a white starchy material, and mentioned that the surface of these lesions reformed quickly after being broken. Fail to treat this immediately, he said, and most of those affected would die and those who survived would be left with residual purple-black scars. Much later, the Song dynasty paediatrician Qian Yi offered a more detailed account of the illness, clearly distinguishing its symptomatology, diagnosis and treatment. Dong Ji, another noted Song dynasty paediatric specialist, wrote *Xiaoer Banzhen Beiji Fang Lun* (Treatise on Children's Rashes, 1093) that contained a more detailed specialist discussion of smallpox and its treatment. At this time, though, we find no mention of any preventative inoculation techniques.

Chinese authors in relatively modern times, claiming to access documents now lost, made retrospective claims about the early origins of smallpox inoculation in China. *Niudou Xinshu* (New Writings on Smallpox Inoculation, 1884) claimed that inoculations were carried out between +713 and +741 by a Dr Zhao, who reportedly advocated nasal intake of powdered smallpox pustules as a preventative measure. These claims remain un-substantiated and, coming as they do after Jenner, are probably an example of medical chauvinism.

More interesting, though, as it predates Jenner's work by the best part of a century, is a book published in 1713 by Zhu Chun-gu called *Douzhen Dinglun* (Established Principles of Smallpox). This states that in 1014, during the reign of the Song dynasty Emperor Ren Zong, a recluse from Mount Emei inoculated the son of Prime Minister Wang Dan against smallpox using human pox scabs. Unfortunately, no detailed description of the methodology was provided, so this account also remains in doubt. The earliest reliable mention of preventative treatment of smallpox is in Zhang Lu-yu's *Zhangshi Yitong* (Zhang's Medical Compendium) of 1695, and more detailed accounts appear in *Yizong Jinjian* (The Golden Mirror of Medicine, 1742). Here various methods are described, but the most favoured technique involved nasal insufflation of dried finely powdered human pox crusts taken from a patient in the recovery stages of smallpox. The method was described as being only moderately effective. Apart from these descriptions in the Chinese literature, the practice is known to have been taken eastwards to Japan in 1652–1654 by a Chinese refugee doctor called Sai Mun-cho.

By the late 17th century smallpox inoculation had become established in China's court circles from where news of the method spread to the Russian court. During the reign of Emperor Kangxi (1662–1722) the Russian court sent medical emissaries to China to learn the technique, and from Russia the method is believed to have spread to the Balkans.

In 1716 the Duke of Devonshire moved to Turkey to serve as British Ambassador, and in 1718 his wife, Lady Mary Wortley-Montague, had their five-year-old son inoculated against smallpox. Whilst travelling through Turkey she had observed the inoculation of a small child by a method she called 'engrafting' which involved subcutaneous insertion of a tiny amount of scab material taken from a patient who had been infected mildly with the disease. Mary had a keen personal interest in smallpox having herself been scarred from the disease and also having lost her brother to smallpox a few years earlier. In 1721, after her return to Britain and in the midst of a new smallpox epidemic, she arranged to have her five-year-old daughter vaccinated in the same way she had witnessed in Turkey. This was the first child in Britain ever to be inoculated against an infectious disease.

Lady Wortley-Montague mounted a campaign to persuade a reluctant British medical establishment that the technique was safe and effective. She visited smallpox patients with her children to advertise the fact that they were safe from infection. Soon the wife of the future King George II wanted her children protected in the same way, and arranged for six condemned prisoners to serve as volunteers for a safety trial with the promise of a pardon if they survived. All six were released unharmed after the procedure. Later, in another 'clinical trial', 11 orphan children were treated and also suffered no harm, so Princess Caroline allowed her children to be inoculated and the technique quickly became popular amongst high society. In this way smallpox inoculation was introduced into the UK with 845 people having been inoculated by 1730.

Physicians of the time soon caught on to the potential of this new treatment, and posters advertising smallpox inoculation in Gloucestershire have survived dating to the early 1730s. Jenner was born in Gloucestershire in 1749, and advertisements offering to 'inockilate' against smallpox appeared locally when he was eight years old. Jenner began his medical studies under the local surgeon David Ludlow, and it is likely that Lady Mary Wortley-Montague's introduction of inoculation would have been well known both to Ludlow and the young Jenner. Jenner's own first experiments were conducted in May 1796, and he published his discovery in 1798. Jenner's innovation can be viewed as a refinement of an existing Chinese treatment rather than his own revolutionary thinking. He suggested the use of cowpox scabs rather than mild attenuated strains of the human form of smallpox – hence the term 'vaccination' derived from the Latin for cow. But without the fundamental innovation from China, the Russian court's delegation to China and Lady Wortley-Montague's tireless efforts, it seems unlikely that the inoculation concept would have reached medicine in the West for many more years.

Outside influences on Chinese medicine

The earliest known instances of medical ideas entering China from abroad can be traced back as early as the Han and Tang dynasties. Prior to the Yuan dynasty, around the 13th century, though, very little of medical value is believed to have come from the West. Prior to the Yuan dynasty, points of contact between East and West were scant, so early influences on Chinese medicine came predominantly from the Indian subcontinent and later, from the Tang dynasty onward, from the Arabic world.

Marco Polo is famed for his awestruck, exaggerated and partially second-hand accounts of his Eastern travels just prior to the beginning of the Ming dynasty in the 13th century. Although an early traveller, he was not the first Westerner to explore China; Italian merchant pioneers had visited and lived in China in the previous half-century – gravestones bearing Italian names and dates from the late 12th century have been excavated from Nanjing city walls. There was inevitably some exchange of ideas following these overland trade routes in the Yuan and early Ming; indeed the resemblance between the imperial scholar's hat and gown and the academic garb of the early Italian universities may be more than coincidence. Traffic of medical ideas from West to East at this time seems to have been minimal if not entirely absent.

As the Mongol invasions of the late 13th century spread westwards, they introduced some elements of oriental culture, and also their genome, to Europe, along with the mayhem and bloodshed. The introduction of printing to the West in about 1440 is another example of Eastern influence, and Gutenberg is believed to have had communication channels with China. A little later Chinese medicinal rhubarb (*da huang*, rheum palmatum) emerged as one of the precious trade commodities along the Silk Route to become a staple of mediaeval European medical practice. The overland trade route was a dangerous and arduous and expensive one, and communications were slow and restricted until the expansion of links became possible as a result of European sea navigation-based trade.

The end of the Ming and founding of the Qing dynasty in 1644 coincided with the birth of modern economies in the West, a time when new generations of merchant adventurers from Portugal, Spain, Holland and England started to sail to China in large numbers. No longer restricted to camel loads, now shiploads of trade items such as silk and porcelain could be transported to Europe. The associated romance with Chinoiserie also introduced some Chinese medical practices to the West at this time. In addition to a new East–West transmission of medical ideas, the new trade routes made China more accessible to missionaries who, just like the Indian Buddhists a thousand years previously, offered medical skills as a softener to win the hearts and minds of the populace. In 1568 the Portuguese Bishop of Macao set up a small Christian hospital that was the first such endeavour in China, although this existed largely for the benefit of Portuguese merchants. The first missionary to use medicine specifically to help establish Christianity in China was the Italian Jesuit missionary Matteo Ricci (Li Ma Dou, 1552–1610) who, from 1582, preached his religion for 30 years in many parts of the country.

In May 1693 Emperor Kangxi was suffering from malaria and had been treated by his court physicians without effect. Jesuit missionaries offered cinchona bark and some herbs imported from India. Kangxi's symptoms quickly improved, and thus he became convinced of the power of Western medicine. Cinchona was effective in treating the febrile symptoms of malaria. Ironically, Chinese medicine itself had what modern pharmacology has now shown to be much more effective herbal treatments for malaria – *qing hao* (artemsia annua) and *chang shan* (dichroa febrifuga). Had Kanxi's court physicians known these treatments and treated him more skilfully, the acceptance of Western medicine would perhaps have been less enthusiastic. Subsequently, though, the French missionary doctor Bernard Rhodes was allowed to treat Kangxi for his palpitations and for a growth on his upper lip that further helped Western medicine gain credence. Whatever the reasons, at the imperial level the tide was starting to turn against China's traditional medicine, although such high-level contacts had yet to exert a wider influence on medical thinking and practice across China.

Responding to the nascent imperial interest in the possibilities of medicine from the West, a book called *Xi Guo Ji Fa* (Western Countries' Rules and Methods) was published by Matteo Ricci, which gave the first writings on Western medical practice to be published in China. The earliest texts describing anatomy from a Western viewpoint were *Ren Shen Shua Gai* (A Brief Description of the Human Body), translated by Deng Yu-han (1635), and *Ren Shen Tu Shua* (Human Anatomical Atlas), translated by Luo Ya-gu. However, these texts did not present the state-of-the-art anatomy of Versalius; instead the content drew mostly on the antiquated theories of Aristotle and Galen, and consequently included numerous erroneous ideas – for example, that the function of lungs was to cool the heart.

Kangxi went on to develop a personal interest in the anatomical knowledge possessed by the Jesuits, an interest that led him to commission Joachim Bouvet (1656–1730) to produce some anatomical writings. This work was later completed by Dominique Parennin before being personally edited by Kanxi himself for publication in 1710. Unfortunately, its publication in the Manchu language and only in manuscript form meant that it had no influence whatsoever on standard Chinese medicine. Shortly afterwards a policy change occurred in the Qing government attitude to foreigners that led to Emperor Qian Long's imposition of a strict ban on missionary activities in 1757. For the next century these isolationist policies limited the exposure of Chinese medicine scholars to the influx of Western medical knowledge, and so the many advances of Western medicine were kept at bay until the opium wars at the start of Britain's Victorian era.

Much of the medical knowledge that had been introduced to China by the missionaries during the Ming and Qing dynasties was outdated or incorrect. Exceptions to this were the inclusion by Wang Keng-tang of better diagrams than had previously been seen of the human skeleton in his book on classifying ulcers (*Yang Ke Zhun Sheng*). Others such as Wang Ang and Wang Qing-ren all assimilated some Western medical theory into Chinese medicine literature.

Influx of modern Western medicine

If we have to choose a date, the entry of Western medicine into China could be said to have begun in 1805 when the East India Company surgeon Dr Alex Pearson started to offer Jenner's smallpox vaccination to China's poor. Given the nature of smallpox epidemics, this was quickly accepted, although the irony of Western medicine championing its ideas using a method whose origins were probably in China appears to have gone unnoticed. Important to note as well is the fact that vaccination, although an important medical innovation, was not especially representative of a Western system of medicine. It was a strange novelty therapy, with no specific scientific explanation, bolted on to a medicine whose treatment mainstays were substances such as strychnine, opium and cocaine, combined with bloodletting and some crude surgical techniques. So in truth, Western medicine at this time had a very limited repertoire of effective medicines to draw on; in retrospect we can see that many of its methods were, in fact, very toxic, irrational or ineffective. Indeed, a strong case could be made for the overall superiority and sophistication of the therapeutic armoury of China's traditional medicine at that time in history, and this may be one reason why its impact on Chinese medicine thinking and practice was, for some time, very limited. The influx of Western medicine was, therefore, powered more by the arrogant assumption of superiority by the colonials than it was by any true measure of clinical efficacy, although modern medicine was certainly superior in some ways – its understanding of anatomy and its application of technology, such as the microscope, to medicine and, arguably, in the specific powers of some early scientific methodologies to the subject.

Western influence was more firmly stamped on China during the opium wars in 1839 and 1841 when Britain used heavy military force to ensure the continued sale of the drug to the Chinese. This led to humiliation and the imposition of oppressive treaties and territorial concessions. Through the foreign control of Hong Kong and Shanghai, a deluge of Western economic and political culture spread unchecked into China, and Victorian-era medicine began to take a firm hold. Within the space of just a few decades numerous Western medicine hospitals, clinics, medical schools and medical journals had become established.

Founding of clinics and hospitals

As mentioned, medical practice was a convenient vehicle to allow missionaries to settle and become accepted by the Chinese people. Such influence began in 1820 when the English Protestant missionary Robert Morrison and the naval doctor John Livingstone set up a clinic in Macao. They employed a Chinese herbal physician who treated the majority of the patients, so the influence of Western medicine was limited to those patients for whom it was deemed more suitable, but the use of Western medicine gradually increased, and by 1827 their clinic had grown to become a hospital offering more Western medicine. In 1834 the American missionary doctor Peter Parker came to China and established an ophthalmology clinic in Guang Zhou, and then, after the opium wars, large numbers of missionaries and doctors came to China. The treaties imposed after the opium wars specifically sanctioned the building of schools, hospitals and churches that was largely funded by commercial interests that stood to profit from the new trade incursions into China. Fortunes were to be made here.

Between 1842 and 1848 numerous mission hospitals were founded in the five main cities on China's east coast, and by 1905 the number had reached 166 church hospitals and 241 clinics. A famous and enduring example was Bo Ji Hospital in Guang Zhou, which had grown out of ophthalmology; this hospital survived right through to the communist revolution in 1949. In 1862, a London church set up the Double Flagpole Hospital, which in 1906 merged with other hospitals to become Xie He Hospital, the biggest in Beijing. Soon such hospitals were widespread across the country, leading to a general acceptance of Western medicine in China and contributing to a decline in public esteem for Chinese medicine with its old-fashioned and small-scale grubby clinics operated by wizened old scholars wielding calligraphy brushes and dried roots.

The surgeons and physicians working in these hospitals continued to assert their superiority by emphasising those areas where Western medicine had the upper hand, such as anatomy and its application in surgery. There is no question that the Western physicians' detailed mapping of human anatomy was far superior to that which had been recorded in China's traditional medical legacy. This fascination with anatomy had emerged from a social and entertainment phenomenon in the West. From the 1830s Britain had been in the grip of a kind of anatomy fever, with public dissections and numerous museums of anatomy plying a profitable and rather ghoulish trade across the country. This is one reason why Victorian physicians gave anatomy a pivotal position in medicine, one that it did not hold in the minds of educated doctors in China who tended to leave such matters to the more lowly traumatology specialists. Also, British medicine of the time tended to favour the skills needed for surgical interventions because of the need generated by their military pursuits in empire building across the world. China's classical medicine emphasised refined clinical diagnostic skills and orderly readjustment of function over knife skills.

Publication of biomedicine textbooks

The true influence of Western medical science influence in China began when Dr Benjamin Hobson published translations of five Western textbooks through the 1850s. These were later compiled together into a single volume called *Hexin Shi Yi Shu Wu Zhong* (Hobson's Five Medical Works).

Hobson's first text was an outline of anatomy and physiology called *Quan Ti Xin Lun* (New Complete Discussions); this was adopted by the missionary movement as part of their crusade to introduce Western medicine to China. Another of his texts, *Xi Yi Lue Lun* (Discussions on Western Surgery), offered some comparisons of the two medical systems that had traditional practitioners rattled. Previously Chinese literati medical scholars had no particular reason to critically reflect on the fundamental basis of their practice; they were, after all, the inheritors of the middle kingdom's grand medical tradition. Now, as a result of Western medicine's supreme confidence, surgical prowess and unarguably accurate scholarship, the cracks of self-doubt began to widen in the world of traditional Chinese medicine.

Through the 1880s and 1890s many more medical science texts were translated and published in Chinese, including the British *Pharmacopia* and a text on clinical examination that had been translated by John Dudgeon, Professor of Anatomy and Physiology at Tong Wen Guan (Imperial College). Around the same time the scholar Ding Fu-bao translated many Japanese biomedical texts into Chinese, and so from the middle of the 19th century, roughly a hundred Western medicine textbooks became available in Chinese. Medical journals also began to appear. The first came in 1880, although this only ran for two years. In 1887 the journal of the

Broad Medicine Association (Bo Yi Huibao) was more successful and, with various mergers and format changes, has continued through to modern times. These journals contributed to the spread of science-based medicine in China.

Zhang Xi-chun, pioneer of East–West medical integration

Zhang Xi-chun (born in 1860, style name Shou Pu) was a native of Yanshan county in Hebei province and grandson of a distinguished physician. Zhang first followed his father's path by studying literature, but after twice failing the imperial civil service examinations, he turned to medicine. He amassed a large collection of medical texts and, after studying hard for over ten years, Zhang began to attract many patients. Following the nationalist revolution in around 1911, he won acclaim after working as a military doctor, and in 1918 was appointed Dean of the Li Da Chinese Medicine Hospital. He pioneered the integration of classical Han dynasty medicine with later schools and with Western medical knowledge, and his frequent success in treating cases that Western medicine considered very difficult made him famous in China.

Zhang Xi-chun, alongside renowned physicians Lu Jin-sheng and Yang Ru-hou from Jiangsu province and Liu Wei-chu in Guangdong, became known in the early 20th century as the 'four masters of medicine'. Also, with Zhang Sheng-pu and Zhang Shan-lei, he gained fame as one of the country's 'three Zhangs'. In 1926 Zhang Xi-chun founded the Tianjin Institute for Integrated Chinese and Western Medicine and taught hundreds of students from across the country. From 1918 he published many essays on medicine but he died in 1933, shortly after he finished writing teaching materials on the *Shang Han Lun*. Zhang's son edited his writings and these were then published as a compilation, the 30-volume *Yi Xue Zhong Zhong Can Xi Lu* (Medical Essays Esteeming the Chinese and Respecting the Western), in 1934. After liberation, his grandchild gave the rights to the book and various other writings to the Hebei Hygiene Association, and these were first published in 1957. Considered an important modern classic of Chinese medicine, Zhang's writings have been reprinted many times.

Zhang Xi-chun made some significant contributions. Being exposed to Western medicine in his thirties, he saw that there was an opportunity for Chinese medicine to improve from cross-fertilisation with biomedical science, and so he became a passionate integrationist. His view was that many of the insights of modern medicine, were already implicit in Chinese medicine. Welcoming Western medicine, Zhang sought a commonality and agreement between the two, and considered that integration was not difficult. This was reflected in his motto 'esteem the Chinese and respect the Western'. In theory and practice, diagnosis and treatment, Zhang's work to integrate Chinese and Western medicine was inspirational for many traditional doctors and helped establish the idea that the two medicines could work side by side.

Zhang was also notable for being a highly skilled clinician driven by a genuine altruistic impetus to improve Chinese medicine practice. An acute observer, his descriptions of patients are considered to be especially lucid and penetrating. In order to improve his insight into the *bencao*, he often tried consuming the more potent medicinals himself before prescribing them to patients, and his personal experiments included testing many harsh and potentially toxic herbs such as *ba dou, liu huang, gan sui, xi xin, ma huang* and *hua jiao*. His prescription writing demonstrated a focused, adventurous and high-dosage style with a precision that was matched by few of his peers. Of the 189 formulae Zhang discussed in his *Yi Xue Zhong Zhong Can Xi Lu*, 160 were his own compositions including *sheng xian tang* (lift the sunken decoction) and *zhen gan xi feng tang* (curb the liver to extinguish wind decoction). Since Zhang's time many of China's physicians have confirmed the clinical value of these formulas and so they have entered standard modern practice. Zhang was also celebrated for bringing a new stylistic clarity to case history writing; his insightful clinical gaze, accurate use of herbs and lucid style are now viewed as comprehensive and masterful.

Chinese medicine in the modern era

A struggle for survival

During the Republic of China period (1912–1949) Chinese medicine had to fight for its continued survival against drives to modernise by the Beiyang (northern warlords) and Guomindang (nationalist) governments. There were numerous heated conflicts between Chinese medicine organisations and the new government that made repeated moves to make the practice and teaching of traditional medicine illegal. This friction created a difficult time for traditional medicine in China. It grew out of a widespread official disdain for traditional culture and a desperate desire to modernise amongst the political classes. Acumoxa practice continued to suffer neglect, even from Chinese medicine protagonists, to the extent that the newly established technical colleges of Chinese medicine that were opened in the 1910s and 1920s chose to omit acumoxa from the syllabus.

Initial protests

Following Dr Sun Zhong-shan's (Sun Yat-sen) Xinhai democratic revolution of 1911 that overthrew the Qing dynasty, Nanjing was established as the nation's capital whilst the warlords in the north continued to occupy central China. Still fresh in the Chinese psyche were the humiliations that had followed the opium wars and the other conflicts with the Russians and the Japanese. Once full of pride at its long-standing and self-evident cultural superiority, China increasingly began to see itself as a fallen and backward nation, one in desperate need of moving into the modern industrial, scientific and technological world. There was a sudden overwhelming sense that much of the rest of the world had better technology, science, infrastructure and government. Wishing to bring their country into the modern world, the consensus amongst leading politicians and intellectuals was that

China needed to emulate Western styles of administration in order to become a more modern nation. As well as taking inspiration from the West, they also looked to the Japanese Meiji Restoration that had, over the preceding decades, successfully introduced Westernisation into Japan. In relation to healthcare the Meiji model also espoused Western medicine to the exclusion of traditional medical practices, so in Chinese government circles there was a strong feeling that its colleges and practices should simply be banned completely. Already by 1912 the officially approved government curriculum for medical schools included no Chinese medicine content whatsoever, much to the dismay of traditionalists.

Yu Bo-tao and others from Shanghai's Shen Zhou Medical Association were the first to protest; they soon networked with groups across the country to organise lobby groups to save Chinese medicine from extinction. By October 1913, 19 local medical organisations had joined the movement. Traditional pharmacies and manufacturers such as Beijing's esteemed Tong Ren Tang and Xi He Nian Tang pharmacies added their influence to the protest, and representatives were elected to petition the government in Nanjing for traditional medical schools to continue to function. They offered five reasons why Chinese medicine should be retained, and proposed an eight-step plan for modernisation, which included:

- the establishment of new publishing houses for Chinese medicine texts and journals to benefit practitioner education

- founding colleges for the professional development of practitioners so they could be brought up to date on new developments in medicine

- regulating the clinical procedures used in Chinese medicine so that it could be made safer and more coherent

- regulation of the manufacture of prepared medicines to ensure safety and consistency

- setting up libraries, herb repositories and laboratories for the study of Chinese medicine.

The petition paper was submitted to Chief Education Minister Mr Wang, who immediately rejected it, and in a public speech he announced, 'I am determined to abolish Chinese medicine; from now on we will not be using it.' Traditionalists were incensed at Wang's attitude and responded with a strong refutation; daily protests were held across the country attacking the government for its undue acceptance of foreign ideas and for its ill-considered abandonment of China's proud scholarly medical heritage.

Taken aback by this unanticipated strength of feeling from the public, from the media and from Chinese medicine professionals, in 1914 the government education department replied more thoughtfully to Yu Bo-tao's petition document. They now agreed to the requests and the eightfold development plan. In future the traditional medical schools would be permitted to function, but their curriculum content would be subject to review. Implicit in the new response was, at last, some recognition of the contribution that Chinese medicine had made to the health of the populace through history. This was the first time in China's long history that a movement had been mounted in defence of the medical tradition, and it had been a success, albeit, as it turned out, a short-lived one.

In March 1922 a renewed attack on Chinese medicine was launched. The Northern government proposed a bill aimed at regulating medical practice, which required that licences to practise would be given only to those who held a college diploma or who had passed a state exam, an exam that was to be administered by the police. These new proposals also stipulated that practitioners must keep duplicate patient records for official inspection so that any 'inappropriate treatment' could be 'punished accordingly'. This move was strongly resented by the traditional medicine community who saw it as restrictive and heavy-handed. By June the Shanghai Chinese Medicine Association had convened a national conference; delegates urged all practitioners to refuse the licence and voted to demand that the Home Office withdraw the proposed legislation. Instead they proposed that practitioner credentials should be assessed by professional associations and overseen by well-respected doctors who would be elected locally. They did not see any sense in being regulated by the police who were in no position to judge medical matters. All of the nation's Chinese medicine associations agreed with these proposals, and in August, faced with such large-scale and united opposition, the government was forced to abandon its ill-considered legislation.

Then, in 1925, the Northern government enacted new legislation aimed at regulating the profession. This time it was more realistic, being better in line with the current medical realities such as the insufficient numbers of Western-style physicians able to deliver modern healthcare to the populace. The legal status of Chinese medicine schools was also to be recognised, and new more practical regulations were to be put in place in relation to fitness to practise. In reality, though, the battles over professional territory had hardly yet begun.

In February 1929 the central health department of the nationalist Guomindang government held its first conference in Nanjing. Here it was agreed to support an earlier proposal from Yu Yun-you to 'abolish the old medicine and so remove obstacles to medicine and health'. This was done on the grounds that Chinese medicine doctrine amounted to nonsense and crankery, that pulse diagnosis was a form of deception, that its ideas hindered scientific progress and that traditional medicine was powerless to prevent epidemic disease. Presumably legislators were ignorant of the fact that the idea of smallpox inoculation had originated in China and that the *wen bing* advocates had, in the previous few centuries, developed a fairly accurate understanding of the transmission of epidemic disorders from person to person well in advance of Western science. Mr Yu proclaimed that 'as long as the old medicine remains the people's mental outlook will remain unchanged, the new medicine will not develop and the provision of healthcare will not improve', and proposed a new detailed plan to abolish Chinese medicine. The conference resolved to combine Mr Yu's initiatives with regulatory measures aimed at countering the previous proposals to update practice and training in what they now labelled 'old medicine'.

The government now recognised that the old medicine and its advocates could not simply be made to disappear overnight; its destruction would be too disruptive, socially and politically. So they shifted to a gradualist approach using a series of new legal directives. Health departments would be responsible for the registration of old medicine practitioners and that licences to practise should be a requirement by the end of 1930. Also, for a five-year period, institutes would be set up to provide mandatory certificated training in medical sciences for these practitioners; any who failed to gain certification would be banned from practice unless they could demonstrate long experience. All these licences would expire after 15 years and would not be renewable. All advertisements for traditional clinics and the old medicine were to be forbidden, newspapers would be banned from promoting it and the opening of traditional medical colleges was to be prohibited. Plainly, the intent was gradual strangulation of all traditional medical practice over a period of a few decades, and modern medicine would be officially promoted to take its place. All this was at a time when pharmaceutical medicine, for all its bluster, still offered few effective treatments and surgery remained a very risky endeavour. It was ironic, too, that medical texts in the West at that time, such as Taylor's *Practice of Medicine*, were beginning to advocate acupuncture for conditions such as lumbago. Just as China was abandoning acupuncture, Europe was beginning to discover it! It was also around this time that Western pharmacology was pilfering the bronchodilator drug ephedrine from the despised Chinese medicine tradition by extracting it from the herb *ma huang*, thereby providing modern medicine with its first effective asthma treatment.

Faced with this renewed political threat to its survival, the Chinese medicine world reacted once again with fulminating indignation. The Shanghai Chinese Medicine Association instantly telegraphed the health department in Nanjing to express their opposition in the strongest terms. In late February articles were published in the national press calling for opposition to the measures, and a conference of national medical groups was convened in Shanghai to discuss the way forward. On 2 March, Yu Yun-you published a special issue of the Central Health Committee bulletin devoted to the abolition of Chinese medicine which served to inflame feelings even more. The government in Nanjing was deluged with telegrams from across the country expressing opposition to the proposed measures; these came not only from practitioners but also from diverse fields outside of Chinese medicine. On 17 March, the national medical societies' three-day conference took place in Shanghai, with 262 delegates representing 132 regional associations. Banners at the conference declared 'Resist the Cultural Invasion – Support Chinese Medicine!' and 'Long Live Chinese Medicine!' Shanghai's traditional medical world stopped in protest against the government moves. The conference agreed to put three resolutions into action: to set up a general national medical group league, to immediately dispatch a delegation to Nanjing to lobby the government and to inaugurate 17 March as Chinese Medicine Day. The petition group departed immediately for Nanjing and the new league was founded shortly afterwards.

So, having failed simply to ban the old medicine, the government had tried more stealthy and incremental tactics, but with this new backlash from physicians and the media, they were forced again to put their modernising measures on hold. The approach now was to concede as little as possible to the profession's demands whilst at the same time aiming to erode and to gently and consistently denigrate. They announced, for instance, that Chinese medicine colleges were to be downgraded in name and status to *chuan xi suo* (training institutes), and that traditional clinics be banned from using the word *yi yuan* (hospital). The profession simply chose to ignore these directives. In another blatant measure the health department aroused further resentment by banning the use of all Western medical methods and equipment by Chinese medicine practitioners. Another Shanghai conference was arranged in December with additional petitions to Nanjing, but these were side-stepped by the authorities and came to nothing.

The 1929 Guomindang proposals to phase out Chinese medicine practice were withdrawn in response to the protests and, in an attempt to appease the situation, a state-controlled National Medicine Institute was set up in March of 1931 that promised to address the academic and administrative issues involved. In June 1933, at the main Guomindang conferences, there was a proposal to establish new national medicine legislation, but the Chief Minister for Home Affairs, Wang Jing-wei, remained insistent that the old medicine should be completely outlawed:

> Traditional medicine talks about *yin-yang* and five elements but they attach no value to anatomy. There is no scientific evidence, there is no analysis of Chinese herbs and their effectiveness is insignificant. Having experienced it myself I am deeply dissatisfied with the errors contained in this medicine. (Chief Minister Wang Jing-wei, 1933)

At the start of 1934, at a public conference of China's Western-style doctors, Wang gave another long speech attacking Chinese medicine, again on the basis that it was not scientific and could not exist alongside scientific medicine. This was condemned by Shanghai's traditionalists who appealed to the government to improve the status of Chinese medicine, and demanded that the two systems be treated equally. They asked for enactment of the earlier 'national legislation' that had promised legal status to traditional practice. Thousands of protesters lobbied the Guomindang conference in January 1934, chanting impassioned slogans, and the entire Chinese medicine community went on a one-day strike in support. The next day a further petition was made to the conference, but requests for equality were once more rejected.

Wishing to block the implementation of the 'national medicine' legislation, Wang Jing-wei wrote to the head of the legislature Mr Sun, saying: 'The issue not only relates to the lives of those in our country but also the grace in the world. If national medicine were to be given official power I fear it will bring misfortune for China.' He asked Mr Sun to try to alter the legislation so that it would no longer offer official recognition to the traditional professions. These manoeuvres were disclosed in September 1935 in the journal *Spring and Autumn of the Medical World*, where the government tactics were referred to as 'the beating of drums before an attack'. That by doing this they had revealed the truth behind the government's two-year delay in implementation of the legislation, it was clear that the aim was still to have the old medicine removed from the map of modern China. Once again the ire of the Chinese medicine community was raised, and they fought back with a clear rebuttal of government policy; again the traditionalist lobby gained wide support from many of those involved in public life.

In November 1935 lobbyists attending the fifth Guomindang conference again demanded that the government treat the two medicines equally, and thereby ensure future academic standards for the benefit of the people. The National Medicine Legislation Act, that had waited two years, was finally forced into enactment on 22 January 1936. This set required academic standards in Western and traditional medical subjects, but omitted to discuss any standards for acumoxa practice, such was the disdain for this aspect of the medical tradition. Unfortunately, the strength of the medico-political divide being what it was, it only took a few months before new laws were introduced by the health department that were designed to restrict Chinese medicine further. Purporting to simply introduce procedural detail, these amendments in effect completely negated the national medicine legislation.

The original bill had given legal recognition to Chinese medicine college graduates, but the new amendments restricted this to those colleges registered with the education department. This was perhaps reasonable at first glance, until we realise that the education department did not actually have Chinese medicine listed as a subject, so the effect was that no Chinese medical college graduates could be recognised by the legislation. Also, the regulation was to be administered by a health department entirely orientated towards Western medicine. At the end of 1936 the Shanghai Medical Organisation and 18 other medical groups demanded that a senior health department official be appointed specifically to oversee Chinese medicine in order to counter the inherent biases. The very next day this request was rejected. The profession's response was to redouble their unification and campaign efforts for equal treatment and to fight for recognition of Chinese medicine colleges; eventually this recognition came and, on paper at least, the two medicines were to be treated equally in law. At last, after years of struggle, a significant victory had finally been achieved. Unfortunately, though, just weeks later, a Japanese invasion threw the country into turmoil and the Chinese medicine issue was effectively set aside.

A few years later, with the Japanese in retreat, the country remained chaotic and was lurching towards civil war. The Guomindang government continued its campaign against Chinese medicine and so, from the beginning of 1946, traditional medicine had to renew its fight for survival. One sanction imposed against practitioners at this time was the banning by the Hangzhou Health Authority of the use of Western drugs or injection equipment by traditional physicians. Weeks later, in February 1946, the Nanjing government ordered the closure of Shanghai's Chinese medicine colleges, and this was followed by similar closures in Sichuan and Guangdong. In June the government stipulated that traditional physicians should no longer be referred to as 'doctors'.

These measures were vigorously resisted; the two Shanghai colleges refused to close and called for the whole Chinese medicine community to fight the closures, and once again there was organised resistance from traditional professionals across the country. More representations were made to the Nanjing government demanding enactment of the legislation that would give equality to the two medicines in accordance with the earlier 1935 Act. These petitions were completely ignored and officials were dispatched from the state-run Shanghai Medical School to inspect the two traditional schools. As expected, they reported that the quality of teaching, the qualifications of the teaching staff and the equipment, curriculum and students of these two schools did not meet the regulatory standards, and they insisted that the ban should remain. It was probably true that standards at Shanghai's three Chinese medicine colleges were inferior to those of the state medical schools, but this was due to the fact that they were chronically under-resourced. Despite their fiscal neglect, relatively speaking they were still leaders in China's traditional medicine education. It was plain that the government intent behind dispatching rivals as an inspection team was to eliminate Chinese medicine.

In 1947, as the attacks continued to escalate, so did the resolve of the Chinese medicine community to unite and fight using further protests. Protesters in Nanjing fasted for three days in a tactic intended to force a reply from the Guomindang government, but Chairman Jiang Jie-shi (style name Chiang Kai-shek) remained unmoved, and eventually the police removed the protesters. Renewed action took place in May 1948 when the plea to the government for the 'dissemination of our original medicine to keep the nation healthy' was submitted, but it came just as the government was collapsing. In the light of the new political crisis situation, dealing with the gripes of the Chinese medicine community seemed an irrelevance.

Cheng Dan-an (1899–1957) and the acumoxa renaissance

Cheng Dan-an was studying acupuncture in Japan in the early 1930s at a time when it had reached a nadir in China. Returning to Wu Xi in south China in 1933, he helped improve its respectability by discussing the acupuncture points using modern anatomical terminology. He then founded a new acumoxa college and published an acupuncture textbook that incorporated the modern ideas from physiology that had been part of his training in Japan; this scientific gloss was also very helpful in catalysing a new respect for acumoxa. By training a new generation of acumoxa practitioners and teachers, Cheng revitalised this withered limb of Chinese medicine and helped found the new traditional Chinese medicine (TCM) acupuncture lineage. Then, when the communists came to power, he became very influential in forming the health policies of the new government, and in this way helped press for acumoxa to become part of the official healthcare system of modern China.

The Mao era

In 1949 Mao Zedong succeeded in ousting the nationalist Guomindang government that fled to Taiwan, taking with them as much wealth as they could. He was also successful in ending the Japanese occupation and uniting the country again, although deprivation and public health remained a considerable problem. In 1950 the communist government's first working party on the nation's health introduced the idea of bringing Chinese medicine and Western medicine together to tackle the difficulties. In 1955 the health ministry founded the National Academy of Chinese Medicine. The ideal was felt to be East–West medical integration, and with this in mind, doctors of Western medicine were persuaded to supplement their biomedicine studies with formal study of Chinese medicine. The idea was also for Chinese medicine practitioners to develop fluency in Western biomedicine. Officially the two styles of medicine were placed on an equal footing, although many medical students were reluctant to embrace this part of their studies, as they tended to see Chinese medicine as having low status. Nevertheless, by 1959 Chinese medicine had succeeded in being included as one of the government science and technology research priorities. Compared with the situation in the 1920s, this was a triumph for Chinese medicine, which had not only been saved from impending extinction, but was now receiving a massive boost in terms of state recognition and funding.

From one perspective this about-turn must have been a little uncomfortable for Chinese government officials because communism was supposed to be forward-looking – it was about the science of government and about a modern technological industrial state. Its doctrinaire hatred of the past was evident in the mass destruction by Red Guards of most of the country's temples and ancient cultural relics. Acupuncture and herbal medicine were emblematic of an old China that was being swept away to allow the construction of a glorious new utopia, and acupuncture and herbs were a reminder of China's feudalistic past. So, Mao Zedong's instinct would have been to get rid of it; he faced the practical issue of having inherited a country in chaos, a legacy of the Japanese occupation and the failures of the ousted Guomindang government. During the communists' arduous Long March across the country to seize power, his followers were forced to rely on traditional healthcare methods that had proved effective, and so Mao had acquired some respect for Chinese medicine. Indeed, even in 1928 when the communists' access to medicine was blocked by the Guomindang, Mao wrote an article entitled 'Struggles in the Qing Kang Mountains' in which he advocated the use of traditional medicine. Having seen an estimated 182,000 malaria cases in his troops successfully treated with acupuncture and Chinese herbal medicine during his campaign, he formulated his idea of 'making the past serve the present'. In 1944, a few years before the communist takeover, Mao had spoken at a conference in Yunnan where he urged traditional and Western physicians to overcome their differences and to work together for the health of the nation. A year later an acupuncture clinic was opened at Yunnan Peace Hospital, and acupuncture began to be officially taught again.

So, at the start of his rule in the early 1950s, Mao had inherited a stricken country. Millions were sick and dying from cholera, dysentery, starvation and neglect; this was a situation that could not be resolved, with China's meagre supply of Western medicine practitioners. Mao had little choice but to call on the many Chinese medicine practitioners for help. With government support and funding, and driven by revolutionary fervour, the traditional doctors marshalled a battle to restore public health that included the training of an army of 'barefoot doctors' trained in simple forms of acupuncture and herbal medicine and other basic hygiene and healthcare skills. This initiative managed to turn the situation around within the space of two or three years; indeed, so remarkable was the turn-around that the then head of the League of Nations (later the United Nations) declared this the greatest achievement by any government so far in the 20th century. This success helped confirm the communists' view that Chinese medicine was a 'great treasure house' for the benefit of the people.

In 1955 Mao's regime continued its support for acupuncture and Chinese medicine by founding the Beijing Academy of Traditional Chinese Medicine and the Research Centre for Acupuncture and Moxibustion. By 1956 large new colleges of traditional medicine had also been founded in Shanghai, Guandong and Sichuan and, by the 1980s, the number of traditional medicine universities and colleges had grown to more than 30. In 1985 a clause was written into the national constitution that officially gave equal status to the two medicines and pledges to develop both systems, informally referred to as the 'walking on two legs policy'.

Given the communists' inherent modernistic outlook, it was felt that if Chinese medicine was to be retained to serve the people in the new China, then it should be re-examined and organised into a more modern and politically correct body of knowledge, one that was better aligned with the communist dialectic and that was more amenable to incorporation into a standardised teaching curriculum. The vast treasure house of the tradition needed to be re-evaluated, simplified and sanitised; those aspects that were impossible to square with the new political and scientific mindset had to be removed, or at least downplayed. So, in the two decades following the late 1950s, committees of eminent traditional physicians re-worked the tradition, removing references to spirits and Daoist metaphysics, and altering the language so it seemed more in tune with party dogma.

On the positive side there was certainly a need for this re-evaluation; in its two-and-a-half millennium history Chinese medicine had accumulated an overstuffed ragbag of wisdom and nonsense and all points in between. In addition to the committees whose job it was to make the tradition more congruent with current scientific and political beliefs, research programmes were funded that aimed to investigate efficacy and mechanism. In retrospect we can see that the process was heavily coloured by the beliefs and values of 1950s fundamentalist communism, and that the cleansing had perhaps been over-zealous. Nevertheless, the process allowed Chinese medicine to be made more amenable to college education and to be standardised so that its practitioners across China, and later across the world, had a common professional language and core approach. This has been invaluable for the exportation of Chinese medicine and acupuncture to the Western world. With its vast and arcane literature base and a specialist terminology that is difficult to understand even for ordinary Chinese speakers, it would have been much more difficult for Western non-Chinese speakers to evaluate the tradition. Especially useful was the identification of *ba gang* theory (first coined in 1947 by Dr Zhu Wei-ju to label the most commonly used analytical elements of pattern differentiation) as a rational diagnostic and explanatory model at the core of the whole tradition.

Significant research funding was allocated to acupuncture and Chinese herbal medicine with the intent of bringing the medicine better into line with modern science, and large amounts of pharmacology were carried out. This work continues today, perhaps driven now less by the idealist humanitarian orientations of the 1960s and 1970s, and more by the possible financial rewards from novel drug identification. It was anticipated that the application of science would quickly lead to an understanding of the nature of the *jing-luo* – channel system – and understanding of *qi, yin* and *yang,* and so on. And that neurophysiology studies would lead to an understanding of the mechanisms of acupuncture and that clinical studies would demonstrate that Chinese medicine and acumoxa medicine has clinical value. Although a great deal has been achieved, the task has turned out to be much more unwieldy than imagined at that time.

Arrival of acupuncture and Chinese medicine in the West

Trading along the Silk Road and later by sea, alongside insights gleaned from Jesuit missionaries, traders and diplomats, brought a slow trickle of hearsay medical knowledge from China. Then, the increased trade with China at the end of the 17th century brought more exposure of Europeans to Chinese ideas and aesthetics as well as the fine trade commodities such as porcelain, silk and tea. Information on acumoxa treatment also filtered into Europe on the back of the various romances with Chinoiserie that occurred in the 17th and 18th centuries, but the near complete absence of appropriate scholarship meant that understanding was very sketchy until the 20th century. Rumours grew about the acumen, high learning and great diagnostic skills of the traditional physicians of China.

In the 17th century a handful of Chinese texts on acumoxa were translated into European languages, the first being that of the Reverend Hermann Busschof of the Dutch East India Company, whose long-standing gout had been successfully treated in Java using moxibustion. His interest in this therapy was aroused after his daughter had been successfully treated by a female practitioner originating from southwest China who had become known for use of 'fire therapy' to treat local people. One treatment using 20 cones of moxa on Busschof's foot had given him relief of pain and inflammation for over a year. On his return to the Netherlands he translated some writings on moxibustion and published his *Essays on Gout* in Dutch in 1675. At this time the English ambassador in Den Hague, William Temple, was experiencing such severe pain, inflammation and swelling in his foot that his physicians feared that amputation would be his only option. The secretary to the mayor of Den Hague had previously been successfully treated for gout by this newly introduced treatment, and he suggested it to Temple. He, too, was quickly cured and, soon after, a maid of Temple's had her toothache treated, also with good results. Temple wrote an essay on the treatment, and news of this miraculous treatment quickly spread through high society. The interest of the Royal Society of Medicine was aroused, and in 1676 they quickly arranged for Busschof's book to be published in English. As a result the practice of moxibustion quickly became popular amongst London's society physicians, and allowed them to successfully treat an affliction that was especially common amongst their clientele. In the same year the *Essays on Gout* also appeared as an edition in German. This appears to be the first instance of acumoxa therapy in Europe. Shortly afterwards, another early discussion of acumoxa appeared at the hands of the physician Willem Ten Rhyne who had been exposed to *De Acupunctura* in his travels to Japan. In 1683 he published a textbook on arthritis in Latin that devoted 20 pages to acumoxa treatment and which mentions the word 'meridians' almost certainly for the first time in a European language. By 1683 the term 'acupuncture' had made its first appearance in the *Oxford English Dictionary*.

In 1686 Michal Piotr Boym further added to the literature when he published a Latin translation of *Mai Jing* (Pulse Classic). The source text he used was, however, not Wang Shu-hu's famed classic text but another later pulse text with the same name. Boym's book was then further translated into various European languages, initiating a fad for pulse taking amongst Western physicians who wished to emulate the oriental knowing clinical gaze. Unfortunately the explanatory model that the Chinese pulse diagnosis system was designed to feed into was unintelligible to the minds of European physicians, and so any significant appreciation of its value was hindered, and there seems to have been little genuine insight into how pulse diagnosis was carried out or how it was interpreted.

Then, for a period in the 18th century, interest in acupuncture and moxibustion declined until, as a consequence of the ever-increasing exposure to East Asian culture and medicine, in the second half of the 19th century some English physicians began to adopt acupuncture needling techniques for the treatment of back pain. French and British doctors continued to pursue an interest in acumoxa as an exotic novelty therapy and, from here, it first reached the United States through their links with France when Dr Franklin Bache published an article about it in 1825. This interest rumbled on and, in his *Principles and Practice of Medicine*, first published in 1916, the influential 'father of modern medicine', Sir William Osler, recommended acupuncture as a treatment for back pain. It was a French physician, though, who was the first Westerner to take the subject seriously enough to apply genuine scholarship to acumoxa and Chinese medical theory.

George Soulie de Morant

George Soulie de Morant was the pre-eminent figure in the introduction of a more scholarly approach to acupuncture study to the West. Born in 1879, he learned Mandarin from a Chinese intellectual he had encountered in France when he was young. He had intended to study medicine, but these ambitions were frustrated following his father's early death, and instead he worked for a Parisian bank that gave him a posting in China. Here his rare fluency in Mandarin quickly led to his appointment as consul for the French foreign ministry. Fascinated by all aspects of Chinese culture, de Morant was very soon moving in the highest intellectual circles. Whilst travelling in Yunnan province during a Cholera epidemic he noticed that acupuncture seemed to be a more effective treatment than the Western drug treatments in use at the time, and this inspired him to commit to detailed further study with many famous acupuncturists throughout his two decades living in China. He also acquired some classic acumoxa textbooks such as *Zhenjiu Da Cheng* (Great Compilation of Acupuncture and Moxibustion), and he used these as a basis for his own writings.

In the decade following his return to France in 1917, de Morant published many articles that promoted interest in acupuncture, and in this way he successfully inspired a new generation of French physician acupuncturists. In the 1930s and 1940s he published many articles and books, and as a result of his inspirational and scholarly work he was nominated for the 1950 Nobel Prize. He continued his work despite suffering a stroke in 1951, but eventually died in 1955. In 1972 his main writings on acupuncture were compiled into a monumental text, *L'Acuponture Chinoise*, published in English in 1994. This masterwork is notable for many things, but it is especially useful for providing a glimpse of the acupuncture thinking of elite physicians half a century before the introduction of modern Chinese acupuncture. French acupuncture also benefited from their colonial associations with Vietnam and 20th-century Vietnamese practitioners such as van Nghi.

Chinese herbal medicine was largely ignored, mainly confined to the semi-insular Chinese communities in the United States, Europe and Australia; serious interest from occidental practitioners has only developed in the last few decades. In the early 1980s, with a dozen or so practitioners, the UK was ahead of Europe in the study and practice of Chinese herbal medicine but behind the United States. Since then attention to, and scholarship of, this medicine has grown exponentially, with some estimates putting the numbers professionally practising this medicine at around 3000. The liberalisations in China and the increase in global migration have also greatly contributed to its adoption.

President Nixon's trip to China

If the publication of de Morant's *L'Acuponture Chinoise* was a pivotal moment in the exportation of acupuncture to the West, another such moment occurred when the newly elected President Nixon made a historic state visit to China in 1971 accompanied by the world's media. During this trip a *New York Times* reporter, James Reston, developed appendicitis and was successfully treated with acupuncture, a story that was quickly picked up by the other journalists in the entourage. A witness to this incident was President Nixon's physician Dr Walter Tkach, who was impressed enough to set up a National Institutes of Health (NIH) committee to investigate acupuncture, and in 1972 there was a conference presenting preliminary research studies. This episode sparked academic scientific interest in acupuncture, and Western researchers began to be exposed to research from China. Of particular interest was the work of Beijing's Professor Han whose research had suggested that acupuncture raised pain thresholds by stimulating the release of a neuro-humoral substance that was soon identified as the first endogenous opiate – endorphin. Western scientists such as Canadian Professor Bruce Pommerantz continued this research effort through the 1970s and 1980s, and acupuncture began to gain a measure of scientific respectability. Some medical authorities considered that the treatment was simply an elaborate oriental form of hypnosis, thereby purporting to explain one mystery using a different one. The early NIH-sponsored findings were that, contrary to expectation, people who were most easily hypnotised seemed to be the least responsive to acupuncture.

Another interesting effect of Nixon's visit to China came out of his presidential mission statement at the start of his election to the presidency. Previously, at the start of the 1960s, President Kennedy had hit on the idea of a mission for his anticipated decade in power – he announced that America was going to put a man on the moon. By the end of the decade, having achieved this, there was a sense of anticlimax and a feeling that the billions of dollars might have been better directed at a humanitarian cause. With this in mind, Nixon's presidency began with him declaring at a press conference in the Whitehouse Oval Office that America was 'declaring war on cancer'. Billions were allocated to this endeavour, with the implication that the victory would be achieved in that decade. So, Nixon's 1971 visit to China spurred the Chinese to also allocate a large government research budget to researching cancer care. In China, because Chinese medicine was a significant aspect of state-supported medicine, this meant that a large amount of research was funded into the pharmacology and clinical use of Chinese herbs in oncology. Acupuncture also benefited from this work – especially its use in controlling adverse reactions to cancer chemotherapy. This work came to the attention of Western cancer research institutes in the 1990s.

All this attention raised the profile of acupuncture in the West, and Chinese medicine treatments that had generally been contained within Chinese communities in the West began to attract attention. One part of the *zeitgeist* of the time was the 'hippy' explorations of all things Eastern, so through the 1970s, interest in the study of acumoxa, Chinese medicine and the martial arts began to take hold. Younger people in the United States began to seek out instruction from experts in the Chinese community – notably Dr Hong Yen-hsu in California, Dr James Tin Yau-so in New

England, Dr Shen of New York and Dr Henry Lu in Canada, all people who had been trained in the styles of Chinese medicine taught in pre-revolutionary China. A handful of intrepid Americans travelled to China and Taiwan for prolonged study of Chinese medicine, people who were serious enough in their quest to learn Mandarin. These included Dan Bensky, Dr Ted Kaptchuk and John O'Connor who returned in the 1970s with the modern medical school style of Chinese medicine that, although sanitised by the communist regime, gave a more easily comprehensible summary of the medical tradition than had been available previously. Since this time acupuncture and Chinese medicine scholarship in the West has grown exponentially, and much better avenues for understanding have opened up alongside an influx of doctors of Chinese medicine to the West.

In Britain in the 1960s a handful of pioneers had become interested in acupuncture. Most were naturopaths or osteopaths such as J. D. van Buren, Jack Worsley, Mary Austin and Alexander Rose-Neil who, intrigued by this exotic therapy, travelled to France for short courses of instruction with French acupuncturists such as Lavier and van Nghi. One of the very few texts available in English at that time was written by Dr Wu Wei-ping of Taiwan, and some British pioneers travelled to his clinic for short internments and instruction. Another UK pioneer was Dr Felix Mann who, as well as studying with the French practitioners, had access to a sinologist called David Owen, who helped translate material for Dr Mann's introductory books on acupuncture. Worsley, van Buren and Rose-Neil founded acupuncture colleges, each with their own style of practice, and many of the early graduates of these colleges, such as Giovanni Maciocia and Peter Deadman, progressed scholarship further. Exemplary improvements in self-regulation and training for acupuncture and Chinese medicine in the UK, European Union, North America and Australia have created a mature profession with standards comparable with those in traditional medical schools in Mainland China.

Numerous Westerners now live, or have lived, for periods of many years in China and Taiwan, learning the medicine close up and translating its texts and ideas with ever-increasing scholarship and fidelity. Today, only the obstacles presented by the ignorance of legislators and by the resistance of vested medical industry corporations stand in the way of the whole world benefiting from China's remarkable and historic medical system.

POSTSCRIPT

In 1998 I received a wonderful gift from my colleague Dr Han Li-ping, a modern text called *China's Ocean of Herbs*, which is an 18cm-thick 4000-page tome in tiny Chinese script that includes many brief quotes from the wider historical *bencao* tradition. Translated into English this would probably run to 10,000 pages, and a collection of the sources drawn on for this book would fill a library. This helps give dimensions to the *bencao* part of the tradition. Add in the historical writings on prescriptions, on diagnosis, theory and medical specialisms, and the size of the literature base becomes difficult to envisage. Roughly 90,000 pre-modern texts have been listed in imperial library records. One might select almost any area of interest, say dermatology, dietetics or traumatology, and quite literally spend a lifetime attempting to survey the contents of the medical storehouse. With this in mind it should be evident that the story that lies between the covers of this book omits a lot more than it includes. So, although inevitably selective, the narrative I have tried to present is what most take to be the key parts of the tradition – the most famous figures, the milestone texts and some of the key ideas. That said, I deliberately chose not to become too embroiled in attempts to précis the complexities of the *Neijing* and the *Shang Han Lun* as these would consume considerable space and have also been discussed in some detail by others.

What I hope that readers have gained from my work is a clearer sense of how the foundations of classical Chinese medicine came into being, and how its story has unfolded over two millennia. Some commonly held misapprehensions have been questioned – the sense that this is a medicine frozen in the Han dynasty, the idea that it is akin to the folk medicines of old Europe or that it is a metaphysical, quasi-religious form of medicine. Readers will perhaps also have gained the understanding that Chinese medicine is not simply about 'balancing energies' or removing 'stagnation', that it summarises the very considerable efforts that have been made to rationally investigate anatomy, physiology, the aetiology of disease and pathology. In the sections on education we have come to see that the romantic notion of education by apprenticeship fails to include appreciation of the fact that high-level formal institutional medical education existed too, often with thousands of students undergoing formal courses of training, and that even the private mentors often ran mini-training institutes. It is interesting as well that long before the introduction of universities in Europe, government-controlled pharmacies sold standardised products with quality control and expiry dates. All in all, by exploring this subject, we may also have gained a sense of both the genius and humanitarian dimensions to be found in the Chinese intellectual endeavours of the past and, in particular, the sense that there was an ethic of personal excellence underlying the scholarly traditions.

Although not an explicit theme of the text, looking a little deeper readers may even have acquired some sense that a different approach to knowledge from that which we are accustomed to lies behind China's 'proto-science'. What we find at work here is an iterative process of knowledge acquisition where progress is slow and where errors arise, but where gradually through time medicine and its practitioners become more effective. This might be contrasted with the 'sudden breakthrough' mindset of current medical science which is so often followed only a few years later by an 'Oops, sorry – we got it wrong, but here's another breakthrough!'

In pharmacology, drugs are tested for their instant, powerful but generally transient effects. Chinese medicine did this too – a patient can take the purgative *da huang* and see something happen quite quickly. The more interesting investigations in Chinese medicine involved tracking the subtle and often long-lasting changes that happen when medicinals are used over extended periods of time. It is partly this more leisurely perspective, alongside its focus on actual human function in the real world, that gives this medicine its wise gaze.

It is true, though, that Chinese scholars of history, although they remained far ahead of the West in many fields for millennia, never actually reached an understanding that could properly be called 'scientific'. For the brief foregoing remarks we could say that the fruits of the Chinese scholars' methodology produced different, but no less valuable, outcomes. From some perspectives, the differences might be seen as a strength, but still this question, first posed by Needham, remains. One answer is to be found in the realisation that the technical terms used in the Chinese traditions were not subjected to the formally agreed conventions that exist in modern academic and scientific work. Often different authors use the same term in different ways, and key concepts are poorly defined. How different the progress of Chinese medicine might have been if the Chinese scholars had only listened to the founding scholar of the scholarly tradition, Confucius, when he exhorted them to 'First rectify the names…!'

I believe that this is a great era for China's medical tradition because it has the opportunity to advance with the help of the new and sharp tools that science can bring to the examination of truth. The power of scientific investigation and analysis gives us the chance to re-visit the facts and assumptions of ancient doctrine. But central to this is the need to begin such an examination from a perspective of true understanding and insight into what the tradition consists of – science based not on prejudice and superficial assumptions, but a complete, hermeneutic and respectful appraisal of the tradition. This book may help this, first by bringing a little more light on this medicine and, even better, by inspiring others to improve on my work here.

GLOSSARY

Bagang   Eight-principle patterns, a modern term for the most important distinctions used to guide diagnostic thinking, namely *yin-yang*, hot-cold, deficient-excess and internal-external. This system appeared under different names throughout history. *Xie qi–zheng qi* replaces *yin-yang* in some versions.

Bencao   Roots and herbage, the usual name for a *materia medica* that describes the properties, indications, application and doses of medicinals used in Chinese herbal medicine.

Bian zheng lun zhi   Treatment based on pattern differentiation. This describes the fundamental approach used by Chinese medicine where a constellation of clinical information is synthesised by the practitioner to inform the diagnosis and treatment of the patient's complaint.

Bing   Illness, symptom, the presenting main complaint normally used as the point of departure for investigation of the underlying pattern (*zheng*) requiring treatment. Most of these are formally named in classical Chinese medicine, examples being *lin bing* (dysuria) and *beng lou* (menstrual leaking and flooding). Investigation of typical *zheng* patterns that underlie *bing* diseases seen clinically has been a key endeavour throughout history.

Domain   All the various aspects of anatomy and physiology associated with a *zangfu* organ. For example, the Lung domain includes the nose, the skin and the hair on the body as well as the actual anatomical lungs themselves. To signal this technical sense of organ names many English language texts capitalise them when referring to the Chinese medicine usage and use a lower case initial when referring to the anatomical organ.

Fangji xue   The study of medical formulas and their construction. Chinese herbal medicine plays close attention to the manner in which medicinals can be combined in a strategic manner to be more effective than substances used alone. A simple example might be the use of substances to protect the digestion paired with a medicinal that, although effective, tends to irritate the intestinal mucosa. The three hundred or so formulas most commonly prescribed today are the ones that have been found to be most effective and well balanced out of the tens of thousands recorded in *fangji xue* textbooks compiled throughout history.

Initial-stage heat disorders   Acute febrile diseases where the first signs include fever, sore throat, headache, thirst and a floating-rapid pulse all suggestive of a heat pathogen. This is distinct from wind-cold attack that starts with chills and only slight fever, sneezing, rhinitis and muscle aches and a floating-tight pulse.

Luo mai   The various networks of small branches of the *jing-luo* system.

Qi Although often translated as 'energy', this word does not properly convey the true sense of this term, which functions as a qualifier character used alongside other characters to suggest a quality that is evanescent or at the limits of perception. It should perhaps be rendered in English not as a full word itself, but a word fragment such as 'eous' as in 'gaseous'. The term *qi* is used to denote the subtle influences that underlie function, change and transformation in the body and in the world. A fascination to Chinese thinkers since the Warring States period or before, numerous types of *qi* have been labelled and discussed across all fields of investigation and study, from warfare to philosophy.

Qijing ba mai Eight extraordinary vessels. Described in the *Neijing*, this is a channel system that is considered to work in parallel with the 12 main channels. Two of these, the *du mai* and *ren mai*, have their own points that run along the midline of the back and front respectively. The remainder share points with the main channel system. This system may have originated from a different medical tradition that evolved in the centuries prior to the Han dynasty.

San fa Three methods. This refers to the three most basic routes through which pathogenic *qi* can be eliminated: through the 'upper orifices', mainly by induced emesis, through the skin by promoting sweating and through the lower orifices, which most often refers to bowel purgation.

Sanjiao Three heaters. One system for categorising the functions of the body in use since early times in Chinese medicine divides the body into thoracic, epigastric and lower abdominal regions, the upper part relating to the movement and transformation of *qi* and blood, the middle part involving the digestive processes of assimilation and transportation and the lower part being 'in charge of' elimination of wastes. Early physiology and pathology detailed these functions and their associated pathologies and later, in the Qing dynasty, this model was extended to also describe the different stages of febrile disease using a higher level of understanding of *sanjiao* function in relation to *yuan qi* and the totality of *qi* functions in the body.

Shen Spirit-consciousness. In medicine this refers to the spiritedness that is reflected in the signs of clear consciousness and rational behaviour. It is also detectable in the brightness of the complexion, in an animated quality perceived in the pulse, in movement and in the body tissues. It is considered to indicate good function in the heart *zang*. The term is used in many other contexts in Chinese culture, such as in cosmology, where it indicates the sense of a universal consciousness. In modern vernacular Mandarin it is most commonly taken to mean 'God'.

Si qi Four *qi*, a term that describes the four stages used in *wen bing* theory as a basis for differentiation of febrile illness patterns. These are: *wei stage* – a superficial stage with initial fever, chills, sore throat and floating pulse; *qi stage* – a fever with signs that the lungs and stomach have been affected; *ying stage* – fever involving the *qi* of the blood; and *blood stage* – a serious fever in which heat has entered the blood leading to skin rashes, delirium and bleeding disorders.

Three methods Early classical medical theory considered that there are only three main routes through which pathogenic *qi* can be expelled from the body: through the skin, via the 'upper orifices' on the head or via the 'lower orifices'. Substances that induce sweating or vomiting or purgation broadly serve these three functions.

Tui na A traditional Chinese therapeutic massage that uses pressure, rubbing and pinching techniques on *jing-luo* channels and acupoints. Hospitals in China often have departments with specialist *tui na* practitioners. For infant care the technique is considered more appropriate than acumoxa treatment.

Wulun liuqi   Five movements, six *qi*, a system of Chinese medical practice that was developed in the Tang dynasty and written into the *Neijing* by Wang Bing. This system takes the ancient calendrical cycles that chart the cyclic energetic changes in heaven and the climate on earth, and purports to explain and predict their effects on man.

Wu xing   Often mis-translated as 'five elements', the character *xing* implies movement or transition from one state to another. A reasonable translation is five transitions because the model identifies five characteristic phases in cycles of change in nature that are labelled as wood, fire, earth, metal and water. The *wu xing* model came to prominence toward the end of the −3rd century as a political model espoused by the government official Zou Yan. Its popularity over the subsequent two centuries ensured that it was used as a system to classify nature and map change and transformation. In Han dynasty medicine it provided a model for labelling tissues and organs in the body, a model that helped physicians map the links between human physiology and the environment. The *wu xing* model slipped from favour in intellectual circles in the 1st century before re-appearing as part of the cosmological thinking that came to prominence from the latter part of the Tang dynasty. It forms the basis for various contemporary styles of acupuncture.

Xu shi   Emptiness and fullness, two of the eight *bagang* principles. *Xu* denotes a state of lacking sufficient of something that should be in the body. *Shi* describes a situation where something is present that should not be there – this might be pathogenic *qi* that has invaded, a pathological product that has developed such as phlegm or a normal body constituent that has become dysfunctional due to stagnation such as may occur with blood, *qi*, fluids, food, etc.

Yang sheng   Nourishing life, a term that covers the health-preservation practices that have been an important part of healthcare since early times, and which remain important today. These include physical exercises, breathing exercises, diet and lifestyle regulation, sexual practices, strictures relating to confinement after parturition, etc.

Yuan qi   Original *qi* according to context. This refers to the fundamental *qi* that underlies all physiological processes in the body, or, in the context of cosmology, it refers to the basic *qi* that permeates the universe and ultimately underlies all change and transformation.

Xiang huo   Ministerial fire.

Zheng qi   Upright *qi*, the sum total of all the natural forms of *qi* that operate in the human body. *Zheng qi* exists in contradistinction to *xie qi* pathogenic *qi*.

Zhong jiao   Middle body section, primarily a shorthand term for the digestive and metabolic functions ascribed to the stomach and spleen.

Zi wu liu zhu   Midnight–midday ebb and tide. Refers to the branch of Chinese medicine chronobiology that links the time of day or night with activity or inactivity in the 12 main *jing-luo* channels.

CLASSIC TEXTS MENTIONED

Listed here are the main historical texts discussed in this book. They are arranged chronologically, except the works of individual authors, which are grouped together. Readers should bear in mind that compiling lists of this kind is a little awkward. Chinese scholars usually have a given name as well as a literary name and sometimes also a nickname. Some even had to change their name mid-career if it clashed with names in the imperial household. Exact dates of publication or authorship are often approximate or in some cases unknown or disputed. Sometimes the same work has a different title in Chinese and some are reprinted over centuries. Book titles can also be rendered into English in many different ways, which means that cross-referencing between English language sources is best done with reference to the Pinyin and/or characters of the author and title.

Pre-Han dynasty texts

Author(s)	Pinyin title	English title	Date	Notes
Anon	*Zhou Yi*	*Changes of the Zhou Dynasty*	c.–1000 to –500	Aka *Yijing* (Classic of Changes)
Attributed to Li Er	*Dao De Jing*	*The Virtues of the Dao*	c.–500	Founding text of Daoism
Anon	*Chunqiu*	*Spring and Autumn Annals*	c.–450?	History of the state of Lu
Attributed to Zuo Qiu-ming	*Zuo Zhuan*	*Zuo's Commentary*	c.–400	Affairs of the state of Lu in Spring-Autumn period
Commissioned by Lu Bu-wei	*Lushi Chunqiu*	*Lu's Spring and Autumn Annals*	c.–239	
Anon	*Zhouli*	*Rites of Zhou*	c.–230	

Han dynasty texts

Author(s)	Pinyin title	English title	Date	Notes
Liu An	*Huainanzi*	*Book of Huainan*	c.−140	
Ban Gu	*Han Shu*	*Han History*	−111	
Anon	*Huangdi Neijing Suwen*	*Yellow Emperor's Internal Classic – Plain Questions*	c.−100	
Anon	*Huangdi Neijing Nanjing*	*Yellow Emperor's Internal Classic – Difficult Questions*	c.−100	
Si Ma-qian	*Shiji*	*Historical Records*	c.−90	
Anon	*Lingshu*	*The Miraculous Pivot*		
Anon	*Shennong Bencao*	*Shennong's Materia Medica*	c.+100	
Zhang Zhong-jing	*Shang Han Zhabing Lun*	*Essays on Cold Attack and Miscellaneous Disease*	+220	
Hua Tuo	*Hua Tuo Zhen Zhong Jiu Ci Jing*	*Hua Tuo's Central Acumoxa Classic*		Lost; fragments recorded in other texts

Post-Han and Tang dynasty texts

Author(s)	Pinyin title	English title	Date	Notes
Huang Fu-mi	*Zhenjiu Jiayi Jing*	*Systematic Classic of Acumoxa*	259	
Wang Shu-he	*Mai Jing*	*Pulse Classic*	c.310	
Ge Hong	*Baopuzi Nei Pian*	*Inner Writings of Bao Puzi*	c.310?	
Ge Hong	*Baopuzi Wai Pian*	*Outer Writings of Bao Puzi*	c.320?	
Ge Hong	*Zhouhou Beiji Fang*	*Emergency Prescriptions to Keep Up Your Sleeve*	c.330	
Ge Hong	*Shan Xian Zhuan*	*Biographies of the Immortals*		
Gong Qing-xuan	*Guiyi Fang*	*Lui Juan-zi's Ghost Legacy Formulas*	c.490	
Chen Yan-zi	*Furen Fang*	*Formulas for Women*	Eastern Jin dynasty c.400	
Xu Zhi-cai	*Xiaoer Fang*	*Formulas for Children*	+479–502	

Xu Zhi-cai		*Classified Medicinals*	
Lei Xiao	*Leigong Paozhi Lun*	*Leigong's Essays on Herb Processing*	470
Tao Hong-jing	*Ming Yi Bie Lu*	*Appended Records from Leading Physicians*	c.500?
Tao Hong-jing	*Shennong Bencao Jing Jizhu*	*Shennong's Bencao Annotated*	490?
Tao Hong-jing	*Zhouhou Baiji Fang*	*100 Emergency Prescriptions to Keep Up Your Sleeve*	520?
Yang Shang-shan	*Huangdi Neijing Taisu*	*Huangdi Neijing: The Great Innocence*	c.600
Chao Yuan-fang	*Zhubing Yuanhou Lun*	*On the Causes and Symptoms of Illness*	610
Zhen Quan	*Zhen Fang*	*Needling Formulas*	Lived 541–643
Zhen Quan	*Mingtang Ren Xing Tu*	*Illustrations of the Human Form for the Teaching Room*	
Su Jing	*Xin Xiu Bencao/ Tang Bencao*	*Newly Revised Materia Medica*	659
Sun Si-miao	*Beiji Qian Jin Yao Fang*	*Formulas for Every Emergency Worth a 1000 Gold*	652
Sun Si-miao	*Qian Jin Yi Fang*	*Wings to the Thousand Gold Prescriptions*	c.680
Court of Emperor Xuan Song	*Guang Zhi Fang*	*Formulas for Widespread Benefaction*	703?
Wang Tao	*Waitai Miyao*	*Essential Secrets from the Imperial Library*	752
Wang Bing	*Bu Zhu Huangdi Neijing Suwen*	*Annotated Huangdi Neijing Suwen*	762
Emperor De Song	*Chen Yuan Guang Li Fang*	*Satisfying Prescriptions for Widespread Benefit*	796
Anon	*Zhong Zangjing*	*Divinely Responding Classic*	Probably 9th to 14th century

Song dynasty texts

Author(s)	Pinyin title	English title	Date	Notes
Ma Zhi, Liu Han	*Kaibao Qingding Bencao*	*Bencao of the Kaibao Reign*	974	
Wang Huai-yin (editor)	*Taiping Shenghui Fang*	*Taiping Era Formulas from Benevolent Sages*	992	
Wang Wei-yi (editor)	*Tongren Shuxue Zhenjiu Tujing*	*Chart of the Bronze Figure Acumoxa Points*	1026	
Anon	*Ou Xi Fan Wu Zang Tu*	*Chart of the Organs of Mr Ou Xi Fan*	1045	
Wu Jian	*Cun Zhen Tu*	*Collected Truths Chart*	1048	
Song Imperial Medical Bureau	*Wangshi Boji Fang*	*Mr Wang's Formulas for Abundant Relief*	1045	
Song Imperial Medical Bureau	*Qingli Shan Jiu Fang*	*Qingli Reign Formulas for Public Relief*	1046	
Song Imperial Medical Bureau	*Jianyao Jizhong Fang*	*Concise Formulary for Public Relief*	1051	
Zhang Yu-xi et al.	*Jiayou Buzhu Shennong Bencao*	*Jiayou Period Supplemented and Annotated Shennong Bencao*	1060	
Shen Kuo	*Liang Fang*	*Fine Formulas*	1061	
Su Song	*Tujing Bencao*	*Illustrated Bencao*	1062	
Pang An-shi	*Shang Han Zong Bing Lun*	*Discussion on Shang Han and General Disorders*	1090	
Chen Cheng	*Chuangguang Buzhu Shennong Bencao Tujing*	*Expanded, Annotated and Illustrated Shennong Bencao*	1092	
Liu Wan-shu	*Suwen Rushi Yunqi Lun Ao*	*Penetrating the Suwen's Mysterious Yunqi Patterns*	1099	
Tang Shen-wei	*Jingshi Zhenglei Beiji Bencao*	*Bencao for Urgent Needs Classified and Verified from the Classics*	1098	Renamed *Zhenglei Bencao* and reprinted in 1108 as *Jingshi Zhenglei Daguan Bencao*
Chen Shi-wei et al.	*Taiping Huimin Hejiju Fang*	*Taiping Era Prescriptions for Universal Public Relief*	1110	
Yang Jie	*Cun Zhen Huan Zhong Tu*	*Chart of Collected Truths Encompassing the Inside*	1113	

Jin-Yuan dynasty texts

Author(s)	Pinyin title	English title	Date	Notes
Kou zong-shi	*Bencao Yanyi*	*Expanded Bencao*	1116	
Song Imperial Medical Publishers	*Zhenghe Shengji Zonglu*	*Holy Compendium for General Relief*	1117	
Qian Yi	*Xiaoer Yaozheng Zhi Jue*	*Knack of Paediatric Patterns Written*	1119	
Qian Yi	*Shang Han Lun Zhi Wei: Ying Ru Lun*	*Shang Han Lun Interpretations: Essay on Infant's Milk*		Lost
Zhu Gong	*Lei Zheng Huo Ren Shu*	*Pattern Categories Text for Saving Lives*	c.1120	
Xu Shu-wei	*Shang Han Fa Wei Lun*	*Shang Han Lun Annotated*	c.1130	
Xu Shu-wei	*Puji Ben Shi Fang*	*Practical Formulas for Universal Benefit*	1132	
Xu Shu-wei	*Shang Han Jiu Shi Lun*	*90 Essays on Cold Attack*	c.1135	
Cheng Wu-ji	*Shang Han Ming Li Lun*	*Clarification of Cold Damage Principles*	1115	
Cheng Wu-ji	*Yao Fang Lun*	*On Medicinals and Formulas*	1120	
Cheng Wu-ji	*Zhu Jie Shang Han Lun*	*Revised Shang Han Lun*	1144	
Shen Kuo *et al.*	*Su Shen Liang Fang*	*Fine Formulas from Su and Shen*	1126	Update of Shen Kuo's *Liang Fang* of 1061
Wang Zhi-zhong	*Zhen Jiu Zi Sheng Jing*	*Acumoxa Lifegiving Classic*	1165	
Han Zhi-he	*Shang Han Wei Zhi Lun*	*Shang Han Lun's Deeper Meaning*	1186	
Chen Yan	*Yi Yuan Zhi Zhi*	*Treatment Based on Aetiology*	1161	Unpublished
Chen Yan	*San Yin Yi Bing Zheng Fang Lun*	*On Formulas for the Three Categories of Aetiology*	1174	Aka *San Yin Fang*
Zhang Yuan-su	*Yi Xue Qi Yuan*	*Medicine Explained*	1175?	
Zhang Yuan-su	*Zhen Zhu Nang*	*A Pouch of Pearls*	c.1180	Proposed a new approach to the characterisation of medicinals

Zhang Yuan-su	*Zang Fu Biao Ben Han Re Xu Shi Yong Yao Shi*	Use of Medicinals Based on Zangfu, Root-Branch, Cold-Hot, Xu-Shi		
Zhang Yuan-su	*Suwen Bingji Qiyi Baoming Ji*	Protecting Life by Su Wen Pathophysiology	1186	Critically re-appraises *Suwen* theories
Liu Wan-su	*Huangdi Suwen Xuan Ming Lun Fang*	Profound Formulas Inspired by the Huangdi Neijing	1180	
Liu Wan-su	*Huangdi Suwen Xuan Ji Yuan Bing Shi*	Investigating the Profound Truths on Pathogenesis in the Suwen	1182	
Liu Wan-su	*Baoming Ji*	Health Protecting Formulas	1186	Based on *wu yun liu qi* theory
Liu Wan-su	*Yi Fang Jing Yao Xuan Ming Lun*	Interpretation of the Essentials of Medical Prescriptions	1188?	
Liu Wan-su	*Shang Han Zhi Ge Fang Lun*	Direct Investigations of Shang Han Lun Formulas		
Liu Wan-su	*Neijing Yunqi Yao Zhi Lun*	Medical Treatment with Neijing Cosmology		Lost
Liu Wan-su	*Shang Han Zhen Ge*	True Patterns of the Shang Han Lun		
Cui Jia-yan	*Cui Shi Mai Jue*	Master Cui's Knack of the Pulse	1189	
Wang Jie	*Lu Chanyan Bencao*	Steep Mountainsides Bencao	1220	
Zhang Cong-zheng	*Rumen Shi Qin*	A Confucian's Duty to His Parents	1228	
Shi Fa	*Cha Bing Zhi Nan*	Guide for Checking Disease	1241	
Li Dong-yuan (Li Gao)	*Nei Wai Shang Bian Huo Lun*	Differentiating Interior and Exterior Attack	1247	
Li Dong-yuan (Li Gao)	*Pi Wei Lun*	Essays on the Spleen and Stomach	1249	
Song Ci	*Xi Yuan Zhi Lu*	On Washing Away Injustices	1247	
Yan Yong-he	*(Yan Shi) Ji Sheng Fang*	(Master Yan's) Formulas to Aid the Living	1253	
Yan Yong-he	*Ji Sheng Xu Fang*	More Life Preservation Formulas	1267	
Chen Zi-ming	*Furen Daquan Liangfang*	Compendium of Good Formulas for Women	1273	

Wang Hao-gu	*Yi Lei Yuan Rong*	*Medicine from the Army Base*		
Wang Hao-gu	*Yin Zheng Lue Lie*	*On Yin Patterns*		
Wang Hao-gu	*Tang Ye Ben Cao*	*Bencao for Decoctions*	1289	
Wang Hao-gu	*Ci Shi Nan Zhi*	*Hard-won Knowledge*	1308	
Wang Hao-gu	*Ban Zhen Cui Lun*	*On Paediatric Febrile Rashes*		
Zhu Dan-xi	*Ju Fang Fa Hui*	*Clarifying the Peaceful Benevolent Formulas*	1347	
Zhu Dan-xi	*Ge Zhi Yu Lu*	*Prescriptions to Keep up Your Sleeve*	1350	
Zhu Dan-xi	*Dan Xi Xin Fa*	*Heartfelt Methods of Dan-xi*	1381	Zhu's work compiled by later followers appears in *Jin Gui Gou Yuan*
Zhu Dan-xi	*Shang Han Bian Yi*	*Shang Han Differentiations*		
Zhu Dan-xi	*Bencao Yanyi Buyi*	*Appended and Annotated Bencao Yanyi*		
Zhu Dan-xi	*Waike Jing Yao Fa Hui*	*Methods of External Medicine*		
Imperial Medical Bureau	*Sheng Ji Zong Lu*	*General Collection for Holy Relief*		
Du Qing-bu (Du Ben)	*Ao Shi Shang Han Jin Jing Lun*	*Master Ao's Shang Han Golden Mirror Treatise*	1341	
Hua Shou	*Zhen Jia Shu Yao*	*Key Pointers for Diagnosticians*	1359	

Ming dynasty texts

Author(s)	Pinyin title	English title	Date	Notes
Wang Lu	*Yijing Suhui Ji*	*Going Against the Stream of the Medical Classics*	1368	
Wang Lu	*Bai Bing Guo Xuan*	*Hooking the Profundities of a Hundred Illnesses*		
Tai Yuan-li	*Tui Qiu Shi Yi*	*A Thorough Examination of the Master's Medical Opinions*	1378?	

Ni Wei-te	*Yuan Qi Zhi Wei*	*Source of the Qi Mechanism Revealed in Detail*	c.1380	
Teng Hong *et al.*	*Puji Fang*	*Prescriptions for Universal Relief*	1406	
Ming Medical Bureau	*Yongle Dadian*	*Yongle Reign Great Compendium*	1408	
Xu Feng	*Zhen Jiu Da Quan*	*Acumoxa Encyclopedia*	1439	
Wang Lun	*Bencao Zhi Yao*	*Collected Essential Bencao*	1496	
Gao Wu	*Zhen Jiu Ju Ying*	*Gatherings of Outstanding Acumoxa Practitioners*	1529	
Gao Wu	*Zhen Jiu Su Nan Jie Yao*	*Essentials of Suwen and Nanjing Summarised*	1529	
Wang Ji	*Zhen Jiu Wen Dui*	*Acumoxa Questions and Answers*	1530	
Xue Ji	*Zheng Ti Lei Yao*	*Categorised Essentials of Traumatology*	1529	
Xue Ji	*Nei Ke Zhai Yao*	*Essentials of Internal Medicine*	1538?	
Xue Ji	*Nu Ke Cuo Yao*	*Women's Diseases – Proven Essentials*	1548	
Xue Ji	*Li Yang Ji Yao*	*Leprous Sores – Pivotal Essentials*	1550	
Xue Ji	*Chuang Yang Ji Yao*	*Key Essentials of Sores and Ulcers*	1571	
Xue Ji	*Waike Shu Yao*	*External Illnesses – Pivotal Essentials*	1571	Xue Ji's texts were later all merged into *Xue Shi Yi An* (Xue's Medical Cases)
Li Shi-zhen	*Maijue Kao Zheng*	*On the Pulse and Diagnostic Patterns*	1564	
Li Shi-zhen	*Qijing Bamai*	*Extraordinary Channels Pathways Examined*	1578	
Li Shi-zhen	*Bencao Gangmu*	*Categorised Bencao*	1596	
Wu Kun	*Yi Fang Kao*	*Examining Herbal Formulas*	1584	
Wu Kun	*Zhen Fang Liu Ji*	*Six Collected Acupuncture Formulas*	1618	
Li Ting	*Yi Xue Ru Men*	*An Introduction to Medicine*	1575	

Anon (attributed to Sun Si-miao)	Yinhai Jingwei	Essentials of the Silvery Sea	c.1580	Ophthalmology text
Yang Ji-zhou	Zhen Jiu Da Cheng	Great Compendium of Acumoxa	1601	
Wang Ke-tang	Liu Ke Zheng Zhi Jun Sheng	Essential Tools for Delineating Patterns and Treatments	1602	
Wang Ke-tang	Nu Ke Zheng Zhi Zhun Sheng	Delineating Patterns and Treatments in Gynaecology	1602	
Wang Ke-tang	Waike Zheng Zhi Zhun Sheng	Delineating Patterns and Treatments in External Illness	1608	
Chen Shi-gong	Waike Zheng Zong	True Teachings on External Illness	1617	
Miu Xi-yong	Bencao Jing Su	Bencao in Plain Language	1622	
Zhang Jie-bin	Jing Yue Quan Shu	Jing-yue's Comprehensive Text	1624	
Zhang Jie-bin	Lei Jing	Categorised Classic	1624	
Zhang Jie-bin	Lei Jing Fu Yi	Appendix to the Categorised Classic	1624	
Zhang Jie-bin	Lei Jing Tu Yi	Categorised Classic Illustrated Appendices	1624	
Zhang Jie-bin	Zhi Yi Lu	Clearing Doubts with Questions	1624	
Sun Zhi-hong	Jian Ming Yi Gou	Concise Medical Accuracy	1629	
Zhao Xian-ke	Yi Guan	Medical Connections	1687	

Qing dynasty texts

Author(s)	Pinyin title	English title	Date	Notes
Deng Yu-han (translator)	Ren Shen Shua Gai	A Concise Description of the Human Body	1635	
Wu You-ke	Wen Yi Lun	Essays on Warm Diseases	1642	
Wang Ang	Yi Fang Ji Jie	Collected Explanations of Medical Formulas	1682	

Wang Ang	Suling Lei Zuan Yue Zhu	Suwen and Lingshu Categorised and Annotated	1688
Wang Ang	Bencao Bei Yao	Handbook of Bencao Essentials	1694
Wang Ang	Tangtou Ge Jue	Formulas in Verse	
Zhang Lu-yu	Zhangshi Yitong	Zhang's Medical Compendium	1695
Zhu Chun-gu	Douzhen Dinglun	Established Principles in Smallpox	1713
Cheng Guo-peng	Yi Xue Xin Wu	Realisations from Medical Study	1732
Cheng Guo-peng	Waike Shi Fa	Ten Methods in Surgery	
Wu Qian et al.	Yizong Jinjian	The Golden Mirror of Medicine	1742
Ye Tian-shi	Linzheng Zhinan Shang Han Men Fang	Clinical Guide to Shang Han Formulas	
Ye Tian-shi	Wen Zheng Lunzhi	Differentiating Warm Patterns	
Ye Tian-shi	Linzheng Zhinan Yi An	Clinical Case History Guides	1746
Ye Tian-shi	Wen Re Lun	Essay on Warm Disease	1746
Wu Ru-tang	Wenbing Tiao Bian	Systematic Differentiation of Warm Disease	1798
Xu Da-chun	Yi Xue Yuan Liu Lun	Essays on the Original Medical Currents	1757
Yan Xi-ting, Shi Zhan-ning, Hong Ji-an	De Pei Bencao	Bencao Combinations	1761
Zhao Xue-min	Bencao Gangmu Shi Yi	Omissions from the Grand Bencao	1765
Liu Bao-yi	Wen Re Feng Yuan	Encountering the Source of Warm Heat	
Liu Bao-yi	Liu Xuan Si Jia Yi An	Liu's Selected Cases from Four Physicians	
Fei Bo-xiong	Yi Chun Sheng	Pure Medicine Remainders	
Fei Bo-xiong	Yi Fang Ji Jie	Collected Explanations of Medical Prescriptions	
Fei Bo-xiong	Shi Liao Bencao	Diet Therapy Bencao	

Fu Shan	*Fu Qing Zhu Nu Ke*	*Fu Qing's Gynaecology*	1827
Xue Xue	*Shi Re Tiao Bian*	*Systematic Differentiation of Damp Heat*	
Xue Xue	*Yi Jing Yuan Zhi*	*On Original Yi Jing Knowledge*	
Xue Xue	*Shi Re Bing Pian*	*Writings on Damp-Heat Disease*	1852
Wang Shi-xiong	*Wenbing Gangmu*	*Compendium of Febrile Disease*	1852
Tang Zong-hai	*Zhong Xi Wu Zhong Shu Jiao Liu*	*Five Texts to Integrate Western and Chinese Medicine*	1884
Zhang Xi-chun	*Yi Xue Zhong Zhong Can Xi Lu*	*Records of Heartfelt Experiences in Medicine with Reference to the West*	1934

BIBLIOGRAPHY

This is a list of many of the sources that were accessed in the writing of this book, although other incidental data came from general reading, news items and cuttings that have appeared in press sources and journals such as the UK's *New Scientist* magazine over the past three decades. The most important sources I have indicated using bold type for the author name.

Allan, S. (1991) *Myth, Art and Cosmos in Early China*. New York: State University of New York Press.

Anon (1971) *I Ching* (Zhou dynasty c.–1000) (Translated by James Legge). New York: New American Library.

Anon (1985) *The Canon of Acupuncture – Huangti Nei Ching Ling Shu* (Eastern Han dynasty) (Translated by Ki Sunu). Compton, CA: Yuin University Press.

Anon (1993) *Master Hua's Classic of the Central Viscera* (Translation of *Zhong Zang Jing* (Divinely Responding Classic) by Yang Shou-zhong). Boulder, CO: Blue Poppy Press. [Traditionally attributed to Hua Tuo (died +208), but probably written in the Tang dynasty.]

Anon (1997) *Huangdi Neijing* (Western Han dynasty) (Translated by Wu Lian-sheng and Wu Qi). Beijing: China Science and Technology Press.

Anon (1998) *The Divine Farmer's Materia Medica* (Eastern Han dynasty c.+100) (Translation of *Shen Nong Bencao* by Yang Shou-zhong). Boulder, CO: Blue Poppy Press.

Barnes, L.L. (2005) *Needles, Herbs, Gods and Ghosts – China Healing and the West to 1848*. Cambridge, MA: Harvard University Press.

Chace, C. and Yang, S. (1994) *The Systematic Classic of Acupuncture and Moxibustion*. Boulder, CO: Blue Poppy Press. [A translation of Huang Fu-mi's *Jia Yi Jing*, Jin dynasty.]

Chen, P. (1999) *History and Development of Traditional Chinese Medicine*. Beijing: Science Press.

Daly, N.P. (1999) 'Hybridising the Human Body: The Hydrological Development of Acupuncture in Early Imperial China.' MA Thesis. Montreal: McGill University.

de Bary, W.T. (1960) *Sources of Chinese Tradition Vols 1 & 2*. New York: Columbia University Press.

Eckman, P. (1996) *In the Footsteps of the Yellow Emperor – Tracing the History of Traditional Acupuncture*. London: Cypress Books.

Farquhar, J. (1994) *Knowing Practice – The Clinical Encounter of Chinese Medicine*. Boulder, CO: Westview Press.

Fu, Wei-kang (1985) *Traditional Chinese Medicine and Pharmacology*. Beijing: Foreign Languages Press.

Fu, Wei-kang (ed.) (1989) *Zhongguo Yixue Shi* (History of Chinese Medicine). Shanghai: Publishing House of Shanghai College of Chinese Medicine.

Gascoigne, B. (2003) *The Dynasties of China*. London: Robinson.

Goldschmidt, A.M. (1999) 'The Transformation of Chinese Medicine during the Northern Song Dynasty.' PhD Thesis. Philadelphia, PA: University of Pennsylvania.

Gernet, J. (1970) *Daily Life in China on the Eve of the Mongol Invasion 1250–1276.* Redwood City, CA: Stanford University Press.

Granet, M. (1934) *La Pensee Chinoise.* Belgium: Rennaisance du Livre.

Granet, M. (1975) *Festivals and Songs of Ancient China.* New York: Gordon Press. [Reprint of 1932 edn.]

Hall, D.L. and Ames, R.T. (1998) *Thinking from the Han – Self, Truth and Transcendence in Chinese and Western Culture.* New York: State University of New York Press.

Harper, D. (1998) *Early Chinese Medical Literature – The Mawangdui Medical Manuscripts.* London: Kegan Paul.

Harper-Parker, E. (reprint of 1908 edn) *Ancient China Simplified.* Alexandria, MN: Echo Press.

Hoizey, D. and Hoizey, M.-J. (1988) *A History of Chinese Medicine.* Edinburgh: Edinburgh University Press.

Hsu, E. (2000) *The Transmission of Chinese Medicine.* Cambridge: Cambridge University Press.

Hsu, E. (2001) *Innovation in Chinese Medicine.* Cambridge: Cambridge University Press.

Hsu, Hong-yen and Wang, Su-yen (1985) *The Theory of Feverish Diseases and its Clinical Applications.* Long Beach, CA: Oriental Healing Arts Institute.

Journal of Traditional Chinese Medicine (Beijing) Various short articles on Chinese medical history, published between 1979 and 2006.

Jullian, F. (1999) *The Propensity of Things – Towards a History of Efficacy in China* (Translated from French by Janet Lloyd). Cambridge, MA: Zone Books.

Jullian, F. (2004) *A Treatise on Efficacy* (Translated from French by Janet Lloyd). Honolulu: University of Hawaii Press.

Kuriyama, S. in D. Bates (ed.) (1995) *Knowledge and the Scholarly Medical Traditions.* Cambridge: Cambridge University Press.

Lau, D.C. and Ames, R. (1998) *Yuan Dao – Tracing Dao to its Source.* New York: Ballantine Press.

Lehman, H. (2013) 'Acupuncture in ancient China: How important was it really?' *Journal of Integrative Medicine 11*, 1.

Li, Dong-yuan (Li Gao) (1993) *Treatise of the Spleen and Stomach* (Translation of *Pi Wei Lung* by Yang Shou-zhong and Li Jian-yong). Boulder, CO: Blue Poppy Press.

Liu, Guo-zhun (1985) *The Story of Chinese Books.* Beijing: Foreign Languages Press.

Luo, Guo-jun and Zheng, Ru-su (1985) *The Story of Chinese Books.* Beijing: Foreign Languages Press.

Ma, Kan-wen (2000) 'Acupuncture: Its place in the history of Chinese medicine.' *Acupuncture in Medicine 18*, 2, December.

Needham, J. (1972) *Science and Civilisation in China.* Vol. II. Cambridge: Cambridge University Press.

Needham, J. (ed.) (2000) 'Nathan Sivin.' *Science and Civilisation in China VI*, 6.

Neem, G. (2009) 'Thoughts and methods of the Huo Shen school.' *The Lantern 6*, 3. [Provided my main source of this school in Chapter 8 (Qing and modern times).]

Paludan, A. (2008) *Chronicles of the Chinese Emperors – The Reign-by-Reign Record of the Rulers of Imperial China.* London: Thames & Hudson.

Pines, Y. (2009) *Envisioning Eternal Empire – Chinese Political Thought of the Warring States Era.* Honolulu: University of Hawaii Press.

Sawyer, R.D. (2004) *The Tao of Spycraft – Intelligence Theory and Practice in Traditional China.* Boulder, CO: Westview Press.

Scheid, V. (2002) *Chinese Medicine in Contemporary China – Plurality and Synthesis.* Durham, NC: Duke University Press.

Scheid, V. (2007) *Currents of Tradition in Chinese Medicine 1626–2006.* Seattle: Eastland Press.

Schwartz, B. (1985) *The World of Thought in Ancient China.* Cambridge, MA: Harvard University Press.

Sung, Tzu (1981) *The Washing Away of Wrongs* (Translation of *Xi Yuan Zhi Lu* (Jin-Yuan dynasty) by Brian McKnight). Ann Arbor, MI: University of Michigan Center for Chinese Studies.

Temple, R. (1999) *The Genius of China.* London: Prion Books.

Unschuld, P. (1985) *Medicine in China – A History of Ideas.* Oakland, CA: University of California Press.

Unschuld, P. (1986) *Approaches to Traditional Chinese Medical Literature.* Dordrecht: Kluwer Academic Publishers.

Unschuld, P. (1986) *Medicine in China – A History of Pharmaceutics.* Oakland, CA: University of California Press.

Unschuld, P. (1986) *Nan-Ching – The Classic of Difficult Issues.* Oakland, CA: University of California Press.

Unschuld, P. (1988) *Introductory Readings in Classical Chinese Medicine.* Dordrecht: Kluwer Academic Publishers.

Unschuld, P. (1990) *Forgotten Traditions of Ancient Chinese Medicine.* Taos, NM: Paradigm Publications.

Unschuld, P. (2003) *Huangdi Neijing Suwen.* Oakland, CA: University of California Press.

Unschuld, P. (2009) *What is Medicine? Western and Eastern Approaches to Healing* (Translated by Karen Reimers). Oakland, CA: University of California Press.

Verwaal, R. (2009) 'Hippocrates Meets the Yellow Emperor.' Master's Thesis. Utrecht: Utrecht University.

Wang, Ai-he (2000) *Cosmology and Political Culture in Early China.* Cambridge: Cambridge University Press.

Wang, Qing-reng (2007) *Correcting Errors in the Forest of Medicine* (Translation of *Yi Lin Gai Cuo* by Chung, Oving and Becker). Boulder, CO: Blue Poppy Press.

Wen, Jian-min and Seifert, G. (2000) *Warm Disease Theory – Wen Bing Xue.* Taos, NM: Paradigm Publications.

Wong, K.C. and Wu, L.T. (1985) *History of Chinese Medicine.* Taipei: Southern Materials Center, Inc. [Reprint of 1932 edn.]

Wu, R.S., Wang, H.F. and Huang, Y. (1997) *Sunzi's Art of War and Healthcare.* Beijing: New World Press.

Zhang, Cong-zheng (Zhang, Z.-H., 1156–1228) (1996) *Zi He Yi, Medical Writings of Zi He* (Edited by Deng Tie-tao). Beijing: 5 Beijing Publishing House.

Zhang, Zhong-jing (1981) *Shang Han Lun* (Eastern Han dynasty) (Translated by Hong Yen-hsu). Long Beach, CA: Oriental Healing Arts Institute.

Zhang, Zhong-jing (1986) *Shang Han Lun* (Eastern Han dynasty) (Translated by Luo Xi-wen). Beijing: New World Press.

Zhang, Zhong-jing (1987) *Jin Gui Yao Lue* (Eastern Han dynasty) (Translated by Luo Xi-wen). Beijing: New World Press.

Zhang, Zhong-jing (1999) *Shang Han Lun* (Eastern Han dynasty) (Translated by Mitchell, Feng and Wiseman). Taos, NM: Paradigm Publications.

Zhang, Zhong-jing (2009) *Shang Han Lun* (Eastern Han dynasty) (Translated by Young and Marchment). Oxford: Churchill-Livingstone.

Zhao, Ruan-jin (2004) *From Legend to Science – A History of Chinese Medicine.* London: Vantage Press.

Zhu, Dan-xi (1993) *Extra Treatises Based on Investigation and Enquiry* (Translation of *Dan Xi Zhi Fa Xin Yao* by Yang Shou-zhong). Boulder, CO: Blue Poppy Press.

Zhu, Dan-xi (1993) *The Heart and Essence of Dan-xi's Methods of Treatment* (Translation of *Ge Zhi Yu Lun* by Yang Shou-zhong). Boulder, CO: Blue Poppy Press.

INDEX

CLASSIC TEXTS INDEX